LANGE

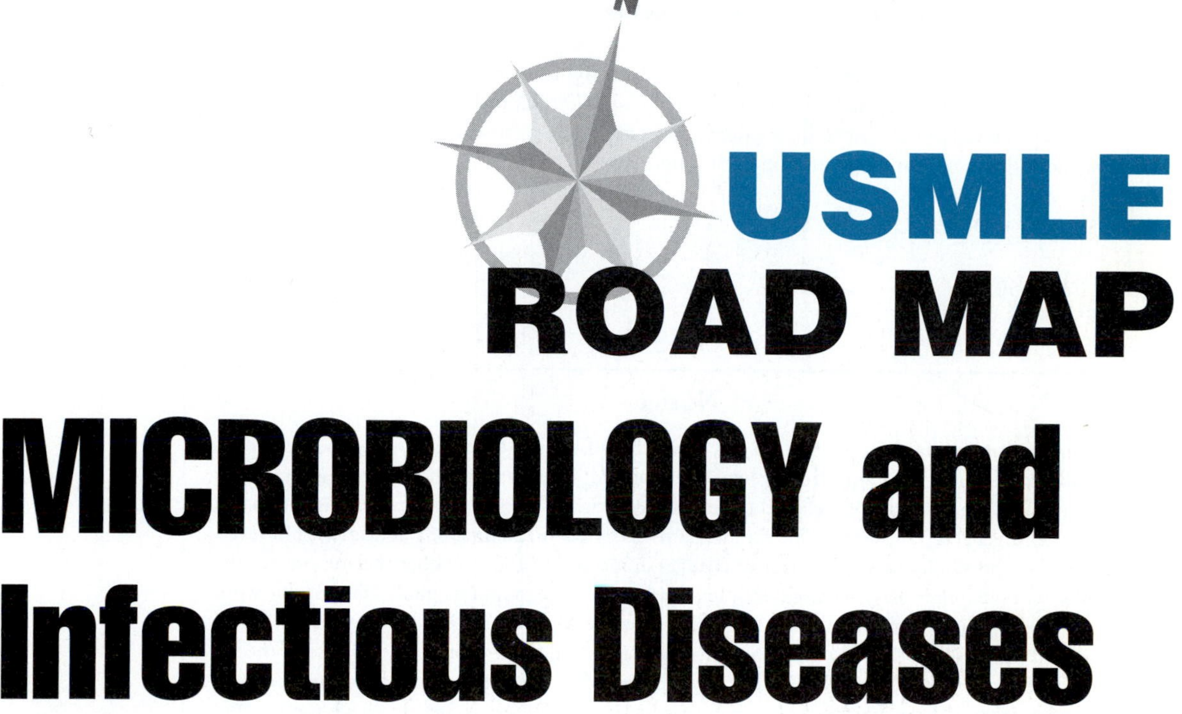

USMLE ROAD MAP MICROBIOLOGY and Infectious Diseases

TIMOTHY J. BOS, PHD

Professor, Department of Microbiology and Molecular Cell Biology
Eastern Virginia Medical School
Norfolk, Virginia

KENNETH D. SOMERS, PHD

Professor, Department of Microbiology and Molecular Cell Biology
Eastern Virginia Medical School
Norfolk, Virginia

Lange Medical Books/McGraw-Hill
Medical Publishing Division

New York Chicago San Francisco Lisbon London Madrid Mexico City
Milan New Delhi San Juan Seoul Singapore Sydney Toronto

The McGraw·Hill Companies

USMLE Road Map: Microbiology and Infectious Diseases

1 2 3 4 5 6 7 8 9 0 DOC/DOC 0 9 8 7 6 5 4

ISBN: 0-07-143507-7
ISSN: 1550-7025

Notice

Medicine is an ever-changing science. As new research and clinical experience broaden our knowledge, changes in treatment and drug therapy are required. The authors and the publisher of this work have checked with sources believed to be reliable in their efforts to provide information that is complete and generally in accord with the standards accepted at the time of publication. However, in view of the possibility of human error or changes in medical sciences, neither the authors nor the publisher nor any other party who has been involved in the preparation or publication of this work warrants that the information contained herein is in every respect accurate or complete, and they disclaim all responsibility for any errors or omissions or for the results obtained from use of the information contained in this work. Readers are encouraged to confirm the information contained herein with other sources. For example and in particular, readers are advised to check the product information sheet included in the package of each drug they plan to administer to be certain that the information contained in this work is accurate and that changes have not been made in the recommended dose or in the contraindications for administration. This recommendation is of particular importance in connection with new or infrequently used drugs.

This book was set in Adobe Garamond by Pine Tree Composition, Inc.
The editors were Janet Foltin, Harriet Lebowitz, and Karen W. Davis.
The production supervisor was Richard C. Ruzycka.
The illustration manager was Charissa Baker.
Graphics and illustrations created by Dragonfly Media Group.
The index was prepared by Andover Publishing Services.

RR Donnelley was the printer and binder.

This book is printed on acid-free paper.

ISBN: 0-07-111686-9 (international)
Exclusive rights by The McGraw-Hill Companies, Inc., for manufacture and export. This book cannot be re-exported from the country to which it is consigned by McGraw-Hill. The International Edition is not available in North America.

CONTENTS

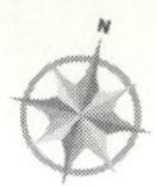

To my wife, Kari, my children, Jacqueline and Eric, my mother, Josephine, and to the memory of my father, Dr. Jacob K. Bos, Jr., who are all a constant source of love, support, and inspiration.

TJB

To my wife, Elizabeth for her encouragement in writing this book; to my children, Kara, Lynn, and Christopher for their love and support over the years; and to the many students who have inspired and challenged me.

KDS

ACKNOWLEDGMENTS

Special thanks to Janet Foltin, Harriet Lebowitz, Grace Caputo, Caitlin Duckwall, and Karen Davis for their help in preparing this manuscript.

USING THE USMLE ROAD MAP SERIES FOR SUCCESSFUL REVIEW

What is the Road Map Series?

Short of having your own personal tutor, the USMLE Road Map Series is the best source for efficient review of major concepts and information in the medical sciences.

Why Do You Need A Road Map?

It allows you to navigate quickly and easily through your microbiology course notes and textbook and prepares you for USMLE and course examinations.

How Does the Road Map Series Work?

Outline Form: Connects the facts in a conceptual framework so that you understand the ideas and retain the information.

Color and Boldface: Highlights words and phrases that trigger quick retrieval of concepts and facts.

Clear Explanations: Are fine-tuned by years of student interaction. The material is written by authors selected for their excellence in teaching and their experience in preparing students for board examinations.

Illustrations: Provide the vivid impressions that facilitate comprehension and recall.

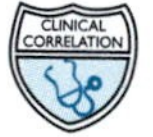

Clinical Correlations: Link all topics to their clinical applications, promoting fuller understanding and memory retention.

Clinical Problems: Give you valuable practice for the clinical vignette-based USMLE questions.

Explanations of Answers: Are learning tools that allow you to pinpoint your strengths and weaknesses.

CHAPTER 1
BASIC BACTERIOLOGY

I. Bacterial Structures

A. The **Gram stain** is used to distinguish two major classes of bacteria based on their **cell wall** structures.

1. **Gram-positive** bacteria contain a single cytoplasmic membrane surrounded by a thick, highly crosslinked layer of **peptidoglycan** (Figure 1–1).
   a. Other cell wall components include **teichoic acid, lipoteichoic acid,** and surface proteins.
   b. Peptidoglycan has pyrogenic activity.
2. **Gram-negative** bacteria contain an inner cytoplasmic membrane, a thin layer of peptidoglycan, a periplasmic space, and an outer membrane (Figure 1–2).
   a. The outer membrane is an asymmetric bilayer in which the outermost layer is composed of lipopolysaccharide (LPS).
   b. Because the outer membrane acts as a barrier, pore proteins play an important role in transport.
   c. LPS consists of 3 parts: **lipid A, core polysaccharide,** and **"O" polysaccharide** (Figure 1–2).
      (1) Lipid A is the component responsible for **endotoxin** activity.
      (2) The "O" polysaccharides are antigenic and used to classify organisms.
      (3) Peptidoglycan is a polymer of alternating ***N*-acetyl glucosamine** (G) and ***N*-acetyl muramic acid** (M) crosslinked by a short peptide bridge (Figure 1–3).
   a. The crosslink is between the terminal **D-alanine** and the penultimate diamino-containing amino acid (lysine or **diaminopimelic** amino acid).
   b. Crosslinking is catalyzed by **transpeptidases** (**penicillin-binding proteins**) that are also the targets of beta-lactam antibiotics.
   c. Crosslinking can be direct (Figure 1–3A) or, as in *Staphylococcus aureus,* through a **pentaglycine** spacer (Figure 1–3B).

B. Several other important structures are involved in transmission and pathogenesis.

1. **Pili,** or **fimbriae,** are involved in adhesion both to other bacteria and to host cells.
2. **Flagella** are the major organelles involved in bacterial motility and are either **polar** or **peritrichous.**
3. **Capsules** surround the cell wall, are usually polysaccharide, and help bacteria escape from phagocytosis.
4. **Spores** allow bacteria to enter a dormant state where they are resistant to harsh environmental influences.

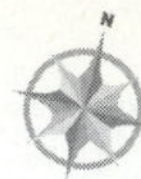

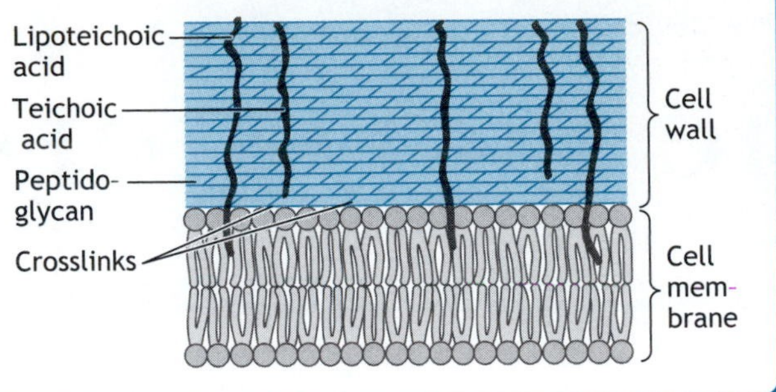

Figure 1–1. The gram-positive cell wall. Structural features include a thick layer of highly crosslinked peptidoglycan, teichoic acid, lipoteichoic acid, and a single cellular membrane.

C. Bacteria do not contain a nucleus.
   1. The genome is contained on a single circular chromosome.
   2. Some bacteria contain self-replicating extrachromosomal DNA, called **plasmids,** that carry genes for virulence factors and antibiotic resistance.
   3. Protein synthesis occurs on bacterial 70S **ribosomes,** which contain 30S and 50S subunits.

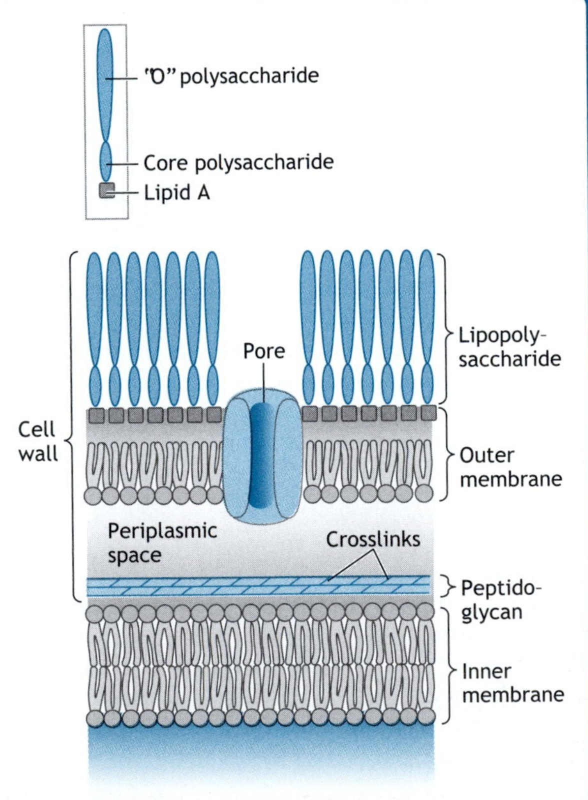

Figure 1–2. The gram-negative cell wall. Structural features include an inner cellular membrane, an outer membrane, a thin layer of peptidoglycan that is lightly crosslinked, and pore proteins. The outer membrane comprises an asymmetric bilayer in which the outer layer is composed of lipopolysaccharide. Lipopolysaccharide has three major components—lipid A, core polysaccharide, and "O" polysaccharide.

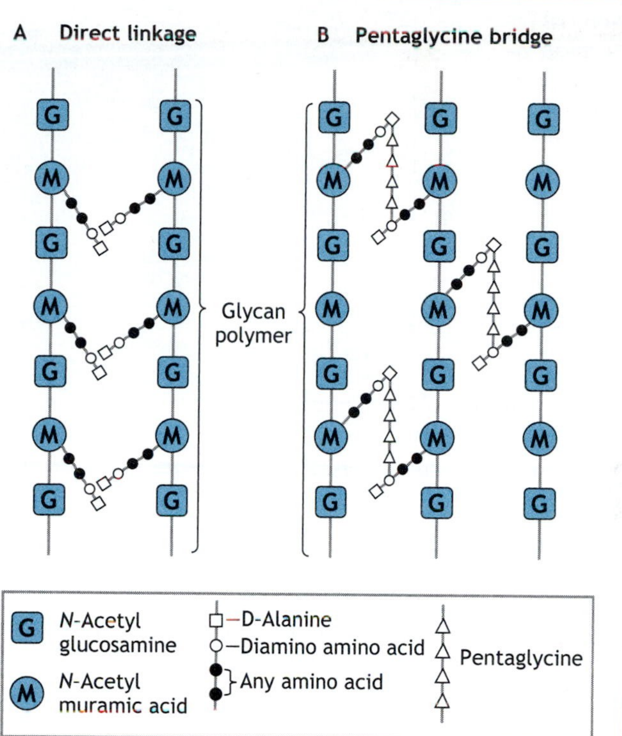

Figure 1–3. Peptidoglycan structure. Peptidoglycan is only found in bacteria and is composed of a glycan polymer with alternating *N*-acetyl glucosamine (G) and *N*-acetyl muramic acid (M). These polymers are crosslinked by a peptide bridge. The peptide linkages always couple the terminal D-alanine to the penultimate diamino-containing amino acid. The linkage can be direct (**A**) or indirect via a pentaglycine bridge (**B**).

II. Bacterial Growth and Metabolism

A. Bacteria reproduce by binary fission.

1. Growth consists of four discrete phases: lag, exponential, stationary, and death (Figure 1–4).
2. Exponential growth kinetics can vary dramatically among bacterial organisms with doubling times from minutes (eg, *Escherichia coli*) to days or weeks (*Mycobacterium leprae*).

B. Pathogenic bacteria are classified as **aerobic, anaerobic,** or **facultative,** depending on the mechanism by which they obtain energy from various carbon sources.

1. Obligate aerobes utilize aerobic respiration pathways.
2. Obligate anaerobes utilize fermentation pathways.
3. Facultative bacteria can utilize either.

III. Bacterial Genetics

A. **Mutation** is a source of genetic variation that occurs at random and at low frequency.

1. Genotypic variation always occurs.
2. Phenotypic variation sometimes occurs but generally affects only a single trait, which can manifest as loss of function or gain of function.

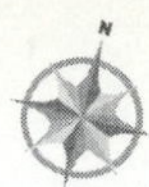

Figure 1–4. Bacterial growth phases. Typical graph shows the 4 different phases of bacterial growth. Doubling times can vary dramatically.

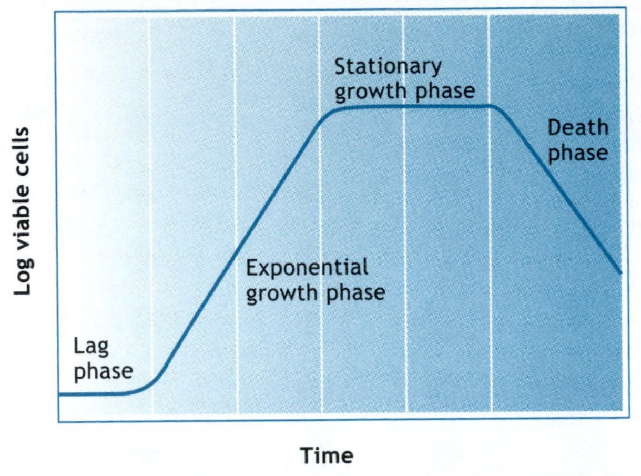

B. **Gene transfer mechanisms** result in the acquisition of new genetic material, occur at high frequency, and can affect both single and multiple traits.

1. **Transformation** is the uptake of naked DNA fragments by living bacteria.
2. **Conjugation** is the transfer of genetic material from one living bacterium to another living bacterium through direct contact (Figure 1–5).
   a. Transfer by conjugation is mediated by ***Tra*** genes encoded on a fertility or **F plasmid.**
      (1) Bacteria that contain the F plasmid are considered F+, or male.
      (2) *Tra* genes encode a specialized structure called the **sex pilus,** which serves to physically connect an F+ cell with an F– cell.
      (3) During conjugation, one strand of the F plasmid is transferred across the sex pilus to the recipient cell, making it F+ as well.

Figure 1–5. Conjugation. A bacterium containing an F plasmid is considered to be a male cell. The *Tra* genes on the F plasmid initiate sex pilus formation and transfer of DNA from the F plasmid to an F– recipient cell. Following transfer, the F– cell becomes F+.

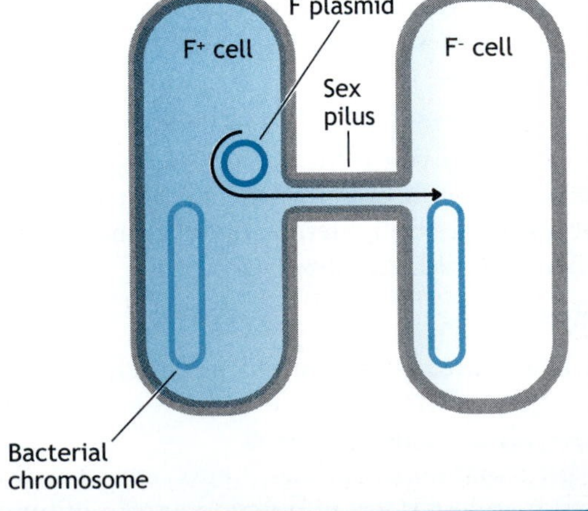

(4) F plasmids contain and transfer other genes, such as virulence factors and antibiotic-resistance genes.

b. During conjugation, other plasmids in the cell can also be transferred through a process called **mobilization.**

c. A bacterium that contains an F plasmid that is incorporated into the bacterial chromosome is called an **Hfr** (high-frequency transfer) because the bacterial chromosome can be transferred to other bacteria at much higher frequency than would normally occur.

3. **Transduction** refers to bacteriophage-mediated gene transfer.

a. When a bacteriophage infects a bacterium, it can either incorporate its genome (bacteriophage) into the bacterial chromosome (**lysogeny**) or replicate, package new bacteriophage particles, and lyse the bacterial host cell (**lytic cycle**).

(1) A lysogenized bacteriophage becomes part of the bacterial chromosome and is replicated during cell division.

(2) Lysogenized bacteriophages can excise from the chromosome and undergo a lytic cycle under adverse conditions by a process called **induction.**

(3) Many virulence factors are carried by lysogenic bacteriophages.

b. **Generalized transduction** begins when random pieces of bacterial chromosome DNA (instead of bacteriophage DNA) are packaged into a bacteriophage particle during a lytic cycle.

(1) The generalized transducing bacteriophage can infect a bacterium and inject the random chromosomal DNA.

(2) This injected DNA can incorporate into the new host by homologous recombination.

c. **Specialized transduction** (Figure 1–6) begins with a lysogenized bacteriophage.

(1) During induction, the bacteriophage DNA is imperfectly excised from the bacterial chromosome such that an extra piece of chromosomal DNA is attached to the bacteriophage DNA.

(2) This specialized transducing phage is thus able to transfer a very specific piece of DNA while retaining all of its infectivity.

4. **Transposons** are segments of DNA that are able to physically move from one DNA location to another (eg, from plasmid to chromosome).

IV. Mechanisms of Antibiotic Action (Figure 1–7)

A. Inhibition of Cell Wall Synthesis

1. **Penicillins** and **cephalosporins** are beta-lactam–containing antibiotics that target the crosslinking of peptidoglycan by binding to and inhibiting the action of transpeptidases (penicillin-binding proteins).
2. **Vancomycin** inhibits crosslinking by binding terminal D-alanine–D-alanine precursors, preventing transpeptidation.
3. **Cycloserine** inhibits the formation of the D-alanine–D-alanine linkage on the peptidoglycan precursor.
4. **Bacitracin** inhibits transport of peptidoglycan precursors through the cell membrane.
5. **Isoniazid** and **ethionamide** inhibit the synthesis of mycolic acids found in the cell walls of *Mycobacterium* species.

B. Inhibition of Protein Synthesis

1. **Aminoglycosides** (eg, streptomycin, neomycin, and kanamycin) irreversibly bind to target proteins on the 30S ribosomal subunit.

Figure 1–6. Specialized transduction. A bacterium containing a lysogenized bacteriophage is induced to undergo a lytic cycle. On induction, the phage DNA is imperfectly excised from the bacterial chromosome. A piece of bacterial DNA is packaged along with the phage DNA. The cell is lysed, and bacteriophages infect new cells.

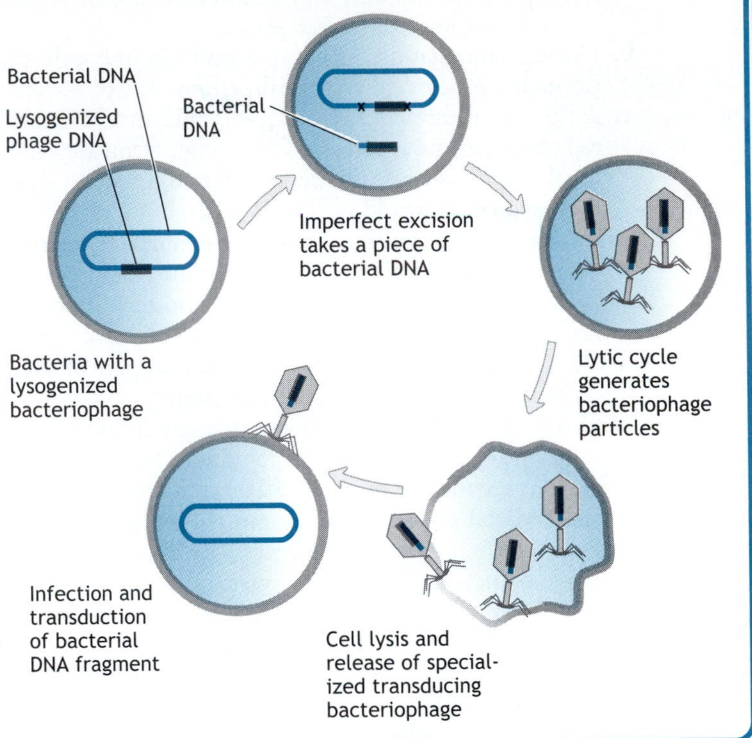

2. **Tetracyclines** also target the 30S subunits through a reversible interaction.
3. **Chloramphenicol** and **macrolides** (eg, erythromycin, azithromycin, and clarithromycin) target the 50S ribosomal subunit.

C. Inhibition of Nucleic Acids

1. The **quinolones** and **fluoroquinolones** (eg, ciprofloxacin and levofloxacin) inhibit bacterial DNA synthesis by inactivating DNA gyrase.
2. **Rifampin** inhibits DNA-dependent RNA polymerase.
3. **Metronidazole** is active against anaerobes, causing breaks in DNA.

D. Alterations of Cell Membranes

1. **Polymyxin** increases cell membrane permeability, especially the outer membrane of gram-negative organisms.

E. Antimetabolites

1. **Sulfonamides** inhibit folic acid synthesis.
2. **Trimethoprim** inhibits dihydrofolate reductase.

V. Antibiotic Resistance (Table 1–1)

A. Inactivation of the antibiotic can occur by **hydrolysis** (eg, beta lactamase).

B. Inactivation of the antibiotic can occur through **chemical modification** by acetylation, phosphorylation, or adenylylation.

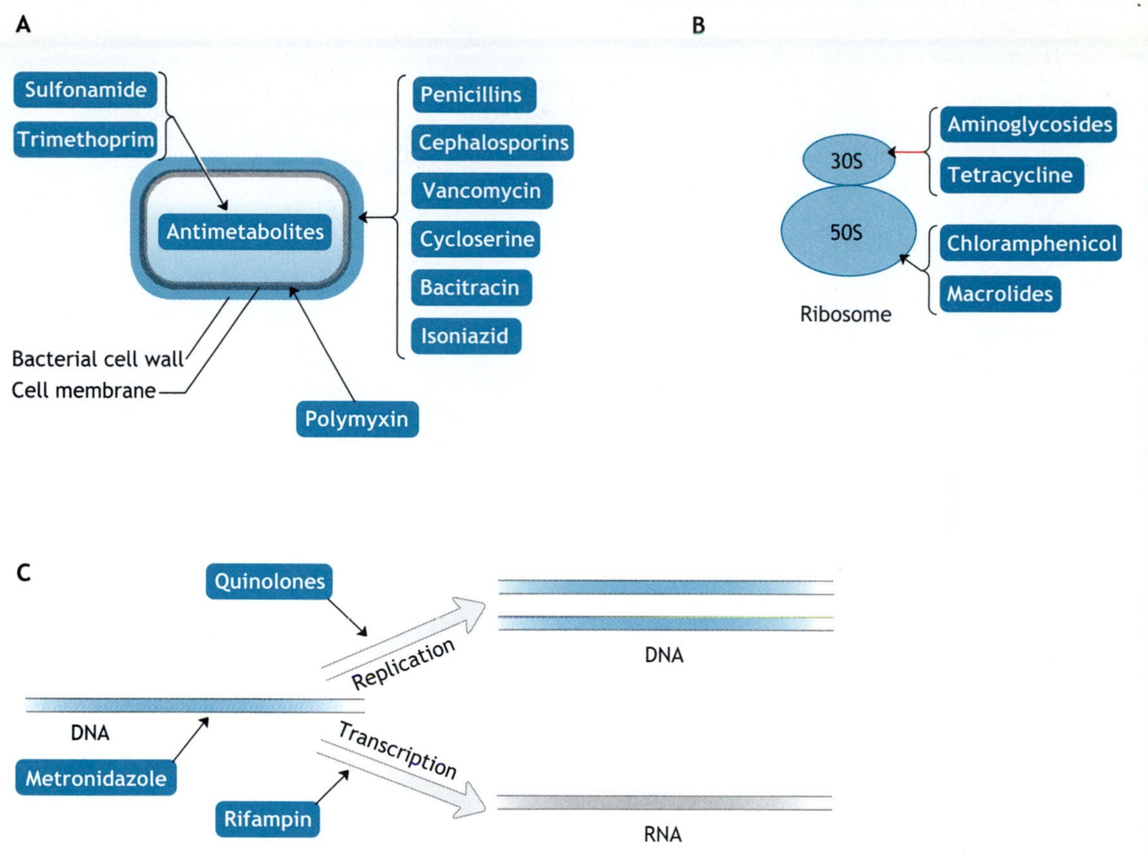

A

Sulfonamide
Trimethoprim
Antimetabolites
Penicillins
Cephalosporins
Vancomycin
Cycloserine
Bacitracin
Isoniazid
Bacterial cell wall
Cell membrane
Polymyxin

B

30S
50S
Ribosome
Aminoglycosides
Tetracycline
Chloramphenicol
Macrolides

C

Quinolones
Replication
DNA
DNA
Metronidazole
Transcription
Rifampin
RNA

Figure 1–7. Mechanisms of antibiotic action. **A:** Schematic showing cell wall–active, membrane-active, and cytoplasm-active antimetabolites. **B:** Antibiotics that inhibit protein synthesis by binding different ribosome subunits. **C:** Antibiotics that inhibit nucleic acids.

C. Mutations or gene acquisitions can result in the **alteration of antibiotic targets.**

D. Altered **permeability,** decreased **influx,** or increased **efflux** from the bacterial cell prevents accumulation of the antibiotic at the site of action.

VI. Mechanisms of Pathogenesis

A. Pathogenic bacteria produce a variety of **virulence factors** that facilitate the pathogenic process.

B. The 4 mechanisms by which virulence factors help **evade the host immune system** are

1. Prevention of phagocytosis (eg, capsules).
2. Facilitation of survival in phagosomes (eg, listeriolysin O).

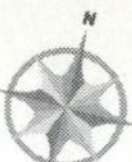

Table 1–1. Mechanisms of antibiotic resistance.

Antibiotic	Antibiotic Hydrolysis	Antibiotic Modification	Altered Target	Altered Permeability, Influx, or Efflux
Penicillins	+		+	+
Cephalosporins	+		+	+
Vancomycin			+	+
Cycloserine			+	+
Isoniazid			+	+
Bacitracin				+
Aminoglycosides		+	+	+
Tetracycline		+	+	+
Chloramphenicol		+		
Macrolides	+		+	+
Fluoroquinolones			+	+
Rifampin			+	+
Metronidazole				+
Sulfonamides/trimethoprim				+

3. Destruction of immune molecules or cells (eg, IgA proteases, leukocidins).
4. Evasion of immune clearance (eg, antigenic variation, phase variation, intracellular invasion).

C. Virulence factors that facilitate **adhesion, invasion,** and **spread** include flagella, pili, cell wall–associated proteins, slime layers, and a variety of enzymes (eg, urease, mucinase, and hyaluronidase).

D. The production of **bacterial toxins** is a common mechanism of pathogenesis.
1. **Endotoxin** (LPS) is an integral component of the cell wall of gram-negative bacteria that stimulates the release of inflammatory cytokines, including interleukin-1 and tumor necrosis factor alpha.
2. Many pathogenic bacteria secrete **exotoxins** that affect a variety of different cellular processes. Mechanisms of toxins are discussed in later chapters with individual organisms (Table 1–2).

Table 1–2. Bacterial exotoxins.

Protein Synthesis Inhibitors	Adenylate Cyclase Activity	Superantigen Stimulation	Neurotoxins	Cytotoxins
Shigella toxin	Cholera toxin	TSST-1	Botulism	Alpha toxins
Diphtheria toxin	*E coli*–labile toxin	Group A *Streptococcus* Spe A, B, C	Tetanus	Streptolysins
Pseudomonas exotoxin A	*Bacillus cereus*–labile toxin	*Staphylococcus* enterotoxins		
	Pertussis toxin			
	Anthrax edema factor			Anthrax lethal factor

CLINICAL PROBLEMS

Strain A of *E coli* contains an ampicillin resistance gene on an F plasmid. Strain B of *E coli* contains a tetracycline resistance gene on a lysogenized bacteriophage. When mixed together, a new strain emerges, strain C, that is resistant to both ampicillin and tetracycline.

1. What mechanism is most likely involved in the generation of this new strain?
   A. Strain B transfers tetracycline resistance to strain A by transposition.
   B. Strain A transfers ampicillin resistance to strain B by conjugation.
   C. Induction of a specialized transducing phage from strain A infects strain B.
   D. A spontaneous mutation in strain A confers resistance to tetracycline.

2. Cell wall–active antibiotics include:
   A. Macrolides, penicillins, and vancomycin
   B. Aminoglycosides, cephalosporins, and macrolides
   C. Penicillins, bacitracin, and cephalosporins
   D. Bacitracin, aminoglycosides, and vancomycin

3. Exotoxins that act as superantigens include:
   A. *S aureus* enterotoxin, pertussis toxin, and diphtheria toxin
   B. SpeA, TSST1, and *S aureus* enterotoxin
   C. Exotoxin A, pertussis toxin, and TSST1
   D. Diphtheria toxin, SpeA, and exotoxin A

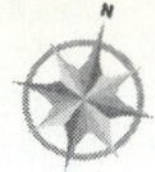

4. Resistance to chloramphenicol is most often caused by:
   A. Antibiotic hydrolysis
   B. Alteration of the cellular target
   C. Antibiotic modification
   D. Efflux of antibiotic out of the cell

A Gram-negative rod is isolated from the blood culture of a 28-year-old man who is exhibiting signs of bacterial sepsis.

5. A close examination of the cell wall of this organism would be expected to reveal:
   A. Teichoic acid, LPS, and a thick peptidoglycan layer
   B. LPS, a periplasmic space, and an outer membrane
   C. Teichoic acid, lipoteichoic acid, and a thin peptidoglycan layer
   D. A periplasmic space, a thin peptidoglycan layer, and crosslinks containing pentaglycine bridges

ANSWERS

1. The answer is B. Ampicillin resistance is carried on the F plasmid. F plasmids initiate conjugation and transfer this gene to strain B. Strain B becomes F+, ampicillin resistant, and tetracycline resistant, and is therefore a new strain.

2. The answer is C. Macrolides and aminoglycosides are protein synthesis inhibitors. All of the others act on the cell wall. Another cell wall–active antibiotic is cycloserine.

3. The answer is B. The *S aureus* enterotoxins and TSST1 as well as the *Streptococcus pyogenes* Spe toxins are all superantigens. Pertussis toxin activates adenylate cyclase, whereas exotoxin A and diphtheria toxins are protein synthesis inhibitors.

4. The answer is C. Chloramphenicol is modified by acetylation by an enzyme called chloramphenicol acetyl transferase. This modification inhibits the ability of chloramphenicol to bind to the 50S subunit.

5. The answer is B. Gram-positive walls have teichoic and lipoteichoic acids and a thick peptidoglycan layer, and some strains have pentaglycine crosslinking. Gram-negative cell walls have a double-membrane structure, a periplasmic space between, LPS, and a thin layer of peptidoglycan.

CHAPTER 2

AEROBIC GRAM-POSITIVE RODS

I. Key Concepts

A. The 5 medically important species in this **diverse group** of organisms encompass 4 genera: ***Bacillus, Corynebacterium, Erysipelothrix,*** and ***Listeria.***

B. The organisms in this group are a rare cause of disease in humans, but several members are highly pathogenic.

C. Key physical properties of each are summarized in Table 2–1.

D. *Bacillus* is one of the two medically important genera (the other is *Clostridium*) known to generate spores.

1. Spores form under conditions of decreased vegetative growth.
2. Spores provide a means of bacterial survival in a dormant state for decades and represent an important avenue to perpetuate spread.

II. *Bacillus, Corynebacterium, Erysipelothrix,* and *Listeria*

A. *Bacillus anthracis*

1. **Clinical manifestations:** *B anthracis* causes three different forms of anthrax: cutaneous, inhalation, and gastrointestinal.
   a. **Cutaneous anthrax** is the most common naturally occurring form of the disease and is characterized by local inflammatory necrotic lesions (**eschar**) at the site of inoculation.
   b. **Inhalation anthrax** (also called **woolsorter's disease**) is a highly fatal form of the disease characterized by rapid and massive edema in the chest followed by cardiovascular shock and death.
   c. **Gastrointestinal anthrax,** which results from ingestion of spores, is very rare but highly fatal.
2. **Transmission/epidemiology:** Anthrax is transmitted almost exclusively through contact with spores.
   a. Anthrax is mainly a disease of cattle, sheep, and horses.
   b. Human infection occurs on contact with infected animals or animal products.
      (1) Raw animal products include hides, wool, hair, and bone.
      (2) Finished animal products include shaving brushes and wool sweaters.
   c. The different disease manifestations of anthrax are related to the site of entry.
      (1) Cutaneous anthrax results from contact with spores through breaks in skin.
      (2) Inhalation anthrax results when spores are inhaled.
      (3) Gastrointestinal anthrax results when spores are ingested.

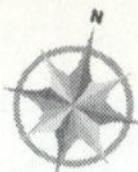

Table 2–1. Physical properties of aerobic gram-positive rods.

Organism	Size	Spores	Motility	Interesting Properties
Bacillus anthracis	Large	Yes	No	End-to-end chains
Bacillus cereus	Large	Yes	No	
Corynebacterium diphtheria	Small	No	No	Pleomorphic Chinese characters
Erysipelothrix rhusiopathiae	Small	No	No	
Listeria monocytogenes	Small	No	Tumbling	Low-temperature growth Intracellular

d. Weaponized anthrax particles designed to promote inhalation anthrax have been developed for biological warfare.

3. **Pathogenesis/virulence factors:** *B anthracis* contains several virulence factors (Table 2–2).
   a. A capsule of D-glutamic acid is antiphagocytic and helps the organism evade the immune system.
   b. Three exotoxins are produced (Figure 2–1).

Table 2–2. Summary of virulence factors.

Organism	Virulence Factor
Bacillus anthracis	Capsule of D-glutamic acid 3 exotoxins Protective antigen Edema factor Lethal factor
Bacillus cereus	2 exotoxins Heat-labile toxin (diarrhea) Heat-stable toxin (vomiting)
Corynebacterium diphtheria	1 exotoxin (diphtheria toxin)
Erysipelothrix rhusiopathiae	Hyaluronidase
Listeria monocytogenes	Listeriolysin O Internalin

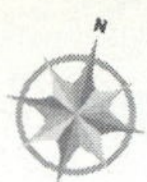

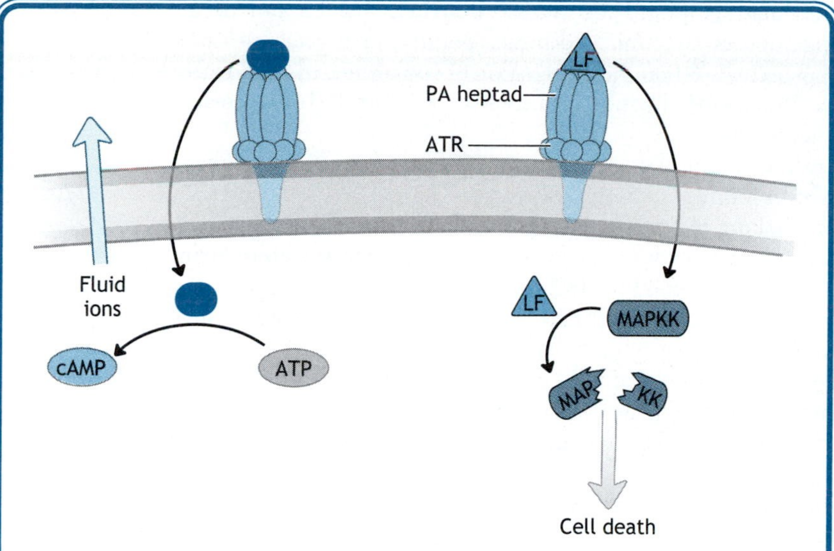

Figure 2–1. Mechanism of action of anthrax toxins. The protective antigen toxin (PA) binds to the anthrax toxin receptor (ATR) on the surface of host cells as a heptamer. Edema factor (EF) or lethal factor (LF) associates with the PA and is internalized. The EF toxin is an adenylate cyclase that catalyses an increase in intracellular cAMP, resulting in an efflux of fluids and ions from the cell into the extracellular space (edema). The LF toxin cleaves MAPKK, effectively shutting off signal transduction through the MAP kinase–signaling network, resulting in cell death.

(1) Protective antigen (PA) binds the anthrax toxin receptor (ATR) on the surface of host cells and facilitates the translocation of the 2 other exotoxins, edema factor (EF) and lethal factor (LF), into the cell.

(2) EF is an adenylate cyclase that increases intracellular cAMP, stimulating an efflux of fluids and ions that results in edema.

(3) LF is a mitogen-activated protein kinase kinase (MAPKK) protease that disrupts cell signaling, causing cell death and tissue necrosis.

4. **Treatment:** Current guidelines should be consulted but, in general, antibiotics such as ciprofloxacin, doxycycline, rifampin, and others are used for treatment. A variety of antitoxin strategies are currently being developed.
5. **Prevention:** Human vaccination with the anthrax vaccine adsorbed (AVA) vaccine targets the PA toxin subunit and is given as 6 shots over 18 months with yearly boosters.

ANTHRAX EXPOSURE

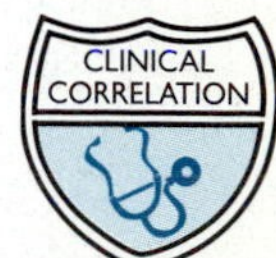

- *Because symptoms can develop 2–43 days after exposure, a 60-day course of antibiotics such as ciprofloxacin is given when exposure to anthrax is suspected.*

B. *Bacillus cereus*

1. **Clinical manifestations:** The main diseases caused by *B cereus* are food poisoning and traumatic eye infections.

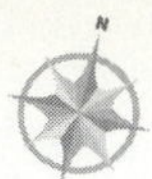

a. Common food poisoning symptoms are **watery diarrhea**—which can occur 6–24 hours after ingestion of contaminated meats, poultry, or vegetables—and **vomiting,** which may occur 1–6 hours after ingestion of contaminated **fried rice.**
b. Opportunistic manifestations include **traumatic eye and intravenous catheter-related infections.**

2. **Transmission/epidemiology:** Food poisoning is by **"intoxication"**—the ingestion of preformed toxin in food.
   a. Spores survive usual cooking temperatures and germinate at room temperature.
   b. The bacteria then produce two different exotoxins: a heat-labile enterotoxin and a heat-stable "vomiting" toxin (Table 2–2).
      (1) The heat-labile enterotoxin is associated with contaminated meats, poultry, and vegetables.
      (2) The heat-stable toxin is associated with contaminated fried rice.
3. **Pathogenesis/virulence factors:** The heat-labile toxin stimulates cellular adenylate cyclase leading to diarrhea. The heat-stable toxin induces vomiting through a mechanism that is not clear.
4. **Treatment:** Food poisoning is self-limited, whereas eye and blood infections may require antibiotics.
   a. Food poisoning is treated with fluid replacement.
   b. Because many of the organisms involved in eye and blood infections are resistant to multiple antibiotics, therapy may involve antibiotics such as vancomycin.
5. **Prevention:** Food poisoning is prevented through good food-handling practices, such as refrigerating foods after cooking and heating foods above 56 °C before eating (heat-labile toxin only).

B CEREUS–RELATED FOOD POISONING

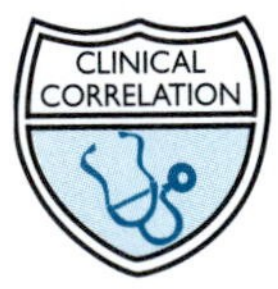

- *The emetic manifestation of B cereus food poisoning is associated with the ingestion of contaminated rice.*
- *The heat-stable toxin responsible for vomiting appears to require something in rice extracts in order to be expressed.*
- *Preparation of fried rice involves cooking, cooling, and recooking. This process inactivates the heat-labile toxin associated with diarrhea but not the heat-stable toxin associated with vomiting.*

C. *Corynebacterium diphtheriae*

1. **Clinical manifestations:** Diphtheria, caused by *C diphtheriae,* is most commonly associated with an infection of the nasopharynx.
   a. One prominent characteristic of pharyngeal diphtheria is the presence of a pseudomembrane made of necrotic dead cells, fibrin, and bacteria.
   b. The pseudomembrane acts as a platform for bacterial growth and toxin production.
   c. Death can result from mechanical obstruction of the airway by the pseudomembrane or by toxemia-induced myocardial and neurologic damage.
2. **Transmission/epidemiology:** Humans are the only natural host.
   a. Transmission is by respiratory droplets.
   b. Although diphtheria has been effectively controlled by immunization, it still remains a threat to unimmunized individuals.
3. **Pathogenesis/virulence factors:** The major virulence factor (Table 2–2) of *C diphtheriae* is an exotoxin encoded on a lysogenized bacteriophage.
   a. The diphtheria toxin is a classic A-B toxin that ADP ribosylates cellular translation elongation factor 2 (EF2) (Figure 2–2).

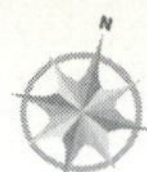

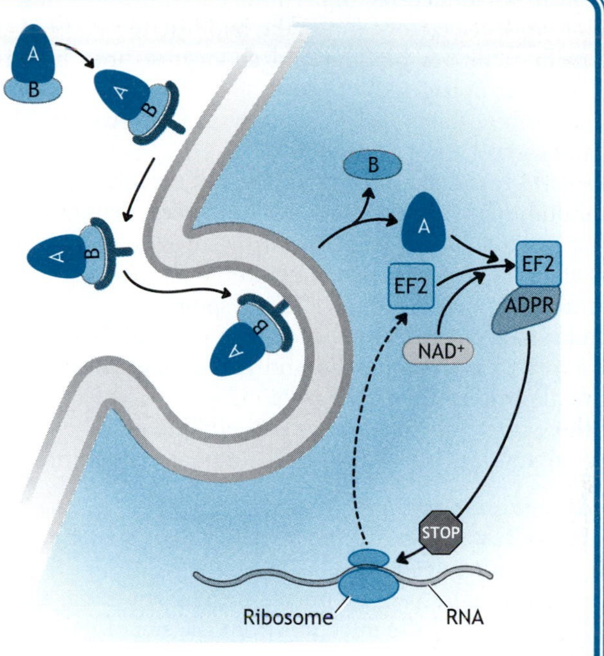

Figure 2–2. Mechanism of action of diphtheria toxin. Diphtheria toxin is a prototype A-B bacterial toxin. The B subunit binds receptors on the surface of host cells, facilitating internalization by endocytosis. The low pH of the endosome triggers cleavage of the two subunits, releasing the catalytic A subunit into the cytoplasm. The toxin A subunit ADP ribosylates elongation factor 2 (EF2), resulting in its inactivation and a complete shutdown of protein synthesis and cell death.

   b. This action shuts down protein synthesis and kills the cell.
4. **Treatment:** The treatment strategy involves a combination of antitoxin administration and antibiotics such as penicillin or erythromycin.
5. **Prevention:** Diphtheria is effectively controlled by immunization.
   a. Active immunization against toxoid induces antibodies directed against the diphtheria toxin B subunit.
   b. These antibodies prevent receptor binding by the toxin.

D. *Listeria monocytogenes*

1. **Clinical manifestations:** There are three categories of listeriosis.
   a. Fetal listeriosis can manifest as meningitis, pneumonia, or septicemia, with severe cases resulting in stillborn births, spontaneous abortion, or an overwhelming disease known as granulomatosis infantiseptica.
   b. Listeriosis in pregnant women is typically **asymptomatic.**
   c. Adult bacterial meningitis caused by *L monocytogenes* is rare in healthy individuals but is a leading cause of meningitis in patients with cancer and those who have received transplants.
2. **Transmission/epidemiology:** Transmission is from ingestion of contaminated foods and through person-to-person spread.
   a. Sources of infection include domestic animals and birds; contaminated soil, water, and sewage; and contaminated meats, cheese, milk, poultry, and seafood.
   b. Food contamination is accentuated by the organism's ability to grow at low temperatures (under refrigerated conditions).
   c. Person-to-person spread can occur through in utero infections, colonization of the birth canal, and nosocomial transmission by hospital workers.

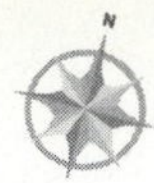

3. **Pathogenesis/virulence factors:** Pathogenesis involves host cell invasion using two major virulence factors: internalin and listeriolysin O (Table 2–2).
   a. Internalin facilitates binding and endocytosis into host intestinal epithelial cells and macrophages.
   b. A pore-forming toxin called listeriolysin O allows organisms to escape from the endosome.
   c. *L monocytogenes* replicates in the host cell cytoplasm, where it escapes the humoral immune system and spreads to adjacent cells or blood.
   d. Transplacental spread is mediated by invasion of placental endothelial cells from an asymptomatic bacteremia in the mother.
   e. Immune clearance requires a T-cell response.
4. **Treatment:** Current guidelines should be checked, but in general *Listeria* infections are treated with ampicillin and an aminoglycoside such as gentamicin or with trimethoprim-sulfamethoxazole.
5. **Prevention:** Infection control involves elimination of animal reservoirs, care in handling infants, and early diagnosis and treatment of infected mothers.

E. *Erysipelothrix rhusiopathiae*

1. **Clinical manifestations:** *E rhusiopathiae* causes a zoonotic, localized, and self-limiting soft tissue infection.
   a. Inflammation results in red-purple, swollen, burning, and itching skin.
   b. The slow spread of the infection from the site of inoculation occurs over approximately 3 weeks.
2. **Transmission/epidemiology:** Erysipeloid is an occupational disease of fishermen, butchers, and veterinarians. Transmission is from direct inoculation into skin abrasions from handling infected animals or animal products.
3. **Pathogenesis/virulence factors:** The major virulence factor (Table 2–2) is hyaluronidase.
   a. Production of hyaluronidase facilitates spread through tissue.
   b. Disease results from the host inflammatory response to infection.
4. **Treatment:** Antibiotics such as penicillin and erythromycin are used for treatment.
5. **Prevention:** Prevention involves care in handling infected animals.

CLINICAL PROBLEMS

Two employees of the microbiology department ordered take-out food from a local Chinese restaurant. Two hours after lunch, one of the individuals experienced severe abdominal cramps, nausea, and vomiting. On questioning, she indicated that the only thing she had eaten that day was fried rice.

1. Which of the following organisms is most likely to have contributed to this illness?

   A. *B anthracis*

   B. *B cereus*

   C. *C diphtheriae*

   D. *L monocytogenes*

2. The virulence factors associated with pathogenesis induced by *B anthracis* include:
    A. Heat-labile and heat-stable exotoxins
    B. Hyaluronidase and a polysaccharide capsule
    C. Listeriolysin O, internalin, and a capsule of D-glutamic acid
    D. Three exotoxins (EF, LF, and PA) and a capsule of D-glutamic acid

An active immunization program to prevent diphtheria was developed in the 1940s. Because immunization was a requirement to attend public school, cases of diphtheria in the United States are now extremely rare, on the order of 1 in 10 million.

3. The vaccine against diphtheria induces antibodies directed against what part of *C diphtheriae*?
    A. Bacterial cell wall
    B. Toxin subunit required for receptor binding
    C. Capsule of D-glutamic acid
    D. Fimbriae

Meningitis is diagnosed in a 2-week-old infant. Examination of cerebrospinal fluid reveals the presence of neutrophils and gram-positive rods.

4. The virulence factors associated with the most likely causative organism include:
    A. Lipopolysaccharide
    B. An exotoxin that alters intracellular levels of cAMP
    C. Internalin and listeriolysin O
    D. Heat-stable and heat-labile exotoxins

ANSWERS

1. The answer is B. *B cereus* causes food poisoning by production of preformed toxin in contaminated food. The heat-labile toxin causes diarrhea, and the heat-stable toxin causes vomiting.
2. The answer is D. The heat-labile and heat-stable toxins are produced by *B cereus.* Listeriolysin O and internalin are virulence factors of *Listeria,* and hyaluronidase is the virulence factor of *Erysipelothrix.*
3. The answer is B. Active immunization can take place by a number of different mechanisms. In the case of diphtheria, antibodies directed against the toxin are sufficient to prevent disease. Without toxin formation, the *C diphtheriae* organisms cannot establish an infection.
4. The answer is C. The organism most likely to be involved with neonatal meningitis that is also a gram-positive rod is *L monocytogenes.* The internalin protein assists in bacterial invasion, and listeriolysin O helps evade phagocytic killing.

CHAPTER 3
GRAM-POSITIVE COCCI

I. Key Concepts

A. Medically important gram-positive cocci belong to three genera: *Staphylococcus, Streptococcus,* and *Enterococcus.*

B. ***Staphylococcus*** species are catalase-positive and characteristically appear as large or small clusters under microscopic examination (Table 3–1).

C. ***Streptococcus*** species are catalase-negative and categorized by their group-specific carbohydrates (Lancefield group) and hemolysis patterns.

D. ***Enterococcus*** species are closely related to *Streptococcus* and are catalase-negative and Lancefield group D.

II. *Staphylococcus*

A. *Staphylococcus aureus*

1. **Clinical manifestations:** *S aureus* is the most pathogenic *Staphylococcus* species and causes a variety of clinical diseases.
   a. **Food poisoning** by intoxication is characterized by vomiting and diarrhea 1–6 hours after ingestion of *S aureus*–contaminated food.
   b. Cutaneous infections include **staphylococcal scalded skin syndrome** (SSSS); **bullous impetigo; folliculitis, furuncles, styes;** and **carbuncles.**
   c. **Toxic shock syndrome** (TSS) is characterized by fever, erythematous rash, hypotension, multiple organ involvement, shock, and desquamation of skin, including the soles of the feet and the palms.
   d. **Pneumonia** follows bacteremia or aspiration of organisms.
   e. **Meningitis** follows trauma, surgery, or bacteremia.
   f. **Acute endocarditis** and **osteomyelitis** follow bacteremia, surgical trauma, or seeding from other foci of infection.
   g. Along with *Neisseria gonorrhoeae, S aureus* is one of the most common causes of **septic arthritis.**
   h. **Abscesses** can form in any organ in response to infection.
2. **Transmission/epidemiology:** *S aureus* is part of the normal flora in the anterior nares in approximately 10–30% of individuals.
   a. *S aureus* can survive long periods on fomites, facilitating transmission from person to person.
   b. *S aureus* is found as normal flora in the vagina in 5% of women, putting them at higher risk for TSS associated with the use of tampons.

Table 3–1. Physical properties of *Staphylococcus.*

Organism	Hemolysis	Catalase	Coagulase	Novobiocin
S aureus	Beta	Positive	Positive	Sensitive
S epidermidis	Gamma	Positive	Negative	Sensitive
S saprophyticus	Gamma	Positive	Negative	Resistant

3. **Pathogenesis/virulence factors:** *S aureus* has many different virulence factors (Table 3–2), including at least 4 different types of toxins, a variety of enzymes, and several structural components that contribute to different disease manifestations.
   a. Heat-stable **enterotoxins** act as **superantigens** (Figure 3–1) and, when ingested, stimulate vomiting and diarrhea.
   b. **TSS toxin** (TSST1) is also a superantigen that causes systemic release of cytokines into the circulation, leading to symptoms of toxic shock.
   c. Cytolytic toxins such as **alpha-toxin** kill a variety of cells, including leukocytes and macrophages, and are involved in heart damage seen in acute endocarditis.
   d. **Exfoliative toxins** cleave desmosomes, causing epidermal separation as seen in SSSS.
   e. **Protein A** binds the Fc region of immunoglobulin, protecting the organism from humoral immune clearance.
   f. **Penicillinase** confers resistance to penicillin antibiotics by cleaving the beta-lactam ring.

Table 3–2. Virulence factors of *Staphylococcus aureus.*

Toxins	• Enterotoxins (heat stable) A, B, C, D, E, G, H, I • Cytolytic toxins: alpha, beta, delta, gamma, leukocidins • Exfoliative toxins –ETA: heat stable –ETB: heat labile • Toxic shock syndrome toxin: TSST1
Enzymes	• Catalase • Coagulase • Hyaluronidase • Lipase • Fibrinolysin
Structural Components	• Protein A • Capsule • Peptidoglycan

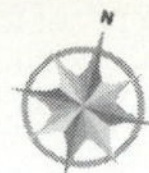

Figure 3–1. Bacterial toxins as superantigens. Superantigen toxins bind directly to MHC class II molecules on antigen-presenting cells and bridge with the Vβ component of the T-cell receptor (TCR), causing nonspecific stimulation of large numbers of T cells and the production of massive amounts of inflammatory cytokines.

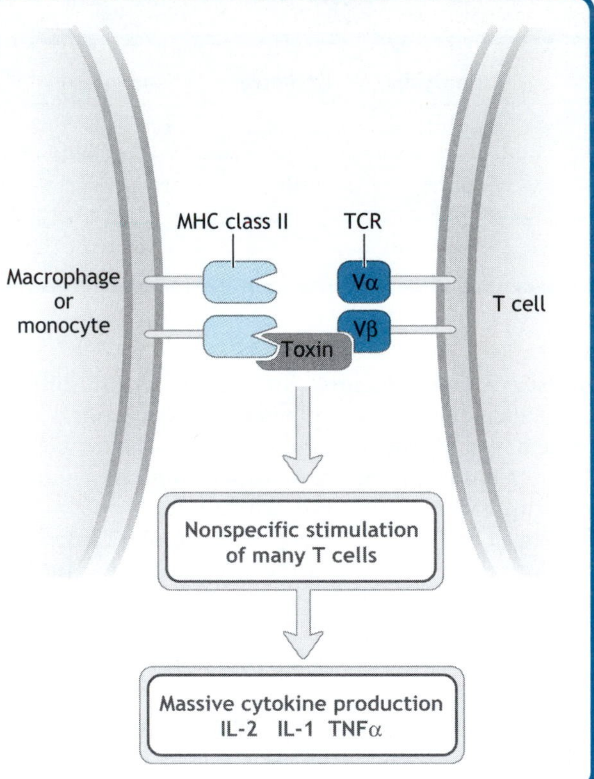

4. **Laboratory diagnosis:** *S aureus* is a catalase-positive, beta-hemolytic, gram-positive coccus that grows in clusters.
   a. *S aureus* can be distinguished from other *Staphylococcus* species by its production of coagulase.
   b. When plated on **mannitol salt selective and differential media,** *S aureus* ferments mannitol, leading to bright yellow colonies.
5. **Treatment:** Antibiotic resistance is a big problem for treating *S aureus* infections (see Clinical Correlation below).
   a. Because 90% of isolates carry a penicillinase, penicillin is generally not effective.
   b. Methicillin, oxacillin, nafcillin, dicloxacillin, and vancomycin are effective on some strains of *S aureus.*
6. **Prevention:** *S aureus* infections can be prevented by cleaning wounds properly, washing hands, following good surgical practices, and limiting exposure to patients by healthcare workers with skin infections.

DRUG-RESISTANT *S AUREUS*

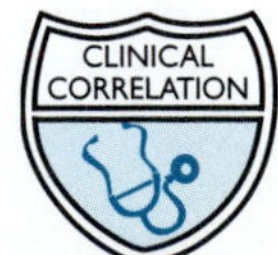

- *Penicillins that are resistant to the action of beta-lactamases and that are effective in penicillinase-carrying strains of* S aureus *have been developed, such as methicillin and oxacillin.*
- *Methicillin-resistant* S aureus *(MRSA) is becoming increasingly common.*

- *MRSA has acquired a gene that codes for a new penicillin-binding protein, making these organisms resistant to virtually all beta-lactam antibiotics.*
- *Vancomycin is effective in many of these MRSA strains. However, some* S aureus *strains are also becoming increasingly resistant to vancomycin, making these organisms extremely difficult to treat.*

B. *Staphylococcus epidermidis*

1. **Clinical manifestations:** *S epidermidis* causes a variety of opportunistic infections, including endocarditis associated with prosthetic heart valves and bacteremia associated with infections around catheters and shunts.
2. **Transmission/epidemiology:** *S epidermidis* is part of the normal resident skin flora and is usually transmitted through surgical placement of valves, catheters, and shunts.
3. **Pathogenesis/virulence factors:** Some strains of *S epidermidis* produce a slime layer that adheres to catheters and shunts, protects organisms from inflammatory clearance, and allows colonization.
4. **Laboratory diagnosis:** Physical properties of *S epidermidis* are summarized in Table 3–1.
5. **Treatment:** *S epidermidis* is often resistant to many antibiotics, including penicillins and methicillin. Vancomycin-resistant strains are emerging.
6. **Prevention:** Removing infected catheters and shunts, following good surgical practices, and washing hands routinely can help prevent infections.

C. *Staphylococcus saprophyticus*

1. **Clinical manifestations:** *S saprophyticus* is a common cause of urinary tract infections (UTIs) in sexually active females.
2. **Transmission/epidemiology:** *S saprophyticus* is normal flora in the lower urinary tract.
3. **Laboratory diagnosis:** Physical properties of *S saprophyticus* are summarized in Table 3–1.
4. **Treatment:** Current guidelines should be consulted, but antibiotics such as norfloxacin and trimethoprim-sulfamethoxazole generally are effective in treating *S saprophyticus*–related UTIs.

III. *Streptococcus*

A. *Streptococcus pyogenes* is a member of the group A streptococci and is further subdivided into more than 80 serotypes based on its M protein.

1. **Clinical manifestations:** *S pyogenes* causes a wide variety of diseases.
   a. **Pharyngitis** ("strep throat") is common in children.
   b. **Scarlet fever** is characterized by a diffuse rash, fever, and "strawberry" tongue.
   c. **Rheumatic fever** is a postinfective sequela that promotes damage to heart muscle and may occur 1–5 weeks after *S pyogenes*–related pharyngitis.
   d. Skin and soft tissue infections include **impetigo** (crusted not bullous) and **erysipelas.**
   e. **Necrotizing fasciitis,** caused by the so-called flesh-eating bacteria, is a more severe soft tissue infection that causes massive tissue destruction and systemic septic manifestations.
   f. Skin infections can progress to **streptococcal TSS,** which is associated with high fatality and disease manifestations similar to toxic shock induced by *S aureus.*

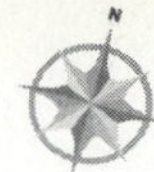

g. Because *S pyogenes* is highly invasive, local infections can become bacteremic, causing **sepsis.**

h. **Acute glomerulonephritis** is a postinfective sequela that may occur 3–6 weeks after either pharyngeal or skin infections with nephritogenic strains of *S pyogenes.*

2. **Transmission/epidemiology:** *S pyogenes* is found in the oropharynx and transiently on skin.
   a. Pharyngeal infections are transmitted by respiratory droplets.
   b. Skin infections occur after direct contact with infected individuals or contaminated fomites, followed by transient colonization and penetration through cuts and breaks in the skin.
3. **Pathogenesis/virulence factors:** *S pyogenes* carries a host of virulence factors (Table 3–3) that contribute to pathogenesis.
   a. Evasion of the immune system involves several structural components and enzymes.
      (1) The hyaluronic acid **capsule** is antiphagocytic.
      (2) **M protein** facilitates C3b cleavage and escape from opsonization.
      (3) **C5a peptidase** destroys C5a, decreasing inflammatory cell infiltration.
      (4) **Streptolysin S** and **streptolysin O** are cytolytic enzymes that destroy leukocytes and other cells.
   b. Tissue spread and invasion are facilitated by **hyaluronidase, streptokinase,** and **DNases.**
   c. The **Spe** toxins act as **superantigens,** resulting in massive release of cytokines that contribute to local and systemic disease manifestations.
   d. Rheumatic fever is caused by autoantibodies to M protein.
      (1) Antibodies cross-react with heart muscle.
      (2) Subsequent infections cause progressive heart damage.
   e. Acute glomerulonephritis is mediated by immune complex deposition.

Table 3–3. Virulence factors of *Streptococcus pyogenes.*

Toxins	• Streptococcal pyrogenic toxin (Spe) –also called erythrogenic toxin (3 types: A, B, C)
Enzymes	• C5a peptidase • Hyaluronidase • Streptokinase • DNase • Streptolysin S • Streptolysin O
Structural Components	• Hyaluronic acid capsule • M protein • F protein • M-like proteins

4. **Laboratory diagnosis:** *Streptococcus* species are all catalase-negative but show different hemolytic and biochemical properties (Table 3–4).
   a. *S pyogenes* is beta-hemolytic and sensitive to **bacitracin.**
   b. Immunologic tests are available against group A antigens (rapid strep test) and are useful for diagnosis of pharyngitis. Depending on the disease manifestation, cultures should be taken from throat, skin, or blood.
   c. Streptolysin O stimulates anti–streptolysin O (**ASO**) antibody.
      (1) Serology to detect ASO titers is useful to document *S pyogenes* infections prior to an episode of rheumatic fever or acute glomerulonephritis.
      (2) ASO titers rise from pharyngeal but not skin infections.
5. **Treatment:** Current guidelines should be consulted, but most *S pyogenes* strains are sensitive to antibiotics such as penicillin and erythromycin.
   a. Skin infections should be cleaned.
   b. Surgical débridement may be necessary, especially for deep infections.
6. **Prevention:** Prompt treatment of primary pharyngeal infections helps prevent rheumatic fever, and individuals who have had rheumatic fever may need prophylactic antibiotics to prevent new infections from stimulating further heart damage.

B. ***Streptococcus agalactiae,*** also known as **group B** ***Streptococcus*** (**GBS**), contains at least 11 different serotypes based on the polysaccharide capsule.
1. **Clinical manifestations:** *S agalactiae* causes both neonatal disease and adult disease.
   a. **Early-onset neonatal disease** (ie, in infants less than 1 week old) presents as **pneumonia, meningitis,** or **sepsis,** with significant mortality and **neurologic sequelae.**
   b. **Late-onset neonatal disease** (ie, in infants 1 week to 3 months old) typically presents as bacteremia and meningitis, with a lower incidence of mortality and sequelae.
   c. Adult disease includes **UTIs** in pregnant women and bacteremia, pneumonia, and skin, joint, and soft tissue infections in compromised individuals.

Table 3–4. Physical properties of *Streptococcus* and *Enterococcus*.

Organism	Lancefield Group	Hemolysis	Catalase	Bacitracin Sensitivity	Optochin Sensitivity
S pyogenes	A	Beta	Negative	Yes	
S agalactiae	B	Beta	Negative	No	
S pneumoniae	Nontypeable	Alpha	Negative		Yes
E faecalis	D	Variable	Negative		No

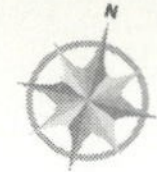

2. **Transmission/epidemiology:** *S agalactiae* colonizes the gastrointestinal (GI) and genitourinary (GU) tracts and can be found as transient flora in up to 30% of pregnant women.
   a. Transmission to neonates can occur in utero or at birth, resulting in early-onset disease.
   b. Late-onset disease results from person-to-person transmission after birth.
3. **Pathogenesis/virulence factors:** The primary virulence factor is the antiphagocytic polysaccharide capsule.
   a. Neonates lack specific protective antibodies that are needed for opsonization.
   b. Pathogenesis results from the inflammatory response.
4. **Laboratory diagnosis:** Physical properties are summarized in Table 3–4.
   a. Culture of blood or cerebrospinal fluid (CSF) is used for diagnosis.
   b. Latex agglutination and other immunologic assays are available for rapid detection of antigen.
   c. Culture is used to determine vaginal colonization.
5. **Treatment:** Current guidelines should be consulted, but, in general, combination therapy with penicillin or vancomycin with an aminoglycoside is used for treatment.
6. **Prevention:** Screening pregnant women for vaginal colonization in the third trimester helps determine risk.
   a. High-risk factors include vaginal colonization, premature birth, and prolonged membrane rupture.
   b. Antibiotic prophylaxis in high-risk pregnancy during labor reduces the incidence of disease.

C. ***Streptococcus pneumoniae*** contains more than 80 serotypes based on its polysaccharide capsule.

1. **Clinical manifestations:** *S pneumoniae* causes a variety of diseases in adults and children.
   a. **Pneumococcal pneumonia** is characterized by an abrupt onset of fever, shaking chills, and productive cough.
      (1) Pneumonia is usually **lobar** but can also be a more diffuse bronchopneumonia.
      (2) Sputum typically contains blood.
   b. *S pneumoniae* is one of the most common causes of **meningitis** in adults and children.
   c. **Bacteremia** often accompanies pneumonia and meningitis.
   d. *S pneumoniae* is a common cause of **otitis media** and **sinusitis.**
2. **Transmission/epidemiology:** Many individuals carry *S pneumoniae* in the oropharynx.
   a. New serotypes can be acquired by direct contact and by respiratory droplet transmission.
   b. Pneumonia results from **aspiration** of endogenous organisms from an oropharynx colonization into the lungs.
   c. Susceptibility to infection results from conditions that disrupt normal clearance mechanisms, such as **viral respiratory infections** and **chronic pulmonary diseases.**
   d. Meningitis can occur following ear and sinus infections, pneumonia, bacteremia, and head trauma.

3. **Pathogenesis/virulence factors:** The primary virulence factor of *S pneumoniae* is its polysaccharide **capsule,** which inhibits phagocytosis. Other factors that help establish infection include
   a. **Secretory IgA protease** and **pneumolysin,** which disrupt mucociliary clearance mechanisms.
   b. Pneumolysin, which inhibits phagocytic killing.
   c. **Phosphorylcholine,** which facilitates invasion and entry into blood.
   d. Cell wall components, including **peptidoglycan** and **teichoic acid,** which activate the alternate complement pathway and stimulate the host inflammatory response–the primary mechanism of pathogenesis.
4. **Laboratory diagnosis:** Physical properties are summarized in Table 3–4.
   a. Gram stain of sputum reveals gram-positive, **lancet-** or bullet-shaped diplococci.
   b. Culture reveals **alpha-hemolytic** colonies sensitive to bile and **Optochin.**
   c. The **Quellung reaction** is used for type-specific identification.
   d. Latex agglutination tests will detect antigen in CSF.
   e. **C-reactive protein,** a nonspecific indicator of acute infection, is bound by a component of the *S pneumoniae* cell wall called **C-substance.**
5. **Treatment:** Resistance to penicillin through changes in penicillin-binding proteins is becoming a major problem. Chloramphenicol, vancomycin, and erythromycin have been effective in some of these penicillin-resistant strains.
6. **Prevention:** A polyvalent polysaccharide vaccine provides protection against 23 different serotypes. A diphtheria toxoid–conjugated vaccine is available for infants and young children against 7 serotypes.

IV. *Enterococcus*

A. ***Enterococcus faecalis*** is a significant cause of nosocomial infections.
1. **Clinical manifestations:** *E faecalis* is not particularly virulent, but infections can be difficult to clear.
   a. **UTIs** and **bacteremia** are the two most common disease manifestations.
   b. *E faecalis*–induced **endocarditis** is associated with previously damaged heart valves.
   c. **Intra-abdominal wounds** often contain *E faecalis* as a component of mixed infection.
2. **Transmission/epidemiology:** *E faecalis* is a normal inhabitant of the GI and GU tracts.
   a. Most infections result from endogenous transmission, but person-to-person spread can occur, especially through the fecal-oral route.
   b. **Indwelling catheters** are common sources for UTIs, and vascular and peritoneal catheters are sources for transmission to blood.
   c. Prolonged hospitalization with antibiotic treatment can promote a selective growth advantage and colonization.
3. **Pathogenesis/virulence factors:** There are no clear virulence factors other than some adhesion proteins and multiple antibiotic resistance.
4. **Laboratory diagnosis:** *Enterococcus* is closely related to *Streptococcus* but can be differentiated based on growth characteristics, including tolerance to high salt and bile and the ability to hydrolyze esculin (Table 3–4).

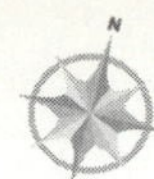

5. **Treatment:** Because of multiple resistance, susceptibility testing should guide therapy.
   a. In general, combination treatment using cell wall–active antibiotics such as ampicillin in combination with aminoglycosides provides synergistic activity.
   b. Vancomycin is used with penicillin-resistant strains.

CLINICAL PROBLEMS

A 20-year-old college student abruptly starts vomiting and exhibits other GI symptoms 2 hours after eating in the dining hall.

1. These symptoms are most likely to have occurred as a result of:
   A. Ingestion of *S aureus* organisms
   B. An ADP ribosylating enterotoxin that elevates intracellular cAMP
   C. A bacterial adenylate cyclase
   D. An enterotoxin superantigen

In the office, a 3-year-old child is seen with a fever, a sore throat, a diffuse rash, and a bright red tongue.

2. What would throat culture most likely reveal?
   A. Gram-positive, catalase-negative, alpha-hemolytic, Optochin-sensitive cocci
   B. Gram-positive, catalase-positive, beta-hemolytic, coagulase-positive cocci
   C. Gram-positive, catalase-negative, beta-hemolytic, bacitracin-sensitive cocci
   D. Gram-positive, catalase-negative, beta-hemolytic, bacitracin-resistant cocci

A 5-year-old is seen in the emergency department with symptoms of meningitis. A Gram stain of CSF reveals many neutrophils and gram-positive, lancet-shaped diplococci.

3. Culture results would be expected to indicate:
   A. Alpha-hemolytic, bacitracin-sensitive colonies
   B. Alpha-hemolytic, Optochin-sensitive colonies
   C. Beta-hemolytic, bacitracin-sensitive colonies
   D. Beta-hemolytic, Optochin-sensitive colonies

A 4-year-old is seen with bullous impetigo. Culture results reveal a beta-hemolytic, catalase-positive, coagulase-positive organism.

4. Based on this information, the organism causing this skin manifestation is most likely:
   A. *S pyogenes*
   B. *S agalactiae*
   C. *S aureus*
   D. *S epidermidis*

5. *S aureus* TSST1 and *S pyogenes* SpeA have in common the fact that they:
   A. Are superantigens
   B. Are cytolytic enzymes
   C. Have identical structures
   D. Are integral components of the cell wall

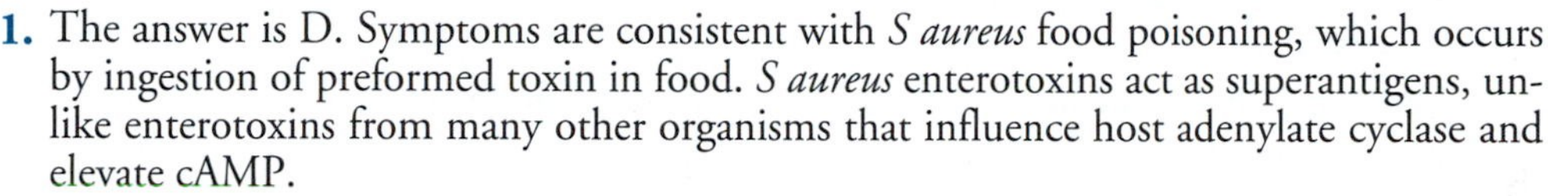

ANSWERS

1. The answer is D. Symptoms are consistent with *S aureus* food poisoning, which occurs by ingestion of preformed toxin in food. *S aureus* enterotoxins act as superantigens, unlike enterotoxins from many other organisms that influence host adenylate cyclase and elevate cAMP.
2. The answer is C. Symptoms are consistent with *S pyogenes*–induced pharyngitis and scarlet fever. The properties listed are characteristic of this organism.
3. The answer is B. The case presentation is consistent with meningitis caused by *S pneumoniae,* which is alpha-hemolytic and Optochin sensitive.
4. The answer is C. Both *S pyogenes* and *S aureus* cause impetigo. *S aureus* is catalase-positive and coagulase-positive.
5. The answer is A. TSST1 and SpeA have different structures but both act as superantigens.

CHAPTER 4
GRAM-NEGATIVE COCCI

I. Key Concepts

A. The two gram-negative cocci of major medical importance are members of the *Neisseria* genus (Table 4–1).

B. *Neisseria* species are typically kidney bean–shaped, oxidase-positive diplococci.

C. Complement plays an important role in immune clearance, so individuals with complement deficiencies are at increased risk for more severe disease.

D. The lipopolysaccharide (LPS) of *Neisseria* is shorter than many other gram-negative bacteria and is called lipooligosaccharide (LOS).

II. *Neisseria*

A. *Neisseria gonorrhoeae*

1. **Clinical manifestations:** Infection with *N gonorrhoeae* results in a variety of diseases, depending on the site of entry.
   - **a.** Infection can be symptomatic or asymptomatic.
   - **b.** Asymptomatic infections represent an important source of spread because individuals do not seek treatment.
   - **c.** In men, the most common symptomatic clinical syndromes are **urethritis, proctitis,** and **pharyngitis.**
   - **d.** In women, urethritis, proctitis, pharyngitis, and **cervicitis** are the most common symptomatic clinical syndromes.
   - **e.** More severe infections result from bacterial dissemination.
     - *(1)* These infections include **pelvic inflammatory disease** (PID), **septicemia, skin and joint manifestations,** and **arthritis.**
     - *(2)* PID can result in scarring of the fallopian tubes, ectopic pregnancy, and infertility.
   - **f. In newborns, conjunctivitis** can lead to blindness.
2. **Transmission/epidemiology:** *N gonorrhoeae* is transmitted through sexual contact and through vaginal delivery to newborns from an infected mother.
   - **a.** Gonorrhea is a human disease with no animal reservoirs.
   - **b.** In women, the incidence of single-exposure infection approaches 50%; in men, it is closer to 20%.
3. **Pathogenesis/virulence factors:** *N gonorrhoeae* has several virulence factors that allow it to evade the host immune system and attach to and invade host cells (Table 4–2).
   - **a.** Binding to mucosal epithelial cells is facilitated by the pilin protein.
   - **b.** Tight binding and invasion are mediated by opa proteins.

Table 4–1. Physical properties of medically important gram-negative cocci.

Organism	Gram Stain	Shape	Spores	Motility	Interesting Properties
Neisseria gonorrhoeae	–	Diplococcus (coffee bean)	No	No	Complex growth requirements Thayer-Martin and chocolate agar
Neisseria meningitidis	–	Diplococcus (kidney bean)	No	No	Growth on blood or chocolate agar

c. Bacteria multiply intracellularly, fuse with the basement membrane, and are discharged into the subepithelial tissue, where they induce a local inflammatory response.

d. Bacteria evade immune clearing through a number of mechanisms.

(1) Antigenic variation and phase variation of pilin and opa proteins allow escape from humoral immune responses.

(2) The Por protein facilitates intracellular survival and replication by inhibiting phagolysosome fusion.

(3) The IgA protease inactivates IgA through proteolytic cleavage, preventing opsonization.

4. **Laboratory diagnosis: In men,** the presence of intracellular gram-negative diplococci in direct Gram stain of the purulent discharge is diagnostic. **In women,** a positive Gram stain of the vaginal discharge must be confirmed by culture.

Table 4–2. Summary of virulence factors.

Organism	Virulence Factor
Neisseria gonorrhoeae	Antiphagocytic capsule (some strains) Por protein (intracellular survival) Pilin (initial attachment) Opa (tight attachment/invasion) IgA protease Beta-lactamase Lipooligosaccharide (LOS): endotoxin similar to LPS
Neisseria meningitidis	Antiphagocytic polysaccharide capsule (A, B, C, Y, W135) LOS (endotoxin) IgA protease Attachment pili

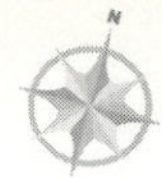

5. **Treatment:** Because of antibiotic resistance, current guidelines should be consulted, and susceptibility testing may be necessary.
   a. In general, third-generation cephalosporins, such as ceftriaxone and cefixime, and fluoroquinolones, such as ciprofloxacin and ofloxacin, are effective for uncomplicated gonorrhea.
   b. Combination therapy with doxycycline or azithromycin is used to treat dual infections with *Chlamydia.*
6. **Prevention:** Silver nitrate eye drops are effective chemoprophylaxis against gonococcal eye infections of newborns.

GONORRHEA

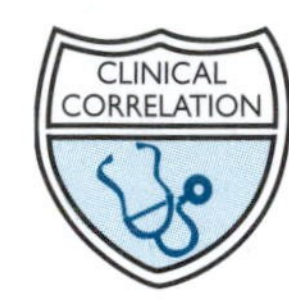

- *Because of its effectiveness and availability, penicillin was the drug of choice for many years.*
- *However, selective pressure contributed to changes in penicillin-binding proteins, requiring greater doses for effectiveness.*
- *Because some strains now also carry beta-lactamases, penicillin is no longer recommended.*

B. *Neisseria meningitidis*

1. **Clinical manifestations:** Infection with *N meningitidis* causes two major clinical syndromes—meningitis and septicemia.
   a. **Meningitis** is characterized by combinations of fever, headache, stiff neck, lethargy, photophobia, confusion, and even coma.
   b. **Septicemia** caused by *N meningitidis* (**meningococcemia**), is often associated with the presence of **petechiae** on the trunk and appendages.
   c. Severe cases can progress to yield widespread **ecchymoses** and disseminated intravascular coagulation (**DIC**).
2. **Transmission/epidemiology:** There are 5 medically important serogroups based on the polysaccharide capsule of *N meningitidis:* A, B, C, Y, and W135.
   a. Outbreaks of *N meningitidis* meningitis arise when mixed populations carrying different serogroups are brought together under crowded conditions, such as in military barracks and university dormitories.
   b. *N meningitidis* is a human disease with no animal reservoirs.
   c. The main mode of transmission is by respiratory droplet.
3. **Pathogenesis/virulence factors:** *N meningitidis* has 4 major virulence factors (Table 4–2).
   a. The polysaccharide capsule is antiphagocytic and important in evading the host immune response.
   b. Cell wall endotoxin (LOS) induces a strong host inflammatory response, which is responsible for many of the symptoms of meningitis and septicemia.
   c. IgA protease and attachment pili facilitate colonization of mucosal surfaces.
   d. Immune clearance requires a specific IgG and IgM response against the polysaccharide capsule.
      (1) Complement-mediated lysis of bacteria by the classical pathway is important to immune clearance.
      (2) Individuals with complement deficiencies are at a much higher risk for disease development.
4. **Laboratory diagnosis:** Gram stain of cerebrospinal fluid and direct agglutination tests can be used to diagnose *N meningitidis* infections.

5. **Treatment:** Suspected *N meningitidis* infections should be treated as a medical emergency. Current guidelines should be consulted, but in general, penicillin or third-generation cephalosporins are the antibiotics of choice.
6. **Prevention:** Acquired immunity, vaccination, and chemoprophylaxis are preventive methods.
   a. Acquired immunity relies on the production of complement-fixing IgG and IgM antibodies from previous infections.
   b. A vaccine directed against serogroups A, C, Y, and W135 is available.
      (1) The B serogroup polysaccharide is a poor immunogen and not covered in the current vaccine.
      (2) A high percentage of cases involve serogroup B.
   c. Chemoprophylaxis with rifampin is used for high-risk individuals who have been in close contact with an index case.

CLINICAL PROBLEMS

A patient presents with fever, stiff neck, and vomiting. Petechial lesions are present on the arms and chest. A Gram stain of cerebrospinal fluid reveals the presence of bean-shaped, gram-negative diplococci.

1. The virulence factors associated with the most likely causative organism of this disease include:

   A. Exotoxin, polysaccharide capsule, and opa

   B. Endotoxin, exotoxin, and attachment pili

   C. Polysaccharide capsule, endotoxin, and IgA protease

   D. Por, opa, and pilin

A college freshman is admitted to the emergency department with symptoms of meningococcemia. Blood culture and latex agglutination identify *N meningitidis* serogroup B. Six months before entering college, she had received the meningitis vaccine.

2. What is the most likely reason to explain her lack of protection?

   A. She has a B-cell immunodeficiency.

   B. Six months is not long enough to develop immunity.

   C. The serogroup B is a poor immunogen not covered in the current vaccine.

   D. The vaccine is not effective for this age group.

A 24-year-old man reports a painful purulent urethral discharge. Direct Gram stain reveals the presence of intracellular gram-negative diplococci. He tells his physician that he has had gonorrhea three times.

3. What is the most likely explanation for his lack of protective immunity from these previous infections?

   A. Antigenic and phase variation have altered surface proteins.

   B. Pilin and opa proteins are poor immunogens.

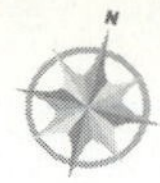

C. The patient has an immunodeficiency disorder.

D. Protective immunity is best achieved through vaccination.

4. Further tests indicated that this patient was also infected with *Chlamydia.* The treatment strategy would most likely include:

A. Penicillin alone

B. A third-generation cephalosporin, such as cefixime alone

C. A fluoroquinolone, such as ciprofloxacin alone

D. A combination of a third-generation cephalosporin with doxycycline

ANSWERS

1. The answer is C. The most likely causative agent is *N meningitidis.* The major virulence factors are LOS (endotoxin), IgA protease, an antiphagocytic polysaccharide capsule, and attachment pili.

2. The answer is C. The current vaccine protects only against serogroups A, C, Y, and W135. Because serogroup B is a poor immunogen, effective vaccination has not yet been developed.

3. The answer is A. Antigenic variation through gene rearrangements create thousands of antigenically different pilin and opa surface proteins. Phase variation turns each of these genes on and off, allowing escape from humoral immune responses.

4. The answer is D. Penicillin is no longer recommended because of widespread resistance. Third-generation cephalosporins and fluoroquinolones are effective against uncomplicated gonorrhea. Dual infections of *N gonorrhoeae* with *Chlamydia* require combination therapies.

CHAPTER 5
ENTERIC GRAM-NEGATIVE RODS

I. Key Concepts

A. Gram-negative rods make up the largest and most diverse group of bacterial human pathogens.

B. Genera within this group can be subcategorized based on common physical, clinical, and epidemiological properties.

C. Enteric pathogens constitute the largest group and include members of the Enterobacteriaceae family as well as the *Vibrio, Campylobacter,* and *Helicobacter* genera.

D. Most bacterial enteric infections are caused by *Escherichia coli, Salmonella enterica, Salmonella typhi, Shigella* species, *Yersinia enterocolitica, Vibrio cholerae, Campylobacter jejuni,* and *Helicobacter pylori.*

II. *Escherichia, Salmonella, Shigella, Yersinia, Vibrio, Campylobacter,* and *Helicobacter*

A. *Escherichia coli*

1. Medically important strains of *E coli* include enterotoxigenic *E coli* (ETEC), enteroinvasive *E coli* (EIEC), enteropathogenic *E coli* (EPEC), enteroaggregative *E coli* (EAEC), enterohemorrhagic *E coli* (EHEC), uropathogenic *E coli* (UPEC), and *E coli* K1.
2. **Clinical manifestations:** *E coli* causes a wide range of disease, including **watery diarrhea** (ETEC, EPEC, EAEC), **dysentery** (EIEC), **hemorrhagic colitis** (EHEC), **hemolytic uremic syndrome** (EHEC), **urinary tract infections** (UPEC), **neonatal meningitis** (*E coli* K1), and **sepsis**.
3. **Transmission/epidemiology:** *E coli* infections are acquired by a variety of mechanisms.
   a. *E coli* is part of the normal intestinal flora; however, endogenous spread to the bloodstream (eg, following bowel perforation, urogenital infection, or trauma) is a major cause of sepsis.
   b. Ingestion of contaminated food or water is the main route of transmission of most pathogenic *E coli* strains associated with gastrointestinal manifestations.
      (1) ETEC is a common cause of **traveler's diarrhea.**
      (2) Outbreaks of EHEC (strain O157 H7) have occurred from a wide variety of sources, including undercooked hamburger, unpasteurized apple juice, and contaminated water in swimming pools.

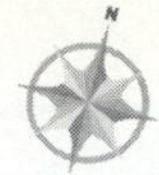

   (3) **EHEC infection** is facilitated by the **low infectious dose,** which can be as few as 50–100 organisms.

   (4) EPEC and EAEC are associated with **infant diarrhea,** especially in developing countries.

  c. UPEC is generally associated with endogenous spread to the urinary tract by poor hygiene, insertion of urinary catheters, and sexual intercourse.

  d. Neonates can acquire *E coli* K1 through fecal contamination during vaginal delivery.

4. **Pathogenesis/virulence factors:** Each of the different strains of *E coli* uses a unique mechanism for pathogenesis (Table 5–1).

  a. ETEC adheres to intestinal epithelial cells and secretes heat-labile and heat-stable enterotoxins (Figure 5–1).

   (1) The heat-labile toxin is an AB toxin that ADP ribosylates a regulatory G protein, resulting in constitutive activation of host adenylate cyclase and elevation of cAMP.

   (2) The heat-stable toxin targets host guanylate cyclase, causing cGMP elevation.

  b. EPEC attachment to enterocytes causes a host cell actin rearrangement, resulting in pedestal formation, destruction of microvilli, and decreased fluid absorption (**attachment/effacement pathogenesis**) (Figure 5–1).

  c. EAEC is characterized by adherence factors that result in large aggregates and a mucous biofilm that block fluid absorption (Figure 5–1).

Table 5–1. Summary of pathogenesis of *Escherichia coli* infections.

Organism	Major Clinical Manifestation	Virulence Mechanism
Enterotoxigenic *E coli* (ETEC)	Watery diarrhea	Heat-labile toxin (LT) Heat-stable toxin (ST)
Enterohemorrhagic *E coli* (EHEC)	Hemorrhagic colitis Hemolytic uremic syndrome	Shiga-like toxin
Enteroinvasive *E coli* (EIEC)	Dysentery	Plasmid-mediated invasion
Enteropathogenic *E coli* (EPEC)	Infant watery diarrhea	Attachment and effacement
Enteroaggregative *E coli* (EAEC)	Infant watery diarrhea	Plasmid-mediated aggregative adherence
Uropathogenic *E coli* (UPEC)	Urinary tract infections	P pili adherence to uroepithelial cells Endotoxin
E coli K1	Neonatal meningitis	Antiphagocytic capsule Endotoxin
Host flora *E coli*	Sepsis	Endotoxin

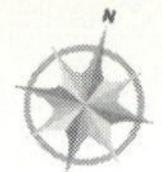

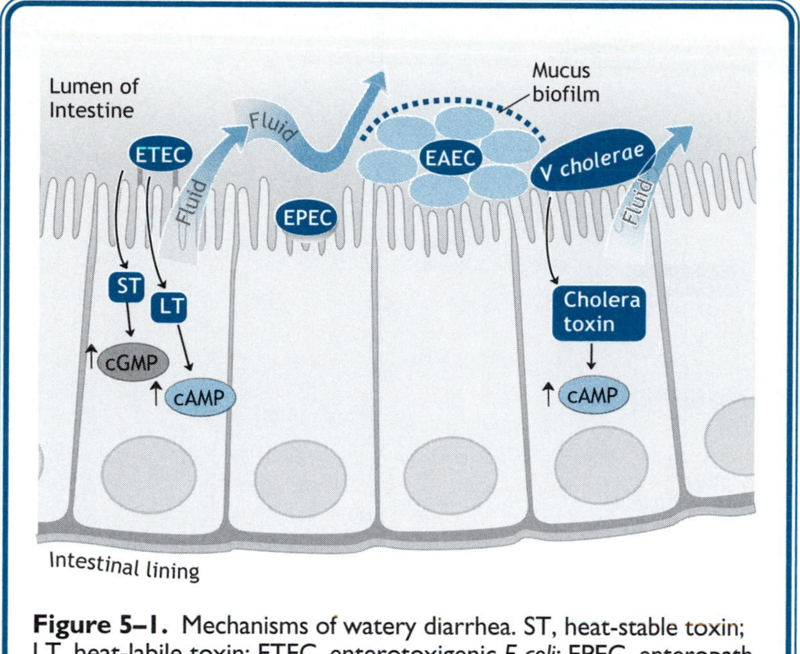

Figure 5–1. Mechanisms of watery diarrhea. ST, heat-stable toxin; LT, heat-labile toxin; ETEC, enterotoxigenic *E coli;* EPEC, enteropathogenic *E coli;* EAEC, enteroaggregative *E coli.*

   d. EIEC attaches and invades into intestinal epithelial cells in the colon, causing cell death and inflammation (Figure 5–2).
   e. EHEC adheres to colonic epithelial cells in a manner similar to EPEC and secretes a Shiga toxin that cleaves 28S RNA, resulting in inhibition of protein synthesis and cell death (Figure 5–2).
   f. P pili adhere to receptors on uroepithelial cells and facilitate establishment of infection by UPEC strains that have ascended from the urethra to the bladder and kidney.
   g. The K1 capsule is identical to that carried by *N meningitidis* type B and is antiphagocytic as well as a poor immunogen.
   h. Because of their gram-negative cell wall, all *E coli* carry **endotoxin** that is responsible for sepsis when organisms penetrate the bloodstream.

5. Laboratory diagnosis: Many *E coli* strains ferment lactose and sorbitol and can be grown on a variety of **selective and differential** media.
   a. Identification is based on serotype analysis of O, H, and K antigens.
   b. EHEC can be enriched from other *E coli* on the basis of their inability to ferment sorbitol.
   c. Latex agglutination is used to detect the K1 capsule in spinal fluid in neonates with meningitis.
   d. Polymerase chain reaction and hybridization can be used to detect toxin and other virulence genes.

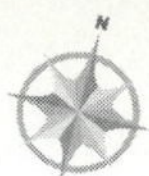

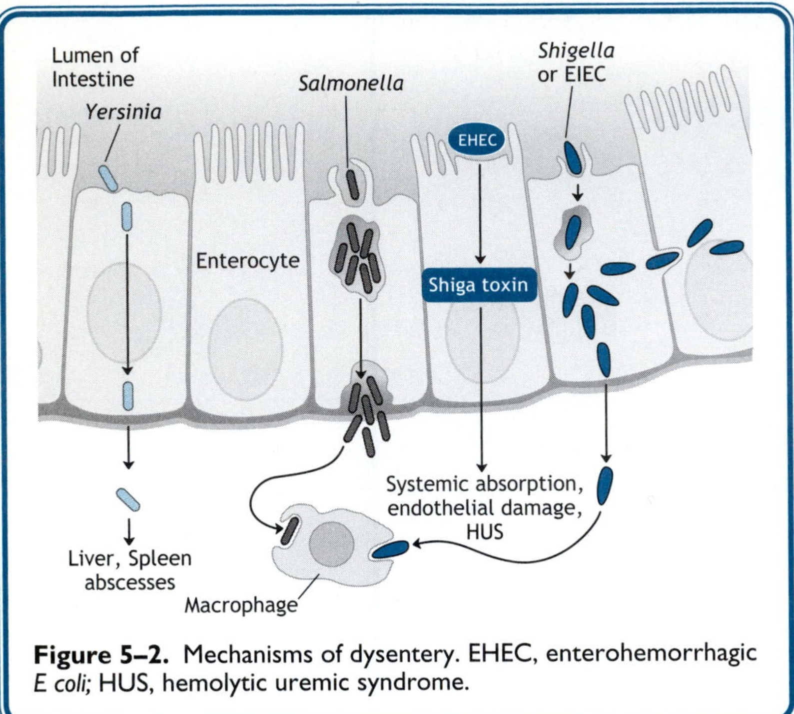

Figure 5–2. Mechanisms of dysentery. EHEC, enterohemorrhagic *E coli;* HUS, hemolytic uremic syndrome.

6. **Treatment:** Treatment is guided by clinical findings and varies depending on the manifestation, so current guidelines should be consulted.
   a. Generally self-limiting, diarrhea is treated with fluid replacement.
   b. Urinary tract infections are treated with sulfonamides or trimethoprim alone or in combination with nitrofurantoin, fluoroquinolones, and sulfamethoxazole.
   c. Treatment for sepsis involves third-generation cephalosporins, often in combination with aminoglycosides.
   d. Neonatal meningitis is often treated with a combination of cefotaxime and ampicillin.
7. **Prevention:** Diarrheal disease is best prevented by avoidance of improperly cooked foods or unpurified water.
   a. Prompt removal of urinary and intravenous catheters can lower the incidence of urinary tract infections and sepsis.
   b. Cranberry juice is thought to inhibit the ability of UPEC strains to bind uroepithelial cells and establish infection.

B. *Salmonella enterica*

1. The several thousand serotypes of *S enterica* induce a similar range of gastrointestinal disease.
2. **Clinical manifestations:** Infection with *Salmonella* most often causes an uncomplicated dysentery.
   a. Blood and pus are often seen after microscopic examination of stool.
   b. Particularly virulent strains are able to penetrate into the bloodstream, causing endotoxin-mediated sepsis.

3. **Transmission/epidemiology:** *Salmonella* species are common flora in a wide variety of animals, especially reptiles, poultry, and birds.
   a. Human infection comes from ingestion of improperly prepared foods.
   b. Insufficient washing after handling colonized animals, such as pet turtles, can lead to ingestion of organisms.
   c. Fecal-oral transmission, especially in food handlers, is facilitated by the fact that *Salmonella* can be shed in human stool for weeks after resolution of diarrheal disease.
4. **Pathogenesis/virulence factors:** *Salmonella* species carry a series of genes involved in facilitating invasion and survival in host cells (Table 5–2; Figure 5–2).
   a. A moderate infectious dose, about 100,000 organisms, is required to establish disease.
   b. Bacteria bind and are endocytosed by intestinal M cells.
   c. Once internalized, bacteria replicate in the endosome and eventually penetrate into the subepithelial tissue and stimulate an inflammatory response.
   d. Most infections remain localized to the intestinal mucosa and submucosa but some strains can penetrate further and enter the bloodstream.
5. **Laboratory diagnosis:** *Salmonella* organisms are readily isolated from stool cultures on common selective and differential media.
   a. *Salmonella* species are differentiated from *E coli* by their inability to ferment lactose.

Table 5–2. Summary of pathogenesis of other enteric gram-negative rods.

Organism	Major Clinical Manifestation	Virulence Mechanism
Salmonella enterica	Dysentery	Endotoxin Invasion
Salmonella typhi	Typhoid fever	Endotoxin Vi polysaccharide capsule
Shigella flexneri *Shigella dysenteriae* *Shigella boydii* *Shigella sonnei*	Dysentery HUS	Virulence plasmid (attachment, invasion, intracellular replication) Shiga toxin
Yersinia enterocolitica	Dysentery Hepatic abscesses	Invasion Heat-stable enterotoxin Endotoxin
Vibrio cholerae	Watery diarrhea	Cholera toxin
Campylobacter jejuni	Dysentery Watery diarrhea	Invasion Enterotoxin
Helicobacter pylori	Gastritis Ulcers	Cytotoxin

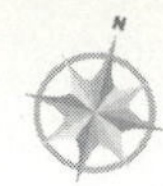

b. H_2S production and motility are features used to distinguish *Salmonella* from other non–lactose fermenters, such as *Shigella.*

6. Treatment: For any diarrheal disease, fluid replacement is essential. Current guidelines should be consulted, but antibiotics generally are not used for *Salmonella*-induced enteritis because they can prolong the carrier state.

7. Prevention: Proper food preparation and handwashing can prevent most infections.

C. *Salmonella typhi*

1. *S typhi* is the causative agent of typhoid fever.

2. Clinical manifestations. The incubation period for *S typhi* is 7–21 days.

a. Infection starts with gastrointestinal symptoms and gradually progresses to systemic disease manifested by fever, malaise, myalgia, and headache.

b. Fever symptoms can last 3–4 weeks.

c. Rose spots on the abdomen are associated with typhoid fever.

3. Transmission/epidemiology: In contrast to *S enterica,* the only reservoir of *S typhi* is humans.

a. Infection occurs after ingestion of contaminated food or water.

b. Humans can become chronic carriers and serve as endemic reservoirs, shedding bacteria in the stool for years.

4. Pathogenesis/virulence factors: The two major virulence factors of *S typhi* are the Vi polysaccharide capsule and endotoxin (Table 5–2).

a. After ingestion, *S typhi* invade M cells above Peyer's patches.

b. Bacteria replicate in endosomes and are transported to the subepithelial layer, where they are engulfed and survive in macrophages.

c. Organisms enter the blood and lymphatics, then replicate in the liver and spleen, resulting in long-term release of endotoxin.

d. Colonization of the gallbladder is associated with the carrier state.

5. Laboratory diagnosis: *S typhi* can be isolated from blood culture in the first week of illness.

6. Treatment: Current guidelines should be consulted, but in general a variety of antibiotics can be used to control the course of infection, including ampicillin, chloramphenicol, trimethoprim, ceftriaxone, and ciprofloxacin.

7. Prevention: Proper sanitation is the main method of control.

a. Carriers should not handle food.

b. Vaccines against the Vi capsule are protective.

D. *Shigella*

1. The four *Shigella* species that account for most infections leading to disease are *S dysenteriae, S flexneri, S boydii,* and *S sonnei.*

2. Clinical manifestations: Infection with *Shigella* causes dysentery clinically similar to that caused by EIEC.

a. Typical symptoms include fever, abdominal cramps, and blood- and mucus-containing diarrhea.

b. *S dysenteriae* also produces a Shiga toxin associated with more serious disease and development of hemolytic uremic syndrome (HUS).

3. Transmission/epidemiology: Fecal-oral spread is the most common mode of transmission.

a. Very few organisms (100–200) are required for infection.

b. Outbreaks often occur in daycare centers and other situations in which fecal-oral spread is common.

4. **Pathogenesis/virulence factors:** The major virulence factors of *Shigella* are genes required for invasion, Shiga toxin, and endotoxin (Table 5–2; Figure 5–2).
   a. *Shigella* organisms invade through intestinal M cells.
   b. After replication in the cytoplasm, they spread laterally to enterocytes.
   c. Cell destruction induces a host inflammatory response.
   d. The Shiga toxin induces endothelial cell destruction by the same mechanism as the toxin carried by EHEC.
5. **Laboratory diagnosis:** *Shigella* species are isolated from stool cultures on a variety of selective and differential media.
   a. Like *Salmonella, Shigella* species do not ferment lactose and are therefore readily distinguished from *E coli*.
   b. Unlike *Salmonella, Shigella* species do not produce H_2S and are not motile.
6. **Treatment:** Treatment is guided by clinical findings, but fluid and electrolyte replacement is often enough for mild cases, whereas antibiotics such as ciprofloxacin and trimethoprim are used for more severe disease.
7. **Prevention:** Proper sanitation and good personal hygiene are the best methods for prevention.

E. *Yersinia enterocolitica*

1. *Y enterocolitica* exhibits increased metabolic activity and growth at low temperatures (eg, 4 °C), which plays an important role in food contamination.
2. **Clinical manifestations:** Disease cause by *Y enterocolitica* is similar to that caused by Salmonella.
   a. Diarrhea, fever, and abdominal pain are characteristic of enterocolitis.
   b. Complications include septicemia and hepatic abscesses.
   c. Reactive arthritis is an important postinfective sequela most commonly found in individuals with the HLA B27 haplotype.
3. **Transmission/epidemiology:** *Y enterocolitica* is transmitted through ingestion of contaminated food, milk, or water. Infections are most common in Scandinavia and in cold areas of North America.
4. **Pathogenesis/virulence factors:** Pathogenic mechanisms involve host cell invasion and production of a heat-stable enterotoxin (Table 5–2; Figure 5–2).
5. **Treatment:** Enterocolitis is generally self-limiting, not requiring antibiotics; more serious infections can be treated with antibiotics such as tetracycline and gentamicin.

F. *Vibrio cholerae*

1. *V cholerae* is the causative agent of cholera.
2. **Clinical manifestations:** The major syndrome is severe watery diarrhea with flecks of mucus (**rice water stools**), resulting in rapid and extreme dehydration.
3. **Transmission/epidemiology:** The primary modes of transmission are ingestion of contaminated food or water and fecal-oral spread.
   a. *V cholerae* is endemic to many parts of the world, including Africa, Asia, South and Central America, and the Gulf Coast of the United States.
   b. Many stains cause mild symptoms, whereas the O1 and O139 pandemic strains cause serious disease.
   c. Because crustaceans can act as a reservoir, ingestion of raw or undercooked shellfish is a source of infection.
   d. Infection requires a large inoculating dose in the range of a billion organisms.

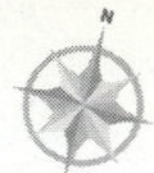

4. **Pathogenesis/virulence factors:** The four primary virulence factors of *V cholerae* are cholera toxin, mucinase, flagellum, and adhesions (Table 5–2; Figure 5–1).
   a. Mucinase and flagella facilitate penetration of the mucous layer that covers intestinal epithelial cells.
   b. Adhesions promote tight binding to the host cell surface.
   c. Cholera toxin is an A-B toxin similar to *E coli*–labile toxin.
      (1) B subunits bind GM1 ganglioside receptors on the cell surface.
      (2) The A subunit catalyses the ADP ribosylation of Gs, resulting in activation of adenylate cyclase, elevation of cAMP, and efflux of fluid and ions into the intestinal lumen.
5. **Treatment:** Fluid and electrolyte replacement is essential because of the rapid and voluminous watery diarrhea. Antibiotics such as ampicillin, tetracycline, trimethoprim, chloramphenicol, and fluoroquinolones may shorten the duration of symptoms.
6. **Prevention:** Proper sanitation, waste disposal, and hygiene are essential for controlling outbreaks. A vaccine is available but short-lived.

VIBRIO CHOLERAE–INDUCED WATERY DIARRHEA

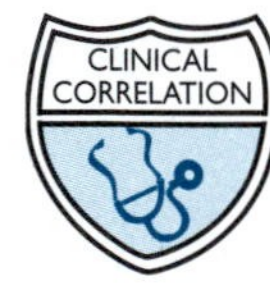

- *Infection with pandemic strains of* V cholerae *lead to rapid and voluminous watery diarrhea in which an individual can lose up to a liter of fluid per hour.*
- *Extreme and rapid dehydration leads to hypovolemic shock, which can result in death if untreated.*

G. *Campylobacter jejuni*

1. *C jejuni* is a small, comma- or S-shaped motile organism thought to be the most common cause of bacterial gastroenteritis.
2. **Clinical manifestations:** Infection with *C jejuni* can present as **watery diarrhea** or **dysentery** accompanied by fever and abdominal pain.
   a. Symptoms are generally self-limiting and last 1–2 weeks.
   b. Autoimmune sequelae include an association with **inflammatory bowel disease** and **Guillain-Barré syndrome.**
3. **Transmission/epidemiology:** Many animals serve as reservoirs for *C jejuni,* including chickens, cattle, swine, dogs, and cats.
   a. Human infection results from ingestion of contaminated food or water.
   b. The infectious dose is high unless stomach acidity is neutralized.
4. **Pathogenesis/virulence factors:** *C jejuni* contains several virulence factors, including an enterotoxin, a cytotoxin, and endotoxin (Table 5–2).
   a. Watery diarrhea is thought to be mediated by the enterotoxin.
   b. Dysentery results from cellular invasion and destruction of mucosal surfaces, which is likely mediated by the cytotoxin and the host inflammatory response.
5. **Laboratory diagnosis:** *C jejuni* is difficult to grow and requires special media, elevated temperature, reduced oxygen, and increased carbon dioxide.
6. **Treatment:** Clinical findings should guide treatment, but fluid replacement in combination with an antibiotic such as erythromycin or ciprofloxacin generally shortens the duration of symptoms.

GUILLAIN-BARRÉ SYNDROME

CLINICAL CORRELATION

- *Guillain-Barré syndrome is a rare neurological disorder of the peripheral nervous system that can be triggered 2–3 weeks after a febrile illness.*
- *Although a rare complication, it is estimated that 20–40% of cases of Guillain-Barré syndrome may be triggered by a* Campylobacter *infection.*
- *Disease is thought to involve antibody production to core lipopolysaccharide sugars present on* Campylobacter *that cross-react with host gangliosides.*

H. *Helicobacter pylori*

1. *H pylori* is a spiral-shaped organism with corkscrew motility that has evolved mechanisms to survive the acid environment of the stomach.
2. **Clinical manifestations:** *H pylori* is the primary agent associated with non-drug-induced gastritis, gastric and duodenal ulcers, and gastric adenocarcinoma.
3. **Transmission/epidemiology:** The mode of transmission is not completely clear.
   a. There are no animal reservoirs, and infection in children is rare.
   b. Infection in adults is more common, suggesting person-to-person spread.

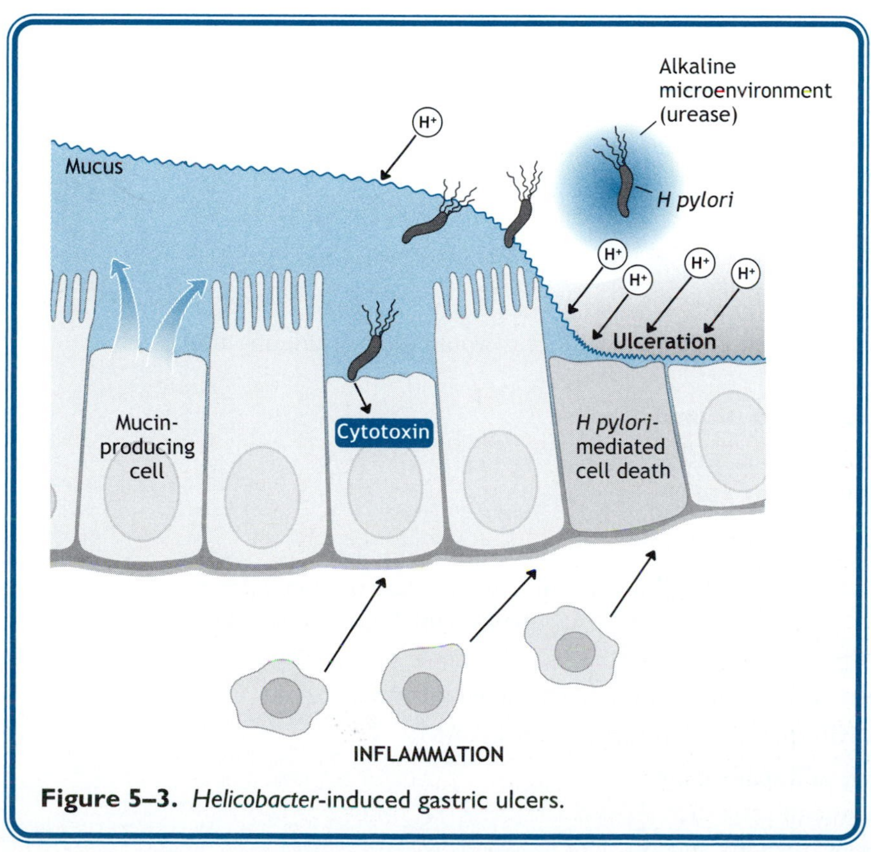

Figure 5–3. *Helicobacter*-induced gastric ulcers.

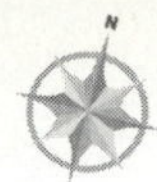

4. **Pathogenesis/virulence factors:** *H pylori* carries several factors involved in virulence, including urease, mucinase, flagella, adherence factors, a vacuolating cytotoxin, and cell wall endotoxin (Table 5–2; Figure 5–3).
   a. Urease catalyses production of ammonia and carbon dioxide from urea, creating an alkaline microenvironment that protects *H pylori* from stomach acidity.
   b. Mucinase and flagella allow *H pylori* to migrate through the thick mucous layer that covers stomach epithelial cells.
   c. *H pylori* secrete a vacuolating cytotoxin that destroys the mucin-producing cells to which the organisms attach and induce an inflammatory response.
   d. The combination of lowered mucous production and inflammation creates areas of ulceration.
5. **Laboratory diagnosis:** Both invasive and noninvasive procedures can be used for diagnosis.
   a. Invasive methods rely on gastric biopsy followed by culture.
   b. Noninvasive methods include serologic testing to detect antibody to *H pylori* and the urea breath test, which is useful for assessing the effectiveness of treatment.
6. **Treatment:** *H pylori*–associated ulcers require therapy with antibiotics such as amoxicillin, tetracycline, and metronidazole in combination with proton pump inhibitors and bismuth.

CLINICAL PROBLEMS

A 28-year-old chicken farmer presented to the emergency department with diarrhea and lower abdominal discomfort. Stool was collected for culture and microscopic examination, which revealed the presence of blood.

1. Based on these results, which of the following organisms would you include in your differential diagnosis?
   A. ETEC, EIEC, *S enterica,* and *Y enterocolitica*
   B. EIEC, *S enterica, Y enterocolitica,* and *Shigella* species
   C. *V cholerae,* ETEC, EPEC, and EAEC
   D. *S typhi, C jejuni, H pylori,* and EHEC

Preliminary laboratory results from stool culture reveal the presence of non–lactose-fermenting colonies. One of these colonies was further tested and found to be H2S-negative and nonmotile at both 22 °C and 37 °C.

2. What virulence mechanism of the organism most likely caused this disease?
   A. Secretion of an A-B toxin that stimulates an increase in cAMP
   B. Secretion of both labile and stable toxins
   C. Attachment and effacement
   D. Invasion through M cells, with basal and lateral spread

The types of dysentery induced by *Shigella* and EIEC are clinically very similar. Infection with *S dysenteriae* will sometimes progress to a condition known as hemolytic uremic syndrome. This syndrome is also a complication of infection with EHEC.

3. The virulence factor shared by *S dysenteriae* and EHEC that is absent from EIEC is:

A. An exotoxin that cleaves 28S RNA in the 60S ribosomal subunit

B. Cell wall endotoxin

C. A heat-stable enterotoxin that results in elevation of cGMP

D. A heat-labile enterotoxin that stimulates host cell adenylate cyclase

4. Urease is considered a virulence factor in *H pylori*–induced gastritis because it:

A. Can bind to mucin-producing cells, resulting in cell destruction and inflammation

B. Helps digest the mucous layer covering gastric epithelial cells to facilitate *H pylori* adhesion

C. Converts urea to ammonia and carbon dioxide, creating an alkaline microenvironment

D. Encodes a cell surface adhesion

Both EPEC and EAEC are major causes of infant diarrhea in developing countries.

5. The primary virulence mechanism exhibited by EAEC involves:

A. Attachment followed by intracellular invasion and epithelial cell destruction

B. Attachment and effacement

C. Inhibition of fluid absorption in response to a mass of bacterial organisms covered by a mucous biofilm

D. Secretion of a heat-labile enterotoxin similar to cholera toxin

ANSWERS

1. The answer is B. Each of these organisms is associated with dysentery. Other organisms that might also be included are *C jejuni* and EHEC.

2. The answer is D. Because this appears to be a relatively mild disease, the most likely organism is a nontoxigenic species of *Shigella. Shigella* species are non–lactose fermenters, do not produce H2S, and are nonmotile. Other organisms in the differential diagnosis include EIEC, EHEC, *S enterica, C jejuni,* and *Y enterocolitica.* Both *E coli* strains will likely ferment lactose. *Campylobacter* requires special media and growth conditions and would therefore not be detected on normal laboratory media. *Yersinia* is conditionally motile and *Salmonella* produces H2S and is motile.

3. The answer is A. The virulence factor shared by *S dysenteriae* and EHEC is a Shiga toxin. All three are gram-negative rods and therefore have endotoxin. The heat-labile and heat-stable toxins are components of ETEC, not EIEC, EHEC, or *Shigella.*

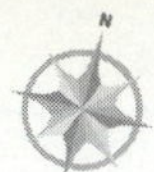

4. The answer is C. One of the reasons *H pylori* can survive the acid environment of the stomach is its ability to neutralize acid in its immediate surroundings.

5. The answer is C. EAEC organisms attach but do not invade. They form a bricklike layer of bacteria on the surface of enterocytes with a mucous biofilm. Attachment and effacement are characteristic of the EPEC strain, whereas secretion of heat-labile and heat-stable enterotoxins is a hallmark of the ETEC strain.

CHAPTER 6
NONENTERIC GRAM-NEGATIVE RODS

I. Key Concepts

A. Nonenteric gram-negative rods can be subcategorized based on common clinical or epidemiologic properties.

B. *Haemophilus, Legionella,* and *Bordetella* are all respiratory pathogens.

C. *Francisella, Pasteurella, Brucella, Yersinia,* and *Rickettsia* are all zoonotic pathogens.

D. *Pseudomonas* and *Klebsiella* are both opportunistic pathogens.

II. *Haemophilus, Legionella,* and *Bordetella*

A. ***Haemophilus influenzae*** is divided into 6 serotypes (a, b, c, d, e, f) based on its polysaccharide capsule.

1. **Clinical manifestations:** The **type b** serotype of *H influenzae* is the most common pathogen and is associated with a variety of disease manifestations.
   - **a.** Mild nasopharyngeal infections can progress to bacteremia, causing metastatic spread to different organs and resulting in **pneumonia, septic arthritis, epiglottitis, sinusitis, otitis media, cellulitis,** and **conjunctivitis.**
   - **b.** **Meningitis** in young children, caused by *H influenzae* type b, is associated with a high incidence of neurologic morbidity that can range from hearing loss to mental retardation.
2. **Transmission/epidemiology:** Nonencapsulated *H influenzae* is a normal inhabitant of the upper respiratory tract.
   - **a.** Encapsulated strains are normally found only in small numbers.
   - **b.** Sporadic outbreaks result from direct contact with respiratory secretions containing encapsulated *H influenzae.*
   - **c.** Before the development of an effective vaccine, *H influenzae* type b was the most common cause of meningitis in children.
3. **Pathogenesis/virulence factors** (Table 6–1): *H influenzae* contains several virulence factors that help it evade immune clearance and stimulate inflammation.
   - **a.** Immune clearance requires formation of protective antibodies to the polysaccharide capsule for opsonization.
   - **b.** The primary pathogenic mechanism is the host inflammatory response to infection.
4. **Laboratory diagnosis:** Rapid diagnosis is critical for *H influenzae*-induced meningitis.
   - **a.** *H influenzae* type b can be detected directly from cerebrospinal fluid using an immunologic latex agglutination test.

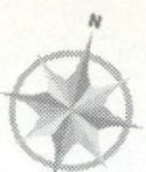

Table 6–1. Summary of pathogenesis of nonenteric gram-negative rods.

Organism	Virulence Factors	Major Clinical Syndrome
Haemophilus influenzae	Endotoxin Capsule IgA protease Attachment pili	Pneumonia Meningitis
Legionella pneumophila	Endotoxin Intracellular survival	Pontiac fever Legionnaires disease
Bordetella pertussis	Endotoxin Pertussis toxin Cyclolysin Tracheal cytotoxin Filamentous hemagglutinin	Whooping cough
Francisella tularensis	Endotoxin Capsule Intracellular survival	Tularemia
Pasteurella multocida	Endotoxin Capsule Hyaluronidase	Cellulitis
Brucella species	Endotoxin Intracellular survival	Brucellosis
Yersinia pestis	Endotoxin Protein capsule Yops Plasminogen activator protease	Bubonic plague Pneumonic plague
Rickettsia rickettsii	Endotoxin Intracellular parasite	Rocky Mountain spotted fever
Rickettsia prowazekii	Endotoxin Intracellular parasite	Epidemic typhus
Pseudomonas aeruginosa	Endotoxin Exotoxin A Exoenzyme S Adhesins Capsule	Pneumonia Wound/burn infections Swimmers ear Urinary tract infections
Klebsiella pneumoniae	Endotoxin Capsule Proteases	Pneumonia Urinary tract infections

b. *H influenzae* requires **X and V factors** for growth and therefore grows on chocolate agar or as satellite colonies around *Staphylococcus aureus* on blood agar.

5. **Treatment:** Antibiotic choice depends on susceptibility testing but includes ampicillin and cephalosporins. Rifampin is used for chemoprophylaxis in susceptible family members.
6. **Prevention:** Vaccination against *H influenzae* type b is an extremely effective strategy for prevention.

B. ***Legionella*** contains more than 60 species and serogroups, although most human disease is caused by 2 or 3 serogroups of ***Legionella pneumophila.***

1. **Clinical manifestations:** There are 2 primary forms of disease caused by *L pneumophila.*
   a. **Pontiac fever** is a mild disease characterized by an "influenza"-like illness.
   b. **Legionnaires disease** is a more severe disease characterized by fever, a dry cough, and a multifocal necrotizing **"atypical"** pneumonia.
2. **Transmission/epidemiology:** *L pneumophila* is an aquatic saprophyte found contaminating many environmental water sources, such as air conditioning systems, hot tubs, hospital showers, and devices used for inhalation therapy.
   a. Because the bacteria can parasitize amebae in the water, they are resistant to the effects of disinfectants like chlorine.
   b. Infection results when aerosols containing bacteria are inhaled by susceptible individuals.
      (1) Most cases involve people with weakened pulmonary defenses, such as heavy drinkers, smokers, and the elderly.
      (2) Individuals with compromised cell-mediated immunity, such as patients undergoing immunosuppression due to organ transplantation or chemotherapy, are also susceptible.
3. **Pathogenesis/virulence factors** (Table 6–1): On inhalation, *L pneumophila* bacteria parasitize alveolar macrophages and monocytes.
   a. C3b coating the bacterial organisms facilitates endocytosis by binding to macrophage CR3 receptors.
   b. **Intracellular survival** is mediated by inhibition of phagolysosome fusion.
   c. Lung damage results from the inflammatory response.
4. **Laboratory diagnosis:** *Legionella* stain poorly with Gram stain, especially in clinical specimens.
   a. Special media containing high levels of cysteine and iron are required for growth.
   b. Diagnosis is made with a variety of methods for **antigen detection, serology** to detect specific antibody, direct microscopy with the **Dieterle silver stain,** and culture.
5. **Treatment:** Penicillins are generally not effective because many *Legionella* carry a beta-lactamase. Current guidelines should be consulted, but antibiotics such as erythromycin, tetracycline, azithromycin, and levofloxacin generally are effective.
6. **Prevention:** Identification of contaminated water sources and measures to reduce bacterial loads such as hyperchlorination are the main methods of prevention.

C. ***Bordetella pertussis*** is the causative agent of **whooping cough.**

1. **Clinical manifestations:** Whooping cough is a severe respiratory illness that can last for weeks.
   a. The first stage of disease is similar to the common cold and is the most infectious.

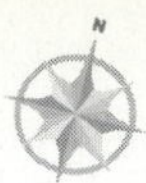

b. The second stage is characterized by **paroxysmal coughing,** exhaustion, and copious mucus production.
c. The disease gets its name from the sharp intake of air between coughing paroxysms that sounds like a "whoop."

2. **Transmission/epidemiology:** *B pertussis* is a highly contagious human pathogen spread by airborne droplets. Whooping cough is most often a disease of young children.
3. **Pathogenesis/virulence factors** (Table 6–1): *B pertussis* carries a number of virulence factors important to pathogenesis.
   a. *B pertussis* binds ciliated cells in the respiratory airway and multiplies on their surface.
   b. Attachment to respiratory epithelial cells is mediated by two proteins: **filamentous hemagglutinin** (Fha) and **pertussis toxin** (Ptx).
   c. The combined action of at least three toxins inhibits normal respiratory clearance mechanisms.
      (1) Ptx is an A-B toxin with a mechanism similar to that of cholera toxin (Figure 6–1).
      (2) **Cyclolysin** is a bacterial adenylate cyclase that is activated by **calmodulin** inside the cell (Figure 6–1).
      (3) Together with Ptx, cyclolysin results in elevated cAMP and increased respiratory and mucus secretions (Figure 6–1).
      (4) **Tracheal cytotoxin** is a peptidoglycan fragment that causes **ciliostasis.**
4. **Laboratory diagnosis:** *B pertussis* is sensitive to drying and requires special media supplemented with nicotinamide for growth.
5. **Treatment:** Treatment is guided by clinical findings, but, in general, erythromycin is used to reduce the number of organisms. Treatment may also re-

Figure 6–1. Activation of adenylate cyclase activity by *Bordetella pertussis.* Pertussis toxin contains 5 nonidentical B subunits (S2, S3, S4, and S5). The A subunit is called S1, and ADP ribosylates an inhibitory G protein (Gi) that regulates cellular adenylate cyclase (AC). Cyclolysin is a bacterial adenylate cyclase that is activated by calmodulin. They work together to increase cAMP, which results in elevated mucus production.

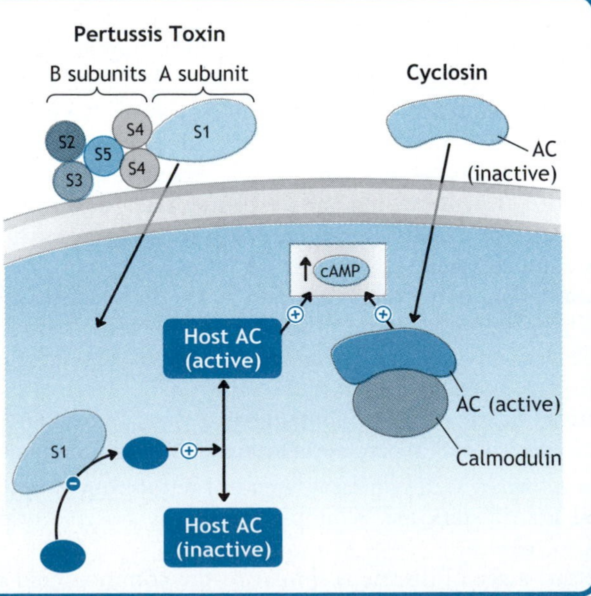

quire supportive care, such as administration of oxygen and suction of respiratory mucus.

6. **Prevention:** Vaccination with killed organisms proved to be an effective means of prevention; however, it did cause side effects. An acellular vaccine based on Fha and Ptx is now available.

H INFLUENZAE TYPE B BACTERIAL MENINGITIS IN CHILDREN

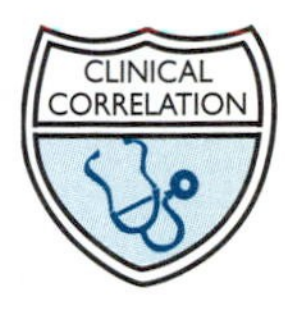

- H influenzae *type b was once one of the most common causative agents of bacterial meningitis in children.*
- *Although passive immunity from maternal antibodies provides protection for newborns, the original vaccine did not adequately protect children younger than age 2.*
- *The original vaccine was based on the polysaccharide type b capsule, which elicited a T-cell–independent response and was therefore a poor immunogen, especially in children less than 2 years old.*
- *The new vaccine couples the type b polyribosylribitol phosphate (PRP) capsule polysaccharide with diphtheria toxoid to elicit a T-cell–dependent response and greater effectiveness in children under 2 years old.*

III. *Francisella, Pasteurella, Brucella, Yersinia,* and *Rickettsia*

A. ***Francisella tularensis*** causes tularemia, also known as rabbit or muskrat fever.

1. **Clinical manifestations:** There are several disease manifestations, all of which are accompanied by acute onset of fever.
   a. **Ulceroglandular** disease is the most common form and is characterized by enlarged lymph nodes and ulcerated necrotic skin lesions.
   b. **Oculoglandular** conjunctivitis results from direct inoculation in the eye.
   c. **Glandular** disease is characterized by lymphadenopathy without ulceration.
   d. **Typhoidal** disease results from sepsis and is highly fatal.
   e. **Gastrointestinal** and **pulmonary** infection may lead to typhoidal disease.
2. **Transmission/epidemiology:** *F tularensis* is a highly infectious organism endemic to many areas of the United States, especially Arkansas, Missouri, and Oklahoma.
   a. Bites from infected **ticks** carried on wild animals, such as rabbits and muskrats, require fewer than 100 organisms to cause infection.
   b. Inhalation of **infectious aerosols** while dressing or skinning infected animals also requires a low infectious dose.
   c. Infection following ingestion of contaminated meats requires a high inoculating dose.
3. **Pathogenesis/virulence factors** (Table 6–1): The two primary virulence factors are an antiphagocytic capsule and endotoxin. Survival in cells and tissues of the reticuloendothelial system is facilitated by its ability to survive in macrophages.
4. **Laboratory diagnosis:** *F tularensis* is slow growing and requires cysteine-rich media.
   a. **Fluorescent antibody** assays on clinical specimens and **serologic analysis** to detect specific antibodies help with diagnosis.
   b. Because *F tularensis* is highly infectious, **laboratories should be notified** of suspected infections.
5. **Treatment:** Some strains produce beta-lactamases, but most are susceptible to streptomycin.

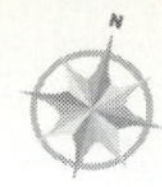

6. **Prevention:** This mainly involves avoiding contact with infected animals, infectious aerosols, and tick vectors. A live attenuated vaccine is available for high-risk individuals.

B. *Pasteurella multocida* is the most common cause of infection from dog and cat bites.

1. **Clinical manifestations:** There are three diseases caused by *P multocida* in humans.
   - a. The most common manifestation is a localized **cellulitis** and lymphadenitis characterized by a painful lesion that develops within 24 hours of infection.
   - b. **Chronic respiratory disease** can develop in patients with pulmonary dysfunction.
   - c. Systemic infection is a rare complication usually restricted to immunocompromised individuals.
2. **Transmission/epidemiology:** *P multocida* is part of the normal flora of animals, including cats and dogs. Human infection occurs through direct inoculation from animal bites.
3. **Pathogenesis/virulence factors** (Table 6–1): The primary pathogenic mechanism of *P multocida* is host inflammation caused by several virulence factors, the most important of which is cell wall endotoxin.
4. **Treatment:** Current guidelines should be consulted, but a variety of antibiotics, including penicillin, tetracycline, and cephalosporins, are generally effective.
5. **Prevention:** Disease prevention is best accomplished by prompt washing of animal bites and scratches.

C. *Brucella* has 4 species that most often result in human disease: *B abortus, B melitensis, B suis,* and *B canis.*

1. **Clinical manifestations:** *Brucella* infections cause a slow-onset, periodic or **undulating fever** with sweats, chills, headache, and fatigue that can become chronic or typhoidal, lasting months.
   - a. Brucellosis is also known by a variety of other names, such as undulant fever, **Malta fever,** and **Mediterranean remittent fever.**
   - b. Severe disease is most often associated with *B melitensis* and *B suis.*
   - c. Disease resulting from infection with *B abortus* and *B canis* is generally more mild.
2. **Transmission/epidemiology**
   - a. Human disease results from contact with infected animals through 2 primary modes.
     - *(1)* One way is direct inoculation of organisms into cuts or breaks in skin.
     - *(2)* The other is ingestion of contaminated unpasteurized milk and cheese.
   - b. Animal infections are species specific.
     - *(1)* *B abortus* infects cattle.
     - *(2)* *B melitensis* infects goats and sheep.
     - *(3)* *B suis* infects swine.
     - *(4)* *B canis* infects dogs.
3. **Pathogenesis/virulence factors** (Table 6–1): The major virulence mechanism stems from the ability of *Brucella* to **survive intracellularly** in cells of the reticuloendothelial system.
   - a. Organisms are sequestered and cause **granulomas** in lymph nodes, spleen, liver, and bone marrow.

b. Replication results in periodic release of organisms and endotoxin into the circulation.
c. Prolonged survival gives rise to chronic disease.

4. **Laboratory diagnosis:** *Brucella* organisms are hard to detect directly in clinical specimens, so diagnosis is based on **clinical** findings confirmed by **culture** and **serologic analysis.**
5. **Treatment:** Current guidelines should be checked, but treatment generally involves an antibiotic such as tetracycline, doxycycline, or trimethoprim-sulfamethoxazole in combination with rifampin or gentamicin over a prolonged course, often 6 weeks or more.
6. **Prevention:** Effective methods of prevention involve pasteurizing milk products, vaccinating animals, and eliminating infected animals.

D. ***Yersinia pestis*** is the causative agent of **plague.**

1. **Clinical manifestations:** There are 2 main manifestations—bubonic plague and pneumonic plague.
   a. **Bubonic plague** is characterized by high fever and the appearance of large, painful, swollen groin or axilla lymph nodes called **buboes.**
      (1) Infection progresses to a bacteremic phase with sudden onset of fever, chills, and **sepsis.**
      (2) Mortality is high when left untreated.
   b. **Pneumonic plague** results from inhalation of infectious aerosols or embolization of bacteremic organisms to the lung.
      (1) Disease development is rapid and highly fatal.
      (2) Infectious aerosols allow person-to-person spread.
2. **Transmission/epidemiology:** *Y pestis* is highly infectious and transmitted through 2 different mechanisms.
   a. Infected **fleas** on wild animal reservoirs (sylvatic plague) or rats (urban plague) are the major vector of transmission of bubonic plague.
   b. Infected humans with pneumonic plague transmit organisms **person to person** through respiratory aerosols.
   c. Endemic areas of sylvatic plague in the United States cluster around the southwestern states.
3. **Pathogenesis/virulence factors** (Table 6–1): A variety of virulence factors contribute to intracellular growth, survival, spread, and pathogenesis.
   a. Bacteria spread from the site of inoculation to local and regional lymph nodes, where they are ingested by macrophages.
   b. *Y pestis* survives in macrophages, replicates, and causes massive inflammatory swelling of the lymph node (ie, bubo).
   c. Organisms spread rapidly from buboes to the bloodstream, causing systemic **endotoxin**-related necrosis of peripheral blood vessels, sepsis, and shock.
   d. **Plasminogen activator protease** facilitates spread, possibly by dissolving fibrin clots.
   e. Embolization of bacteria to the lungs allows person-to-person spread by respiratory droplets.
4. **Laboratory diagnosis:** Organisms can be identified from examination and culture of blood, sputum, and pus from buboes. **Laboratories should be notified** if plague is suspected.
5. **Treatment:** The antibiotic of choice to treat *Y pestis* is streptomycin, with tetracycline, chloramphenicol, and trimethoprim-sulfamethoxazole as alternatives.

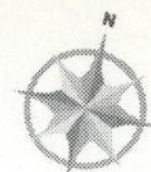

6. **Prevention:** Prevention involves avoiding handling dead wild animals, especially in endemic areas, and controlling rat populations in urban areas. Vaccination with a killed organism vaccine can provide short-term protection for high-risk individuals.

E. ***Rickettsia rickettsii*** is the causative agent of **Rocky Mountain spotted fever** (RMSF).
   1. **Clinical manifestations:** Symptoms of RMSF include acute fever, headache, chills, and myalgia.
      a. A characteristic **petechial rash** usually develops.
      b. Systemic complications include renal failure, encephalitis, and disseminated intravascular coagulation (DIC).
      c. The fatality rate can approach 20–30% if untreated.
   2. **Transmission/epidemiology:** RMSF is transmitted after **prolonged exposure** to **tick** bites. RMSF can be found in most areas of the United States, with the highest focus in the central and mid-Atlantic states of the eastern United States.
   3. **Pathogenesis/virulence factors:** Rickettsiae are obligate intracellular parasites.
      a. After infection, *R rickettsii* replicates in endothelial cells, causing vasculitis and damage to blood vessels.
      b. The petechial rash develops in response to vascular damage.
      c. Systemic infection of the circulatory system causes an increase in vascular permeability and petechial bleeding and can lead to DIC in severe cases.
   4. **Laboratory diagnosis:** The **Weil-Felix test** can be used as an early indicator of rickettsial disease but is not definitive because of its nonspecificity. Common methods of diagnosis are **direct fluorescent antibody** tests from a skin biopsy and **serologic analysis** to detect specific antibody.
   5. **Treatment:** Rickettsial infections can be treated with tetracycline or chloramphenicol.
   6. **Prevention:** Because prolonged exposure is necessary for infection, prompt removal of ticks is a good method of prevention.

F. ***Rickettsia prowazekii*** shares many properties with *R rickettsii,* with the major differences outlined below.
   1. **Clinical manifestations:** *R prowazekii* causes **epidemic typhus.**
      a. Symptoms include acute onset of fever, chills, and muscle aches.
      b. A characteristic **petechial rash** covers the body.
      c. Systemic complications include **meningoencephalitis.**
   2. **Transmission/epidemiology:** Epidemic typhus is primarily a human disease associated with poor living conditions and overcrowding.
      a. The main vector of transmission is the **human body louse.**
      b. **Flying squirrels** can serve as a secondary reservoir.
   3. **Prevention:** Infection with *R prowazekii* is best avoided by improving living conditions, delousing, and removing secondary reservoirs from households and surroundings.

ROCKY MOUNTAIN SPOTTED FEVER AND ENDEMIC TYPHUS

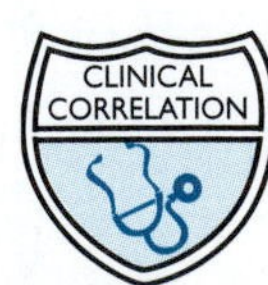

- *The rashes of RMSF and epidemic typhus have distinctive presentations.*
- *RMSF and epidemic typhus are both caused by closely related* Rickettsia *organisms.*
- *Although acute symptoms are similar and both RMSF and epidemic typhus induce a petechial rash, the progression of rash development differs dramatically and is characteristic for each disease.*

- *The rash of RMSF starts at the extremities, can involve the hands and feet, and then spreads inward toward the trunk.*
- *The rash of epidemic typhus starts on the trunk and spreads outward to the limbs, usually sparing the palms of the hands and soles of the feet.*

IV. *Pseudomonas* and *Klebsiella*

A. *Pseudomonas aeruginosa* is a strict aerobe that can live and grow in water, even distilled water, with very few nutrients.

1. **Clinical manifestations:** *P aeruginosa* causes a variety of infections, including swimmer's ear and folliculitis.
   - **a.** *P aeruginosa* is also a major cause of recurring **pneumonia in patients with cystic fibrosis.**
   - **b.** Wound infections, especially in **burn** patients, can lead to sepsis.
   - **c.** Urinary tract infections are usually associated with indwelling catheters.
2. **Transmission/epidemiology:** *P aeruginosa* is a ubiquitous organism in soil, water, food, and plants.
   - **a.** *P aeruginosa* can grow with few nutrients and is found as a contaminant on numerous objects in hospitals.
   - **b.** *P aeruginosa* can survive in many common disinfectants.
3. **Pathogenesis/virulence factors** (Table 6–1): Several virulence factors contribute to pathogenesis.
   - **a.** Conditions that allow colonization play an important role in opportunistic infections.
     - *(1)* Mucus production in cystic fibrosis inhibits ciliated clearance mechanisms.
     - *(2)* Burns and wounds remove skin barriers.
   - **b.** *P aeruginosa* produces several **adhesins** that allow adherence once barriers have been breached.
   - **c. Exotoxin A** is an A-B toxin that inhibits protein synthesis and causes cell death through the same mechanism of action as diphtheria toxin.
   - **d. Exoenzyme S** is an ADP-ribosylating toxin that targets several cellular proteins.
   - **e.** A type III secretion system facilitates direct inoculation of exotoxins into cells, allowing it to evade humoral immune mechanisms.
4. **Laboratory diagnosis:** *P aeruginosa* has a fruity aroma when grown on several different laboratory media and produces several pigments that help in its identification.
   - **a. Pyocyanin** gives a blue color to pus.
   - **b.** The presence of **pyoverdin,** a yellow-green molecule that is fluorescent under ultraviolet light, can be used to monitor infection in burn patients.
5. **Treatment:** *Pseudomonas* species are resistant to many antibiotics, so sensitivity testing is important. They are often sensitive to third-generation cephalosporins, such as ceftazidine and cefepime.
6. **Prevention:** Limiting infection in susceptible individuals through physical isolation and sterile practices is an important method of prevention.

B. *Klebsiella pneumoniae* is a member of the Enterobacteriaceae family and is characterized by its large capsule, giving colonies a mucoid appearance.

1. **Clinical manifestations:** *K pneumoniae* causes an opportunistic necrotizing **pneumonia** and can also cause **urinary tract infections.**
2. **Transmission/epidemiology:** Organisms can be found in soil and water as well as the large intestine.

a. Colonization of the oropharynx is uncommon but can occur in individuals with compromised host defenses, particularly alcoholics, the elderly, and individuals with chronic respiratory illness.
b. Aspiration of organisms from the oropharynx can lead to infection.

3. **Pathogenesis/virulence factors** (Table 6–1): *K pneumoniae* contains a variety of virulence factors involved in mediating tissue destruction.
4. **Treatment:** Because of antibiotic resistance, therapy is guided by sensitivity testing.

CLINICAL PROBLEMS

A 7-year-old girl with cystic fibrosis is hospitalized with pneumonia. Sputum Gram stain reveals gram-negative rods. Culture on blood agar grew colonies with a "fruity" aroma.

1. What organism is most likely causing this child's pneumonia?

   A. *P aeruginosa*

   B. *L pneumophila*

   C. *K pneumoniae*

   D. *H influenzae*

A 24-year-old man is seen in the emergency department with high fever and a large, painful, swollen lymph node in the groin. He just returned from a camping trip in Arizona. Blood and pus were collected from the lymph node and sent for culture and analysis.

2. The laboratory was notified of a suspected infection with:

   A. *R rickettsii*

   B. *B pertussis*

   C. *Y pestis*

   D. *B canis*

A 14-year-old boy scout is seen by the family doctor for fever, headache, muscle aches, and a large rash covering his body. His mother describes the development of the rash, which started on the boy's wrists and ankles, then progressed inward to cover his trunk. The boy mentioned that he had just been on a 4-day campout in rural Virginia, and his mother remembers removing several ticks from his feet after he returned home.

3. What is the most likely cause of this child's disease?

   A. *Y pestis*

   B. *R prowazekii*

   C. *R rickettsii*

   D. *F tularensis*

A 54-year-old man is hospitalized with a dry cough and multifocal pneumonia. Microscopic examination of sputum by Gram stain did not reveal any organisms, but results from a Dieterle silver stain were positive.

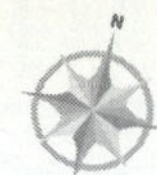

4. The most likely organism is:
   A. *H influenzae*
   B. *L pneumophila*
   C. *P aeruginosa*
   D. *K pneumoniae*

A 3-year-old immigrant from Mexico is seen at the hospital for what appears to be whooping cough. History reveals the child has not received any immunizations.

5. If this diagnosis is correct, the virulence factors associated with pathogenesis include:
   A. Ptx, hyaluronidase, exotoxin A
   B. Cyclolysin, filamentous hemagglutinin, Ptx
   C. Hyaluronidase, exotoxin A, filamentous hemagglutinin
   D. Cyclolysin, hyaluronidase, capsule

ANSWERS

1. The answer is A. *Pseudomonas* is a common cause of opportunistic pneumonia in patients with cystic fibrosis. The fruity aroma is also characteristic of *P aeruginosa.*
2. The answer is C. The clinical symptoms, the large swollen node or bubo, and the travel and camping in an area endemic for plague are consistent with an infection with *Y pestis. R rickettsii* has an associated characteristic rash, *B pertussis* causes whooping cough, and *Brucella* infections cause an undulant fever.
3. The answer is C. The symptoms and development of the rash are all consistent with RMSF caused by *R rickettsii.* The rash for *R prowazekii* occurs in the opposite direction.
4. The answer is B. *Legionella* organisms stain poorly by Gram stain in clinical species, accounting for the different findings with Gram and Dieterle stains. The dry cough and multilobar pneumonia are also characteristic of *L pneumophila.*
5. The answer is B. The virulence factors associated with *B pertussis,* the causative agent of whooping cough, include Ptx, cyclolysin, tracheal cytotoxin, endotoxin, and filamentous hemagglutinin.

CHAPTER 7
ANAEROBIC BACTERIA

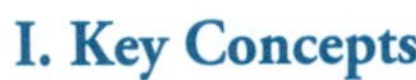

I. Key Concepts

A. Anaerobes are characterized by their inability to grow in the presence of atmospheric oxygen.

1. Some species are extremely sensitive, even to low amounts of oxygen.
2. Other species, including many pathogenic strains, are more aerotolerant, either through the production of catalase and superoxide dismutase or through their ability to form spores under adverse conditions.

B. Medically important anaerobes include both gram-positive and gram-negative organisms.

1. *Bacteroides fragilis* is the most common gram-negative anaerobe.
2. Gram-positive anaerobes include *Clostridium botulinum, Clostridium tetani, Clostridium perfringens, Clostridium difficile,* and *Actinomyces israelii.*
3. All members of the genus *Clostridium* form **spores.**
4. Most infections caused by anaerobes result from endogenous spread or deep wounds.

II. *Bacteroides*

A. *Bacteroides fragilis*

1. **Clinical manifestations:** *B fragilis* can cause a variety of infections, including intra-abdominal abscesses, peritonitis, gynecologic infections, bacteremia, and sepsis.
2. **Transmission/epidemiology:** Because it is part of normal flora of the colon and vagina, *B fragilis* infections most often occur through endogenous spread following trauma.
3. **Pathogenesis/virulence factors** (Table 7–1): *B fragilis* pathogenesis is often associated with mixed infections.
   - a. Local tissue necrosis, causing a decreased blood supply as well as growth of facultative anaerobes such as *Escherichia coli* in the mixed infection, contributes to an anaerobic microenvironment that allows *B fragilis* to proliferate.
   - b. The antiphagocytic capsule assists escape from the innate immune system and may also directly facilitate abscess formation.
   - c. Production of superoxide dismutase contributes to aerotolerance.
4. **Treatment:** Most *B fragilis* organisms produce a beta-lactamase and are therefore often resistant to penicillins and first-generation cephalosporins.
   - a. Treatment involves drainage of abscesses combined with antibiotic therapy using agents such as metronidazole, cefoxitin, chloramphenicol, and clindamycin.

Table 7–1. Summary of pathogenic mechanisms of anaerobes.

Organism	Pathogenic Mechanism
Bacteroides fragilis	Endogenous spread, abscess formation
Clostridium botulinum	Ingestion of preformed botulism toxin (A, C, or E), flaccid paralysis Ingestion and colonization of *C botulinum* organisms by infants with toxin production and flaccid paralysis
Clostridium tetani	Contamination of puncture wounds by spores Germination and tetanospasmin exotoxin production causing spastic paralysis
Clostridium perfringens	Contamination of wounds with spores Germination, rapid growth and production of alpha toxin, causing tissue destruction Ingestion of organisms and diarrheal enterotoxin production upon sporulation
Clostridium difficile	Endogenous spread, colonization, exotoxin A, and exotoxin B
Actinomyces israelii	Endogenous spread and abscess formation

b. Because most *B fragilis* infections contain mixed organisms, several antibiotics are often used to provide broad coverage.

5. **Prevention:** Because *B fragilis* is part of the normal flora, prevention can be difficult. For surgical trauma, prophylactic antibiotics such as cefoxitin are sometimes used.

III. *Clostridium* and *Actinomyces*

A. *Clostridium botulinum*

1. **Clinical manifestations:** *C botulinum* causes 2 major clinical manifestations—**foodborne** and **infant botulism.**
   a. Foodborne botulism results from ingestion of preformed botulism toxin in food.
   b. Infant botulism results from ingestion of *C botulinum* organisms followed by colonization and toxin production in the gut.
   c. Both foodborne and infant botulism cause a **flaccid paralysis** of voluntary and respiratory muscles that can lead to respiratory arrest.
   d. Infant botulism is thought to contribute to some cases of **sudden infant death syndrome** (SIDS).
2. **Transmission/epidemiology:** Spores play a critical role in survival and spread.
   a. Spores in soil contaminate vegetables, survive improper canning, germinate, and produce toxin in the anaerobic environment of the canned foods.
   b. The toxin is heat labile and destroyed by cooking, but because of its potency, suspected contaminated foods should be discarded.
   c. Infant botulism is transmitted by spores contaminating honey.

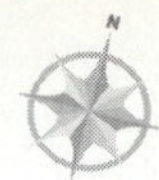

3. **Pathogenesis/virulence factors** (Table 7–1): Botulism toxin is the major virulence factor involved in pathogenesis.
   a. There are 7 or 8 known botulism toxins, but the most common are types A, B, and E.
   b. Botulism toxin ingested from contaminated foods is adsorbed by the gut, enters the bloodstream, and spreads to the peripheral nervous system.
   c. The toxin itself is a protease that degrades proteins necessary for release of acetylcholine at neuromuscular synapses.
   d. The result of this proteolysis is a lack of neuromuscular transmission and flaccid paralysis.
   e. Infant botulism results from ingestion of bacterial spores.
   f. Because the intestinal flora of infants is not fully developed, *C botulinum* can colonize and produce toxin in the gut.
4. **Laboratory diagnosis:** Suspected botulism can be tested by using a mouse bioassay of serum or uneaten food for toxin or by culturing food or feces.
5. **Treatment:** The main treatment strategy is to counter the paralysis using mechanical ventilation and to neutralize the toxin with a trivalent **antitoxin.**
6. **Prevention:** Botulism can be prevented through adequate food preparation, avoidance of suspected contaminated canned foods, and by not feeding honey to infants less than 1 year of age.

B. *Clostridium tetani*

1. *C tetani* has a characteristic tennis racket or drumstick appearance because of its terminal spore.
2. **Clinical manifestations:** *C tetani* causes tetanus, a spastic paralysis characterized by "lockjaw," arching of the back (ie, **opisthotonos**), and respiratory muscle spasms.
3. **Transmission/epidemiology:** Spores of *C tetani* are commonly found in soil and in the intestinal tract of animals and sometimes in humans. Infection is associated with puncture wounds, contaminated injuries, severe burns, and nonsterile surgery.
4. **Pathogenesis/virulence factors** (Table 7–1): The major virulence factor is a neurotoxin called tetanospasmin.
   a. Following infection, spores germinate and produce tetanospasmin toxin.
   b. Tetanospasmin toxin is carried to the central nervous system by retrograde axonal transport.
   c. The toxin itself is a protease that inhibits the docking of inhibitory neurotransmitter vesicles at synapses.
   d. Blocking release of inhibitors at synapses results in continuous firing and severe muscle spasms.
5. **Treatment:** Diagnosis is based on clinical findings.
   a. Treatment involves passive immunization with antitoxin in combination with antibiotics such as penicillin to eradicate organisms.
   b. Supportive measures such as artificial ventilation may also be necessary.
6. **Prevention:** Active immunization with toxoid has been very effective. Boosters are given at 10-year intervals or as prophylaxis after puncture wounds.

C. *Clostridium perfringens*

1. *C perfringens* produces a characteristic double zone of hemolysis when grown on blood agar.

2. **Clinical manifestations:** The 2 major clinical syndromes associated with *C perfringens* infections are **gas gangrene** and **food poisoning.**
3. **Transmission/epidemiology:** Spores play an important role in the spread of organisms.
   a. Spores can be found in soil and the colon of animals and humans.
   b. Wounds contaminated with *C perfringens* spores allow germination and rapid growth of organisms.
   c. Ingestion of food contaminated with *C perfringens* is associated with food poisoning.
4. **Pathogenesis/virulence factors** (Table 7–1): *C perfringens* produces several exotoxins, including **alpha toxin** and an **enterotoxin.**
   a. Spores contaminating a wound germinate and produce alpha toxin.
   b. Alpha toxin is a lecithinase that causes damage to cell membranes, tissue destruction, bleeding, increased vascular permeability, and systemic spread of the toxin.
   c. Food poisoning results from ingestion of contaminated food.
      (1) Spores in the food survive cooking, germinate, and grow rapidly.
      (2) Bacteria are ingested and begin to sporulate in the gut and produce an enterotoxin.
      (3) The enterotoxin causes **watery diarrhea** 8–24 hours after ingestion.
5. **Treatment:** Strategies for treatment vary depending on the clinical manifestation.
   a. Gangrene is life-threatening and usually requires surgical intervention, which may include amputation.
   b. High doses of antibiotics such as penicillin G are used to clear infection.
   c. Food poisoning generally is self-limiting and requires supportive measures and fluid replacement.
6. **Prevention:** For gangrene, timely surgical debridement of traumatic injuries is critical as is sterilization of surgical instruments. Proper food handling is the best prevention for food poisoning.

D. *Clostridium difficile*

1. *C difficile* colonization is associated with use of antibiotics and other chemotherapies that kill other host flora and allow *C difficile* a growth advantage.
2. **Clinical manifestations:** *C difficile* is a common cause of **antibiotic-associated diarrhea, pseudomembranous colitis,** and **toxic megacolon.**
3. **Transmission/epidemiology:** Infection with *C difficile* is most often mediated through **endogenous** spread.
   a. *C difficile* is a minor component of the normal flora in many people.
   b. Fecal-oral spread is rare but can occur in a hospital environment.
4. **Pathogenesis/virulence factors** (Table 7–1): The major virulence factors are 2 toxins referred to as **exotoxin A** and **exotoxin B.**
   a. Once *C difficile* colonizes, it produces exotoxins A and B in the intestine.
   b. Exotoxin A behaves like an enterotoxin, whereas exotoxin B is more cytotoxic.
   c. The result of toxin production is fluid secretion, cell death, and an inflammatory response that can lead to pseudomembrane formation in the colon.
5. **Laboratory diagnosis:** Suspected infections can be confirmed by assaying for toxin in stool, either by enzyme-linked immunosorbent assay or with a cytotoxicity cell culture assay.

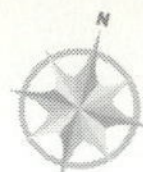

6. **Treatment:** Initial treatment is to discontinue current antibiotics.
   a. For more serious manifestations such as pseudomembraneous colitis, metronidazole or even vancomycin may be necessary.
   b. Toxic megacolon may require surgical resection of the colon.
7. **Prevention:** Because of the potential for endogenous spread, prevention is difficult.
   a. Careful monitoring of antibiotic use and of early signs and symptoms can help prevent more serious manifestations.
   b. Sanitary practices and hand washing can help prevent fecal-oral spread.

C DIFFICILE PSEUDOMEMBRANOUS COLITIS

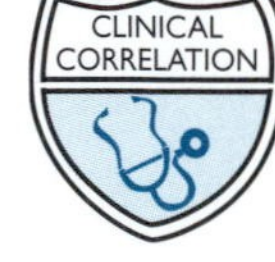

- *Although both metronidazole and vancomycin are effective against* C difficile, *vancomycin use should be approached with caution because of the possibility of enterococci developing vancomycin resistance.*

E. *Actinomyces israelii*

1. ***A israelii*** is a microaerophilic, slow-growing, filamentous organism whose appearance resembles the hyphae of fungi.
2. **Clinical manifestations:** The most common clinical manifestations are **cervicofacial abscesses** associated with **periodontal disease,** poor dental hygiene, and tooth extraction. *A israelii* can also cause abdominal and brain abscesses.
3. **Transmission/epidemiology:** Because *A israelii* is part of the normal oral flora, most infections are caused by endogenous spread.
4. **Pathogenesis/virulence factors** (Table 7–1): The virulence factors for *A israelii* are not clearly defined, and disease is usually associated with the breakdown of mucosal barriers due to trauma and surgery.
5. **Laboratory diagnosis:** Organisms are slow growing but can be cultured.
   a. Diagnosis is generally based on clinical findings and the presence of yellow "sulfur" granules in pus.
   b. Sulfur granules characteristic of *A israelii* are made up of large masses of organisms.
6. **Treatment:** Effective treatment involves surgical drainage of the abscess combined with prolonged therapy with antibiotics, such as penicillin G.
7. **Prevention:** Strategies for prevention include good oral hygiene and prophylactic antibiotics in association with gastrointestinal or oral traumas or surgery.

CLINICAL PROBLEMS

A 30-year-old man has been receiving antibiotic therapy in a hospital environment for 2 weeks. He recently experienced watery diarrhea. The attending physician advises discontinuation of antibiotic use to see whether the diarrhea would resolve. A stool sample is sent to the laboratory for analysis by enzyme-linked immunosorbent assay for exotoxins A and B.

1. What organism does the physician most likely suspect?

   A. *C botulinum*

   B. *C difficile*

C. *C perfringens*

D. *B fragilis*

A 40-year-old woman is experiencing symptoms of flaccid paralysis. History reveals she had eaten some home-canned beans the previous evening. Samples of both the patient's serum and the uneaten beans are sent to the laboratory to test for botulism using a mouse bioassay.

2. Which of the following strategies should be used to treat this patient?

A. Send her home until the results of the bioassay come back

B. Artificial ventilation if needed and injection of antitoxin

C. Immunization with a trivalent botulism toxoid vaccine

D. Begin a course of penicillin G

Following a car accident, an 18-year-old man has an intra-abdominal abscess. Drainage of the abscess reveals a mixture of organisms, including a gram-negative anaerobe.

3. Why would penicillin alone be a poor choice for antibiotic therapy in this individual?

A. Gram-negative organisms do not respond to penicillin because of their cell wall structure.

B. Anaerobes in general are not sensitive to penicillin.

C. The most likely causative agent, *B fragilis,* often carries a beta-lactamase.

D. The pathogenic mechanism of *B fragilis* involves secretion of an exotoxin that must also be neutralized.

A 2-week-old infant is showing signs of flaccid paralysis. On questioning, the mother reveals she fed the child honey.

4. The most likely cause of this child's disease is:

A. Botulism toxin contamination of the honey

B. Clostridial food poisoning as a result of ingestion of *C perfringens*

C. Colonization of the child's intestine with *C botulinum*

D. Contamination of the honey with tetanospasmin

ANSWERS

1. The answer is B. *C difficile* is commonly associated with antibiotic-induced diarrhea. Its mechanism of action involves secretion of an enterotoxin (exotoxin A) and a cytotoxin (exotoxin B).

2. The answer is B. The scenario described is consistent with foodborne botulism, which results from ingestion of botulism toxin. Neutralization of the toxin by passive immunization with antitoxin is the best course to prevent further damage. Supportive measures, such as artificial respiration, may be required to assist in breathing.

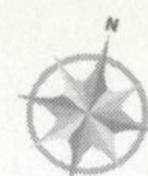

3. The answer is C. The most likely causative anaerobic organism of trauma-induced intra-abdominal abscesses is *B fragilis.* These organisms often carry beta-lactamases that make them resistant to penicillins and first-generation cephalosporin antibiotics. Because this is a mixed infection, combination antibiotics are generally used. *Bacteroides* species do not secrete an exotoxin as part of their pathogenic mechanism.

4. The answer is C. In infants, the intestinal flora is not yet fully developed. *C botulinum* spores in honey can germinate and colonize the infant's intestine, where toxins are produced. The symptoms of flaccid paralysis are consistent with those of botulism.

CHAPTER 8
CHLAMYDIA, SPIROCHETES, AND *MYCOPLASMA*

I. Key Concepts

A. Once thought of as viruses, **Chlamydia** organisms are actually small **obligate intracellular** parasites.

1. They have a cell wall structure similar to that of **gram-negative** organisms, and they lack peptidoglycan but contain lipopolysaccharide.
2. Two distinct forms of Chlamydia are recognized during the organism's life cycle (Figure 8–1).
   - **a.** The **elementary body** is the extracellular infectious form that has sporelike properties.
   - **b.** The **reticulate body** is the intracellular, metabolically active form.
3. Two medically important genera, ***Chlamydia*** and ***Chlamydophila,*** exist.
4. Human infection is most often caused by *Chlamydia trachomatis, Chlamydophila pneumoniae,* and *Chlamydophila psittaci.*

B. **Spirochetes** are thin-walled, spiral, gram-negative bacteria. Medically important spirochetes include *Borrelia burgdorferi, Borrelia recurrentis, Borrelia hermsii, Treponema pallidum,* and *Leptospira interrogans.*

C. ***Mycoplasma*** organisms are unique in that they do not contain a cell wall, their cell membrane contains sterols, and they are the smallest free-living bacteria.

II. Chlamydia: *Chlamydia* and *Chlamydophila*

A. ***Chlamydia trachomatis*** consists of 2 distinct biovars—*trachoma* and *lymphogranuloma venereum*—each with many serotypes.

1. **Clinical manifestations:** *C trachomatis* serovar *trachoma* causes many different clinical diseases, including **trachoma, inclusion conjunctivitis, infant pneumonia, nongonococcal urethritis, Reiter's syndrome,** and **pelvic inflammatory disease.** *C trachomatis* serovar *lymphogranuloma venereum* causes lymphogranuloma venereum.
2. **Transmission/epidemiology:** *C trachomatis* transmission is by direct contact.
   - **a.** For trachoma, transmission to the eye is from contaminated fingers and flies.
   - **b.** Neonatal conjunctivitis is transmitted to the neonate at birth from an infected birth canal.
   - **c.** *C trachomatis* is the most common bacterial sexually transmitted disease in the United States.
   - **d.** Lymphogranuloma venereum is also transmitted by sexual contact.

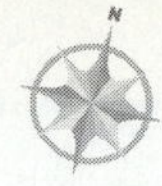

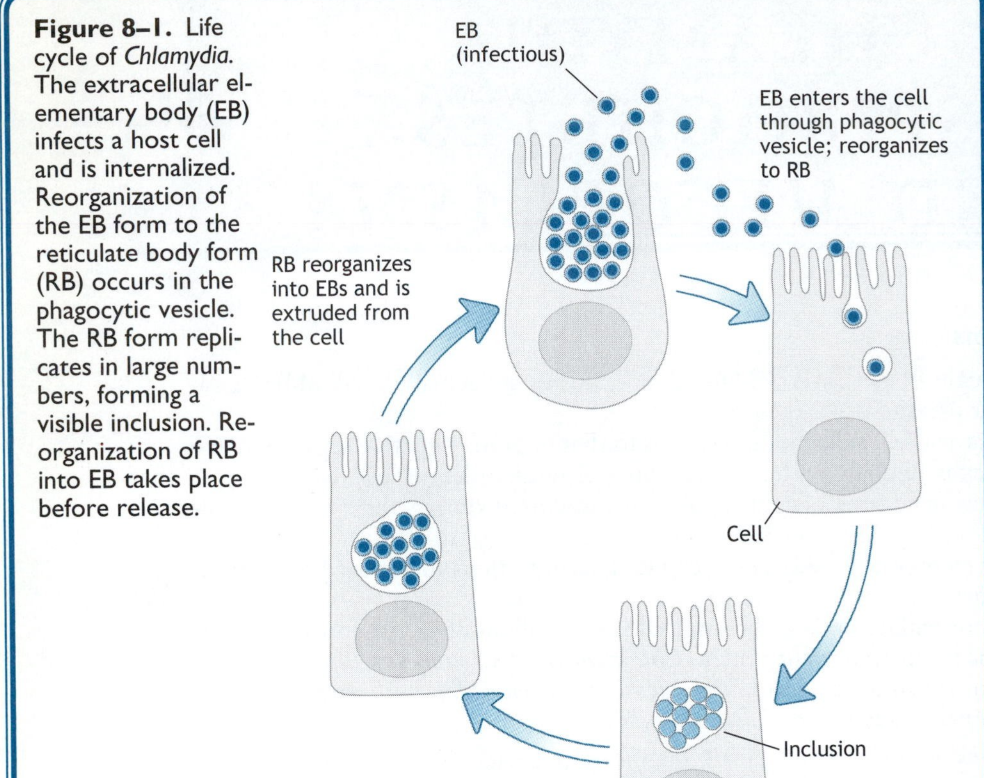

Figure 8–1. Life cycle of *Chlamydia.* The extracellular elementary body (EB) infects a host cell and is internalized. Reorganization of the EB form to the reticulate body form (RB) occurs in the phagocytic vesicle. The RB form replicates in large numbers, forming a visible inclusion. Reorganization of RB into EB takes place before release.

3. **Pathogenesis/virulence factors:** Pathogenesis is due to the host inflammatory response leading to tissue damage.
   a. **Repeated infections** cause progressive inflammation, necrosis, fibrosis, and scarring.
   b. Trachoma is a chronic disease in which repeated infections lead to **blindness.**
   c. Infant conjunctivitis can lead to **corneal scarring** if untreated.
   d. Infant pneumonia follows neonatal conjunctivitis and is characterized by a **staccato** cough and **afebrile** illness.
   e. In women, uterine infections are often asymptomatic and can ascend to cause salpingitis, pelvic inflammatory disease, permanent scarring, and sterility.
   f. In men, urethritis is usually symptomatic.
   g. Lymphogranuloma venereum is characterized by a painless ulcer at the site of infection.
      (1) This is followed by massive swelling of inguinal nodes (**buboes**).
      (2) Systemic symptoms and complications such as abscesses, strictures, and fistulas can follow.

4. **Laboratory diagnosis:** A variety of methods are used in diagnosis, including cell culture, direct fluorescence assays, nucleic acid probes, polymerase chain reaction, and cytologic analysis using Giemsa stains to detect inclusions.
5. **Treatment:** *C trachomatis* is sensitive to tetracyclines, erythromycin, and fluroquinolones.
   a. Specific treatments vary depending on clinical manifestations.
   b. Silver nitrate drops used for prophylaxis of *Neisseria gonorrhoeae* infections have limited effectiveness against *C trachomatis* neonatal eye infections.
6. **Prevention:** Sexually transmitted diseases are best prevented by safe sex practices and prompt treatment of infections.
   a. Treatment of infected mothers late in pregnancy can help prevent transmission to neonates.
   b. Prevention of blindness is accomplished by early treatment and avoiding reinfection.

B. ***Chlamydophila pneumoniae*** was previously called *Chlamydia pneumoniae.*
1. **Clinical manifestations:** *C pneumoniae* causes a variety of respiratory diseases, including **pharyngitis, bronchitis,** and **pneumonia.**
   a. A persistent cough develops that can last for weeks.
   b. **Pneumonia is atypical** and similar to that caused by *Legionella pneumophila* and *Mycoplasma pneumoniae.*
2. **Transmission/epidemiology:** *C pneumoniae* is a human pathogen transmitted by respiratory droplets.
3. **Laboratory diagnosis:** Diagnosis is difficult because *C pneumoniae* is hard to grow in cell culture.
   a. Nucleic acid probe assays are sensitive but not readily available.
   b. Serologic analysis is used to detect a rise in antibody titer.
4. **Treatment**: *C pneumoniae* is sensitive to macrolides and tetracyclines.

C. ***Chlamydophila psittaci*** was previously called *Chlamydia psittaci;* it causes a disease called psittacosis or ornithosis.
1. **Clinical manifestations:** The disease process caused by *C psittaci* can be mild or severe.
   a. Mild manifestations include fever, headache, chills, malaise, myalgia, and bilateral interstitial pneumonia.
   b. Severe manifestations include gastrointestinal symptoms, hepatomegaly, splenomegaly, endocarditis, myocarditis, encephalitis, and even death.
2. **Transmission/epidemiology:** Birds are reservoirs of infection.
   a. Transmission is by inhalation of dried bird droppings.
   b. Persons especially at risk include veterinarians, pet shop workers, and bird handlers.
3. **Pathogenesis/virulence factors:** Organisms enter the respiratory tract and spread to the reticuloendothelial system, causing focal necrosis and systemic organ involvement.
4. **Laboratory diagnosis:** Diagnosis is done serologically.
5. **Treatment:** *C psittaci* is susceptible to macrolides and tetracyclines.

III. Spirochetes: *Borrelia, Treponema,* and *Leptospira*

A. ***Borrelia burgdorferi*** is the causative agent of **Lyme** disease.
1. **Clinical manifestations:** Lyme disease has three stages.

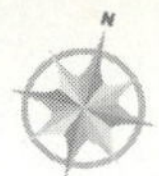

a. Stage 1 is characterized by **erythema migrans,** a **"bull's eye"** rash with a clear center, that may be accompanied by fever, chills, and myalgia.
b. Stage 2 occurs weeks to months later as a disseminated disease with **neurologic** (limb numbness, Bell's palsy), meningitis, encephalitis, and **cardiac** (atrioventricular block, myocarditis) manifestations.
c. Stage 3 occurs months or even years later and is characterized by chronic **neurologic** impairments and **polyarthritis.**

2. **Transmission/epidemiology:** The **reservoirs** for *B burgdorferi* are small mammals such as mice.
   a. The **vector** of transmission is the ***Ixodes*** tick.
   b. One property important to transmission is that prolonged exposure of 24–48 hours is required for infection.
3. **Laboratory diagnosis:** *B burgdorferi* can be grown in culture, but cultures from clinical samples are often negative.
   a. Serologic assays to detect a rise in antibody are the most common methods of diagnosis.
   b. Polymerase chain reaction assays are sensitive.
4. **Treatment:** Treatment varies depending on the stage and severity of symptoms.
   a. Stage 1 is usually treated with doxycycline or amoxicillin.
   b. Late-stage disease with serious neurologic or cardiovascular manifestations is treated with ceftriaxone or penicillin G.
5. **Prevention:** Removing ticks promptly, wearing protective clothing, and using insect repellents are the best methods of prevention. A vaccine is available for high-risk individuals.

VACCINATION AGAINST LYME DISEASE

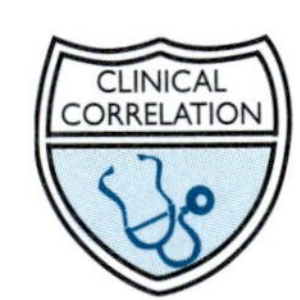

- B burgdorferi *expresses different outer membrane proteins when in the tick than when in the human host.*
- *The vaccine against* B burgdorferi *is designed to stimulate antibody production against the OspA protein that is highly expressed in the tick-associated spirochetes.*
- *During prolonged feeding, antibodies to OspA are ingested by the tick and bind to and inactivate* B burgdorferi *before transmission.*

B. ***Borrelia recurrentis*** and ***Borrelia hermsii*** cause relapsing fever.
1. **Clinical manifestations:** Disease starts with abrupt fever, chills, myalgia, and headache that may be accompanied by splenomegaly and hepatomegaly.
   a. Fever lasts for about a week before resolution, then 3–7 days later a new episode starts.
   b. Cycles of symptom and resolution repeat 1–4 times.
2. **Transmission/epidemiology:** *B recurrentis* is transmitted by the human body louse and usually occurs in epidemics.
   a. *B hermsii* is transmitted by ticks and causes sporadic endemic disease.
   b. In contrast to *B burgdorferi,* only a brief exposure is needed for transmission.
3. **Pathogenesis/virulence factors:** Antigenic variation of outer envelope proteins accounts for recurrence of disease.
   a. Disease manifestations occur when organisms are in the blood by an endotoxin-related mechanism.
   b. After a week of fever, antibodies are produced that clear organisms from the blood.

c. Spirochetes sequestered in the spleen and liver undergo antigenic variation and relapse occurs.

4. **Laboratory diagnosis:** Microscopic diagnosis is made by observing spirochetes by Giemsa stain in peripheral blood.
5. **Treatment:** Tetracycline or erythromycin is used for treatment.

C. ***Treponema pallidum*** is the causative agent of **syphilis.**

1. **Clinical manifestations:** Syphilis is a multistage disease (Figure 8–2).
   a. **Primary syphilis** is characterized by a painless ulcer at the site of infection called a **chancre** that resolves spontaneously and is highly infectious.
   b. **Secondary syphilis** is a disseminated manifestation that occurs 1–3 months after the primary infection.
      (1) Disease is characterized by a maculopapular rash that can cover the body, including the palms and soles of the feet.
      (2) Moist papule lesions occur on mucous membranes and genitals (**condylomata lata**).
      (3) The lesions in secondary syphilis are highly infectious.
   c. **Tertiary syphilis** develops decades later, is usually not infectious, and exhibits multiple organ involvement.
      (1) Granulomas (**gummas**) are present in skin, bone, and other tissues.
      (2) Central nervous system manifestations (**neurosyphilis**) include **chronic meningitis** and dementia.
      (3) Cardiovascular manifestations include **aortic aneurysms.**
   d. **Congenital syphilis** leads to multiple fetal abnormalities, including bone malformations, cardiac abnormalities, mental retardation, and stillbirths.
2. **Transmission/epidemiology:** *T pallidum* is a sexually transmitted disease. Congenital infections are transmitted transplacentally.
3. **Pathogenesis/virulence factors:** Pathogenesis is summarized in Figure 8–2.
4. **Laboratory diagnosis:** Organisms can be seen by dark-field microscopy or direct fluorescence assay.
   a. Because *T pallidum* cannot be grown in cell-free culture (it grows only in rabbit testes), culture is not performed.
   b. Serology involves detection of antibody to **nontreponemal** as well as **treponemal** antigens.
      (1) Nontreponemal tests detect antibody (**reagin**) directed against a cellular protein called **cardiolipin.**
         (a) The test is nonspecific but, because antibody levels rise with syphilis infections, is a good primary screening tool.
         (b) Antibody levels drop with successful treatment.
         (c) Several tests are in use, including the **VDRL** (Venereal Disease Research Laboratory) and the RPR (rapid plasma reagin).
      (2) Treponemal antibody tests (eg, FTAB-ABS and MHA-TP) are used to confirm nontreponemal results.
      (3) **Treponemal antibody titers do not change with treatment but rather stay positive for life.**
5. **Treatment:** Current guidelines should be consulted, but, in general, syphilis is treated with benzathine penicillin.
6. **Prevention:** Safe sex practices and early diagnosis and treatment are the best methods to prevent spread as well as late manifestations of disease.

D. ***Leptospira interrogans*** causes leptospirosis.

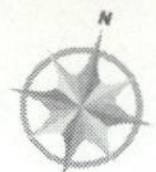

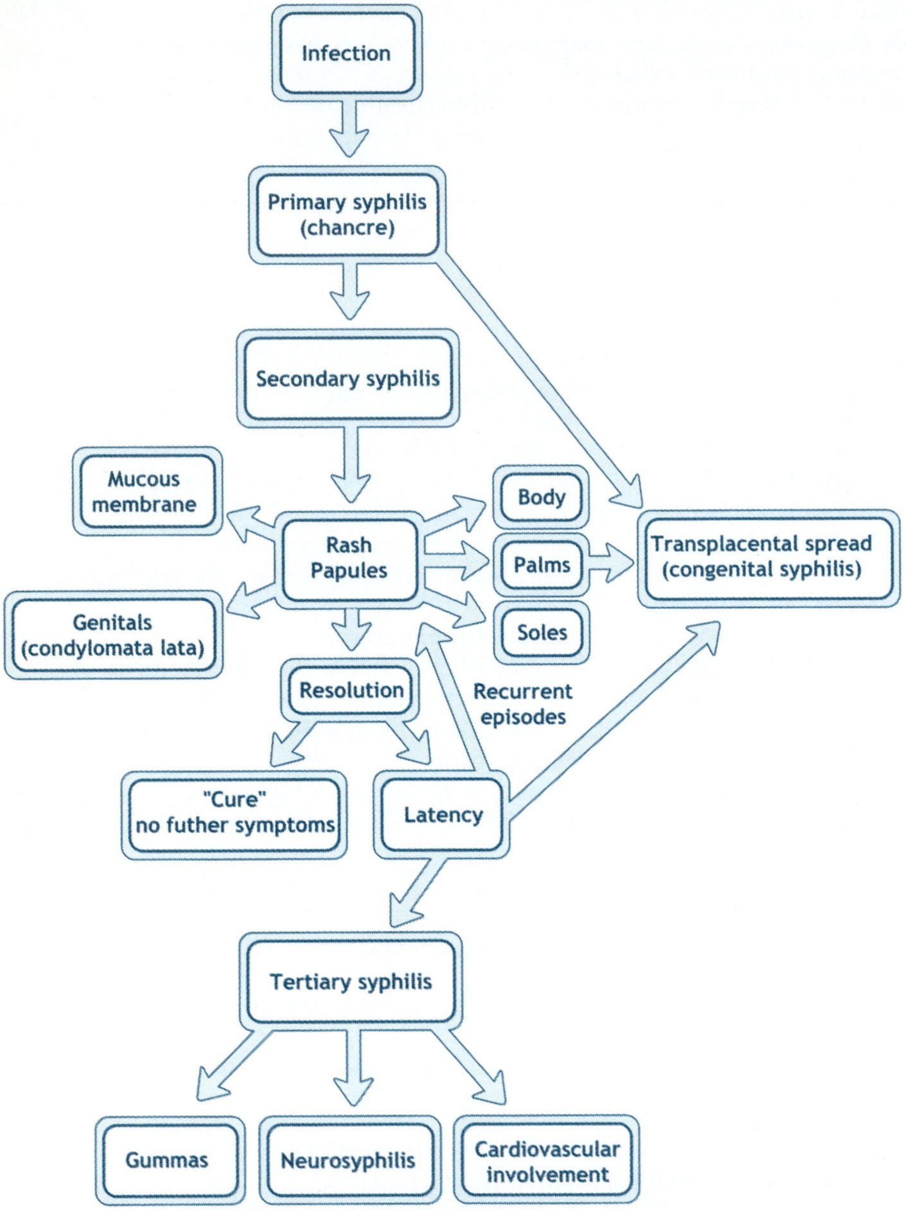

Infection

Primary syphilis
(chancre)

Secondary syphilis

Mucous
membrane

Rash
Papules

Body

Palms

Soles

Transplacental spread
(congenital syphilis)

Genitals
(condylomata lata)

Resolution

Recurrent
episodes

"Cure"
no futher symptoms

Latency

Tertiary syphilis

Gummas

Neurosyphilis

Cardiovascular
involvement

Figure 8–2. Pathogenesis of syphilis.

1. **Clinical manifestations:** *L interrogans* induces a biphasic illness.
   a. The first phase resembles a flulike illness with fever, chills, and myalgia.
   b. The second phase includes **aseptic meningitis** and **iritis.**
   c. A more serious systemic disease (**Weil's disease**), which can lead to death, is characterized by extensive vascular damage, hepatic failure, and renal failure.
2. **Transmission/epidemiology:** Reservoirs include colonized dogs, cattle, rodents, and wild animals.
   a. Transmission is through exposure to water and soil contaminated with animal urine.
   b. *L interrogans* can survive in water for long periods.
3. **Pathogenesis/virulence factors:** Bacteria enter through abraded skin and mucus membranes.
   a. Organisms enter into the bloodstream, multiply, and spread to all tissues.
   b. *L interrogans* is cleared by a humoral immune response, and immune complexes are thought to be involved in the second phase of disease because organisms cannot be cultured from the eye or cerebrospinal fluid.
4. **Laboratory diagnosis:** Organisms are hard to detect.
   a. Culture of cerebrospinal fluid or blood is positive within a narrow window of infection, but organisms grow slowly.
   b. Serologic analysis is most often the diagnostic method of choice.
5. **Treatment:** *L interrogans* is sensitive to various penicillins and tetracyclines. Treatment protocols depend on the severity of disease.
6. **Prevention:** Prophylactic doxycycline can be given to high-risk individuals, and vaccines are available for domestic animals.

THE JARISCH-HERXHEIMER REACTION

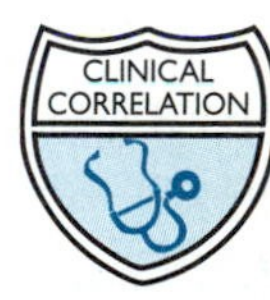

- *Treatment of secondary syphilis and other spirochete diseases (eg,* Borrelia *and* Leptospira*) sometimes results in abrupt fever, chills, headaches, and myalgia.*
- *Because spirochetes are thin-walled, gram-negative organisms, treatment—especially during bacteremic phases—causes cell wall lysis and release of endotoxin, leading to symptoms.*

IV. *Mycoplasma*

A. The most important species that infects humans is ***M pneumoniae,*** also known as **Eaton's reagent.**
   1. **Clinical manifestations:** *M pneumoniae* causes both upper and lower respiratory infections.
      a. Upper respiratory disease includes pharyngitis, otitis media, and tracheobronchitis.
      b. Lower respiratory disease is called primary **atypical pneumonia,** or **"walking pneumonia."**
      c. Infections typically present with a persistent, dry cough.
   2. **Transmission/epidemiology:** *M pneumoniae* is a human pathogen transmitted by infectious aerosols. Long incubation and infectious periods are common.
   3. **Pathogenesis/virulence factors:** The primary virulence factor is the P1 adhesion protein.
      a. *M pneumoniae* remains extracellular but binds to respiratory ciliated epithelial cells via the P1 protein.

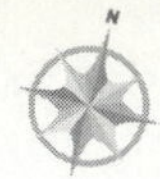

   b. Adherence results in **ciliostasis** and eventual cell destruction, resulting in reduced ciliated clearance.
   c. Bacteria then gain access to the lower respiratory tract.
4. **Laboratory diagnosis:** Diagnosis relies on clinical findings.
   a. *M pneumoniae* can be cultured, but growth is slow.
   b. Serology demonstrating a fourfold rise in titer is diagnostic.
5. **Treatment:** *M pneumoniae* is susceptible to tetracycline and erythromycin.

STRUCTURAL DRUG RESISTANCE OF M PNEUMONIAE

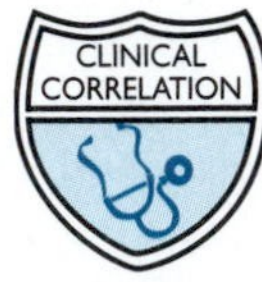

- *The absence of a cell wall in* M pneumoniae *makes it inherently resistant to many different cell wall–active antibiotics, including all of the penicillins, cephalosporins, and vancomycin.*

CLINICAL PROBLEMS

A 5-year-old is diagnosed with primary atypical pneumonia caused by *M pneumoniae.*

1. Which antibiotic is least likely to be effective in treating this child's illness?

   A. Tetracycline
   B. Doxycycline
   C. Erythromycin
   D. Penicillin

An 18-year-old pet shop worker is seen with fever, chills, myalgia, and a bilateral interstitial pneumonia. Her job is to clean the bird cages twice a day.

2. The organism most likely involved in her illness is:

   A. *C trachomatis*
   B. *C psittaci*
   C. *B recurrentis*
   D. *L interrogans*

A 40-year-old with secondary syphilis is given a single dose of benzathione penicillin and experiences fever and chills.

3. What is the most likely explanation for these treatment-induced symptoms?

   A. The wrong antibiotic was used to treat the disease.
   B. The patient had another underlying illness.
   C. Cell wall endotoxin was released upon treatment.
   D. Penicillin stimulates the secretion of bacterial pyrogenic exotoxins.

After being bitten by a tick, a man develops a bull's eye rash with a clear center at the bite site.

4. The organism most likely to have caused this rash is:
   A. *L interrogans*
   B. *B burgdorferi*
   C. *R ricketsii*
   D. *B hermsii*

After spending a weekend in a mouse- and tick-infested cabin, a 14-year-old Boy Scout experiences an abrupt onset of high fever and chills that lasts for 7 days. Three days later, the fever returns.

5. What virulence mechanism is most likely associated with the cyclic nature of this fever?
   A. Antigen variation
   B. Pyrogenic exotoxins
   C. Reinfection
   D. Intracellular invasion

ANSWERS

1. The answer is D. *M pneumoniae* lacks a cell wall and therefore is not susceptible to the beta-lactam antibiotics.
2. The answer is B. *C psittaci* causes a disease consistent with these symptoms and is transmitted as aerosols on dried bird droppings.
3. The answer is C. Treatment-induced fever after treatment for systemic spirochete infections is called the Jarisch-Herxheimer reaction and is related to the release of bacterial cell wall endotoxin fragments after antibiotic-induced cell lysis.
4. The answer is B. *B burgdorferi* is the causative agent of Lyme disease. The bull's eye rash is characteristic of early Lyme disease.
5. The answer is A. The causative agent is most likely *B hermsii,* which causes sporadic, relapsing fever. Antigen variation of outer envelope proteins, while in sequestered sites, allows organisms to escape immune clearance and repopulate the bloodstream.

CHAPTER 9
MYCOBACTERIA

I. Key Concepts

A. *Mycobacterium* species have many properties that set them apart from other bacteria.

B. They possess a unique cell wall that resembles that of gram-positive bacteria but contains high levels of long-chain mycolic acids.

C. The high lipid content of the cell wall prevents uptake of Gram stain but is characteristically **"acid-fast"** by Ziehl-Neelsen or Kinyoun staining methods.

D. The lipid cell wall provides resistance to detergents and many common antibiotics.

E. Mycobacteria are very slow growing, with doubling times in some species (*M leprae*) that approach 2 weeks.

F. A cell-mediated immune response to the protein component of the cell wall (purified protein derivative [PPD] for *M tuberculosis* and lepromin for *M leprae*) is used to monitor infectious exposure.

G. Medically important species include *M tuberculosis, M leprae,* and *M avium-intracellulare* complex.

II. *Mycobacterium* Species

A. ***M tuberculosis*** is the causative agent of tuberculosis.

1. **Clinical manifestations:** The classic manifestation of *M tuberculosis* infection is pulmonary disease.
   - **a.** Active pulmonary disease is characterized by cough, hemoptysis, fever, weight loss, and night sweats.
   - **b.** Lungs contain multiple **granulomas** with extensive **caseation.**
   - **c.** Disseminated (**miliary**) tuberculosis can produce **granulomas** in any organ.
   - **d.** Chronic **meningitis** is a disseminated complication with high fatality.
2. **Transmission/epidemiology:** Tuberculosis is a human disease spread by respiratory aerosols.
   - **a.** Exposure infectivity is high, leading to positive skin test conversion.
   - **b.** Development of active disease is elevated in immunocompromised individuals, such as those with HIV.
3. **Pathogenesis/virulence factors:** *M tuberculosis* organisms survive and replicate in unactivated macrophages.
   - **a.** Primary infection results in granuloma (**tubercle**) formation with caseous necrotic centers.
   - **b.** **Liquefaction** of caseous centers and **cavitation** accompany progression to active disease.

   c. Bacteria can survive for years inside tubercles and become **reactivated** in association with immunosuppression.
   d. Miliary disease can result from tubercle erosion and dissemination via the bloodstream with subsequent involvement of any organ.
4. **Laboratory diagnosis:** Acid-fast bacilli can be detected by direct examination of sputum in individuals with active tuberculosis.
   a. Exposure is monitored by reactivity to the **PPD skin test.**
   b. Culture requires special media and, because of doubling times of 12–24 hours, can take 3–4 weeks.
   c. Biochemical tests, such as production of **niacin** by *M tuberculosis,* are used to distinguish mycobacterial species.
   d. Drug resistance testing is slow but necessary to guide treatment.
5. **Treatment:** Prolonged treatment (6–9 months) with combination antibiotics is necessary.
   a. Treatment recommendations vary depending on susceptibility but include isoniazid (**INH**), ethambutol, rifampin, pyrazinamide, streptomycin, ethionamide, cycloserine, and fluroquinolones.
   b. Multiple-drug–resistant strains are becoming more prevalent.
6. **Prevention:** Chemoprophylaxis can be used in individuals with recent PPD conversions. Vaccination with a live mycobacterium from a related species (**bacillus Calmette-Guérin** or **BCG** vaccine) can provide variable protection.

DRUG RESISTANCE TO *M TUBERCULOSIS*

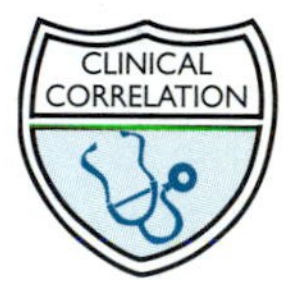

- *Resistance to isoniazid, rifampin, or ethionamide can develop rapidly if used individually for treatment.*
- M tuberculosis *is very slow growing, requiring long-term therapy, (often 9 months or more,) using combinations of 2 or 3 antibiotics.*
- *Long-term therapy often has erratic compliance, leading to selection of drug-resistant strains.*
- *Multiple-drug–resistant strains have emerged that now require combinations of 4 or 5 different antibiotics.*

B. ***M leprae*** is the causative agent of **leprosy.**
1. **Clinical manifestations:** Two forms of leprosy are recognized.
   a. **Tuberculoid** leprosy is characterized by macular skin lesions, peripheral nerve damage, and granuloma formation.
   b. **Lepromatous** leprosy causes extensive tissue and nerve damage and numerous skin lesions containing infectious organisms.
2. **Transmission/epidemiology:** Person-to-person contact is the main mode of transmission with long incubation periods often extending many years.
   a. Lepromatous leprosy is more infectious than tuberculoid leprosy.
   b. Most cases in the United States are in Texas, California, Louisiana, and Hawaii.
   c. Armadillos may act as an endemic reservoir.
3. **Pathogenesis/virulence factors:** *M leprae* replicate and survive in macrophages and **Schwann** cells.
   a. Invasion causes damage to peripheral nerves.
   b. Lepromatous forms lack a specific cell-mediated immune response.
      (1) Organisms replicate and accumulate.
      (2) Extensive skin lesions develop and organisms spread systemically.
   c. Tuberculoid skin lesions contain many granulomas but few organisms.

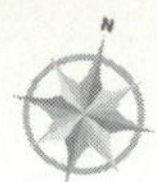

4. **Laboratory diagnosis:** *M leprae* is an obligate intracellular parasite and cannot be grown in cell-free culture.
   a. Lepromin skin tests and microscopic examination of skin lesions for acid-fast organisms aid diagnosis.
   b. Tuberculoid lesions contain few organisms and are lepromin-positive.
   c. Lepromatous lesions contain many organisms and are lepromin-negative.
5. **Treatment:** *M leprae* infections are treated by long-term (up to 2 years) combination therapy.
   a. The drug of choice for tuberculoid leprosy is dapsone in combination with rifampin.
   b. A third antibiotic, clofazimine, is added for lepromatous leprosy.
6. **Prevention:** Dapsone can be used for chemoprophylaxis in exposed individuals.

C. ***M avium-intracellulare*** complex causes an opportunistic pulmonary and disseminated disease in immunocompromised individuals.
   1. **Clinical manifestations:** *M avium-intracellulare* infection is one of the most common systemic infections in patients with AIDS. Resistance to antimycobacterial antibiotics and high mortality are common.
   2. **Transmission/epidemiology:** The organisms are found in water and soil and transmitted by ingestion or inhalation of infectious aerosols.

CLINICAL PROBLEMS

1. Tuberculoid leprosy is characterized by:
   A. A positive lepromin skin test result and few organisms in lesions
   B. A negative lepromin skin test result and many organisms in lesions
   C. A positive lepromin skin test result and many organisms in lesions
   D. A negative lepromin skin test result and few organisms in lesions
2. Why do *M tuberculosis* organisms stain poorly with Gram stain reagents?
   A. Like *Mycoplasma* species, they lack a cell wall.
   B. Their cell wall resembles that of gram-negative organisms.
   C. Their cell walls contain large amounts of mycolic acid.
   D. Their cell walls lack peptidoglycan and consist only of mycolic acid.
3. Which of the following statements about *M leprae* is not true?
   A. It is an obligate, intracellular parasite.
   B. It replicates in macrophages and Schwann cells.
   C. Lepromatous disease is less infectious than tuberculoid disease.
   D. Dapsone is used for treatment.

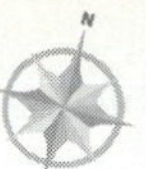

4. Which of the following statements concerning *M tuberculosis* is not true?
   A. Transmission is by respiratory aerosols.
   B. Organisms survive in unactivated macrophages.
   C. Organisms grow slowly, with a doubling time of 12–24 hours.
   D. Treatment regimens generally use single antibiotics for 1–2 weeks.

A 25-year old HIV-positive man is seen in the emergency department with fever, shortness of breath, night sweats, and coughing up blood. A chest x-ray reveals bilateral upper lobe infiltrates. History indicates a 15-lb weight loss and a CD4+ T-cell count of 130. A sputum specimen is positive for acid-fast bacilli.

5. The organism most likely responsible for this infection is:
   A. *Pneumocystis carinii*
   B. *Histoplasma capsulatum*
   C. *M tuberculosis*
   D. *M leprae*

A 30-year-old man from Texas presents with numerous skin lesions on the face that have progressed over the past year. The lesions exhibit loss of temperature and pain sensation. Biopsy of a skin lesion reveals many acid-fast bacilli that failed to grow in culture.

6. The organism most likely responsible for this infection is:
   A. *M tuberculosis*
   B. *M leprae*
   C. *M avium-intracellulare*
   D. *Mycoplasma hominis*

A 45-year-old HIV-positive man is seen in the emergency department with fever, night sweats, chills, and diarrhea. The patient has had progressive weight loss over the past 2 months and was treated previously for *Pneumocystis* pneumonia. His CD4+ T-cell count is 50, a sputum specimen is positive for acid-fast bacilli, and blood culture grows atypical mycobacteria.

7. The most likely diagnosis is:
   A. *M avium-intracellulare*
   B. *M leprae*
   C. *M tuberculosis*
   D. *Mycobacterium marinum*

ANSWERS

1. The answer is A. Tuberculoid leprosy induces strong cell-mediated immune responses and therefore positive lepromin skin test results. Few organisms are present in skin lesions.

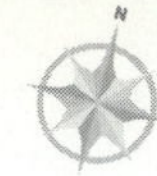

2. The answer is C. High amounts of long-chain mycolic acid prevent penetration of Gram stain reagents. Mycobacteria cell walls resemble those of gram-positive organisms (lots of peptidoglycan) and can be stained with the Ziehl-Neelsen or Kinyoun methods, in which organisms are characteristically "acid-fast."

3. The answer is C. Lepromatous disease is characterized by a lack of cell-mediated immune responses, contain large numbers of organisms in skin lesions, and is therefore more infectious.

4. The answer is D. Treatment is prolonged (9 months or more) with a combination of antibiotics, sometimes as many as 4 or 5 with multiple-drug–resistant strains.

5. The answer is C. *M tuberculosis* causes primary tuberculosis with the above-described symptoms and is an acid-fast bacillus. *P carinii* and *H capsulatum* cause life-threatening pulmonary infections in untreated, immunocompromised patients but are not acid-fast bacteria. *M leprae* typically presents as skin lesions.

6. The answer is B. Slowly progressing skin lesions with nerve damage, associated with loss of temperature or pain sensation, coupled with numerous acid-fast bacilli in the lesions are characteristic of lepromatous leprosy caused by *M leprae.*

7. The answer is A. *M avium-intracellulare* is the most common opportunistic bacterial infection in patients with AIDS, typically occurring as a disseminated infection (positive blood culture) in late-stage disease.

CHAPTER 10
BASIC VIROLOGY

I. Properties of Viruses: Key Concepts

A. Viruses are small, infectious, obligate intracellular parasites.

B. Mature extracellular virus particles, called **virions,** are metabolically inert and mediate the transmission of the virus from host to host.

C. The virion consists of a **genome** that may be either DNA or RNA surrounded by a protein coat, or **capsid.**

D. Intracellular viral replication requires disassembly of the virion, viral genome–directed synthesis of virion components by cellular machinery, and the assembly of progeny genomes and viral proteins to form new virions.

II. Virion Components and Functions

A. Virions are composed of a genome and a protein capsid. The viral genome plus the capsid is termed the **nucleocapsid** (Figure 10–1).

B. Some virions possess a cell membrane–derived lipid **envelope** containing viral glycoproteins that surrounds the nucleocapsid (Figure 10–1).

C. Viruses with envelopes are referred to as **enveloped** viruses; viruses without an envelope are called **naked** viruses.

D. Capsids and envelopes serve to protect the viral genome in its extracellular state from physical and enzymatic destruction.

E. Capsids contain binding sites for attachment to cell receptors and mediate entry of the virion into susceptible cells.

F. Some viruses contain **enzymes** (eg, virion polymerases) or other viral proteins necessary for efficient viral reproduction.

G. The viral nucleic acid genome encodes information needed for viral replication and the synthesis of progeny virions.

H. Virion nucleic acid may be single- (ss) or double-stranded (ds), linear or circular molecules.

I. DNA virus genomes may be ss or ds, linear or circular molecules.

J. RNA virus genomes may be ss or ds, linear or circular, nonsegmented or segmented molecules.

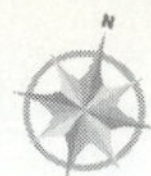

Figure 10–1. Virion components.

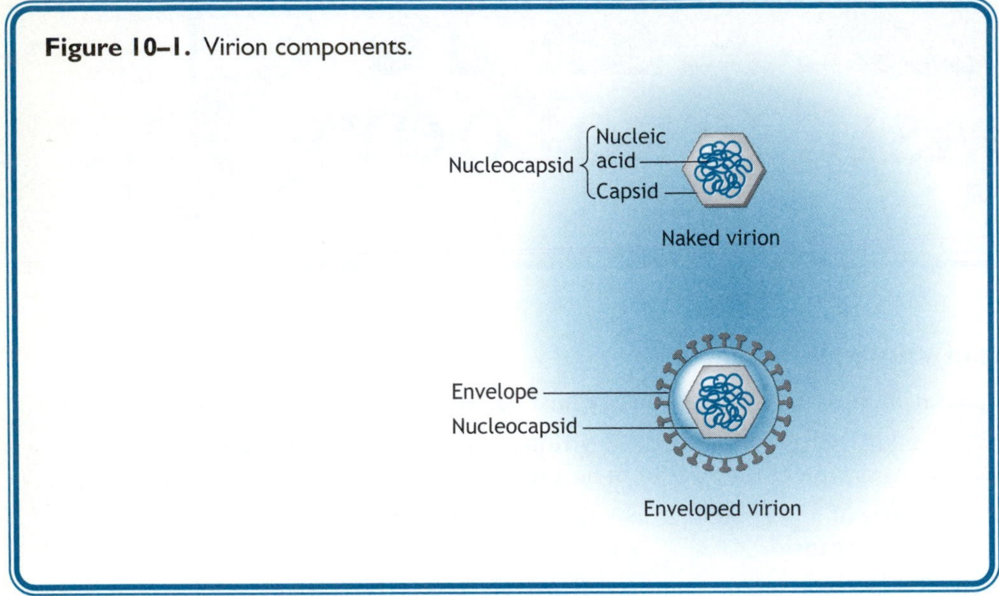

K. The ss viral RNA genomes are classified in 2 ways.
   1. **Positive-strand (+) RNA viruses** denote that the genome is of the same polarity or sense as mRNA.
   2. **Negative-strand (–) RNA viruses** signify that the genome is complementary to mRNA (ie, of negative polarity) and incapable of functioning as mRNA.

III. Virion Structure

A. Viral nucleocapsids have 2 types of symmetry: **helical** and **icosahedral.**

B. Capsid symmetry is based on the arrangement of morphologic subunits called **capsomeres.** Capsomeres are composed of multiple copies of 1 or several different polypeptides that form the capsid.

C. **Helical nucleocapsids** are composed of protein subunits bound to the viral RNA in the form of a helix. ***Note:*** Only RNA viruses have helical symmetry.

D. **Icosahedral nucleocapsids** have protein subunits arranged in the form of an icosahedron with 20 triangular faces and 12 vertices. The viral nucleic acid is located inside the capsid shell.

E. Construction of viruses with icosahedral and helical symmetries is the most efficient and economical means for assembling a virion with limited coding capacity.

F. Some viruses have neither helical nor icosahedral symmetry and are designated structurally as **complex** (eg, poxviruses).

IV. Virus Classification

A. Viruses are classified by nature of the nucleic acid (DNA or RNA), symmetry of the capsid (helical or icosahedral), presence or absence of an envelope, and size of the virion.

B. The taxonomy of viruses uses a Linnaean system as shown:

Taxonomy	**Examples**
Family: viridae	Picornaviridae, Rhabdoviridae
Subfamily: virinae *or*	
Genus: virus	*Enterovirus, Lyssavirus*
Species: virus	Poliovirus, Rabies virus

C. The most recent (2000) taxonomy of medically important human viruses is summarized in Table 10–1.

Table 10–1. Classification of human viruses.

Virus Family	Virus Example	Nucleic Acid	Nucleocapsid Symmetry	Envelope
DNA viruses				
Poxviridae	Smallpox virus	Linear ds DNA	Complex	Yes
Herpesviridae	Herpes simplex, cytomegalovirus	Linear ds DNA	Icosahedral	Yes
Adenoviridae	Adenovirus	Linear ds DNA	Icosahedral	No
Papillomaviridae	Papillomavirus	Circular ds DNA	Icosahedral	No
Polyomaviridae	JC virus	Circular ds DNA	Icosahedral	No
Parvoviridae	B19 virus	ss DNA	Icosahedral	No
Hepadnaviridae	Hepatitis B	Circular, partially ds DNA	Icosahedral	Yes
RNA Viruses				
Retroviridae	HIV-1 & 2, HTLV-1 & 2	Linear ss RNA	Icosahedral	Yes
Reoviridae	Rotavirus	Segmented ds RNA	Icosahedral	No
Paramyxoviridae	Parainfluenza, measles, mumps	Linear ss RNA	Helical	Yes
Rhabdoviridae	Rabies virus	Linear ss RNA	Helical	Yes
Filoviridae	Ebola and Marburg viruses	Linear ss RNA	Helical	Yes

(*continued*)

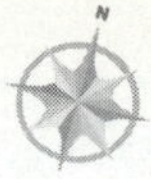

Table 10–1. *(continued)*

Virus Family	Virus Example	Nucleic Acid	Nucleocapsid Symmetry	Envelope
RNA Viruses (*continued*)				
Orthomyxoviridae	Influenza virus	Segmented ss RNA	Helical	Yes
Bunyaviridae	La Crosse virus, Hantavirus	Circular ss RNA; 3 segments	Helical	Yes
Arenaviridae	Lassa fever virus	Circular ss RNA; 2 segments	Helical	Yes
Picornaviridae	Poliovirus, rhinovirus, hepatitis A virus	Linear ss RNA	Icosahedral	No
Caliciviridae	Norovirus	Linear ss RNA	Icosahedral	No
Astroviridae	Astrovirus	Linear ss RNA	Icosahedral	No
Coronaviridae	Coronavirus	Linear ss RNA	Helical	Yes
Flaviviridae	West Nile virus, hepatitis C virus	Linear ss RNA	Icosahedral	Yes
Togaviridae	Eastern equine encephalitis, rubella virus	Linear ss RNA	Icosahedral	Yes

ds, double-stranded; ss, single-stranded.
Derived from van Regenmortel MHV et al. In: *Virus Taxonomy. Seventh Report of the International Committee on Taxonomy of Viruses.* Academic Press, 2000.

V. Viral Replication

A. Steps in Virus Replication Cycle

1. **Attachment:** Viruses **attach or adsorb** to specific cell receptors via **viral attachment proteins (VAPs)** on the viral capsid or envelope.
   a. Examples of VAPs are the hemagglutinin of influenza virus, the fiber protein of adenoviruses, and gp120 of HIV-1.
   b. Examples of cell receptors for viral attachment are sialic acid (influenza virus), acetylcholine receptor (rabies virus), and CD4 (HIV-1).
   c. VAP–cell receptor interactions are complex, often requiring coreceptors for virus entry into the cell.
   d. Both the host range and tissue tropism are determined by VAP–cell receptor interactions.

2. **Penetration and uncoating:** Virus entry into the host cell is energy dependent.
   a. **Direct membrane fusion** and **receptor-mediated endocytosis** are mechanisms of virus entry into cells.
   b. Direct membrane fusion, exemplified by paramyxoviruses and retroviruses, is characterized by fusion of the viral envelope glycoprotein with the cell plasma membrane. The nucleocapsid is then released into the cytoplasm.
   c. Receptor-mediated endocytosis, typified by influenza virus, is triggered by VAP–cell receptor binding, endocytosis of the virus-receptor complex, formation of an endocytic vesicle, and acidification of the endosome. Fusion of the viral proteins and endosomal membranes allows penetration and release of the nucleocapsid into the cytoplasm.
3. **Gene expression and genome replication:** The mission of the virus is to transcribe functional mRNA from the viral genome that encodes viral proteins needed for genome replication and synthesis of progeny virus.
   a. Viruses have evolved several strategies for mRNA synthesis depending on the structure of the viral genome.
   b. Most DNA viruses use cellular DNA-dependent RNA polymerase II to make mRNA. The exception is poxvirus, which replicates in the cytoplasm and carries a DNA-dependent RNA polymerase in the virion.
   c. In (+) RNA viruses (eg, picornaviruses), the genome is mRNA and is translated directly on cell ribosomes.
   d. (–) RNA viruses (eg, orthomyxoviruses) and ds RNA viruses (eg, reoviruses) use a virion-associated RNA-dependent RNA polymerase to synthesize mRNA because the cell has no mechanism to synthesize mRNA from ss or ds RNA templates.
   e. Retroviruses (eg, HIV) have a genome with (+) polarity but replicate via a DNA intermediate. The (+) RNA genome is converted to (–) strand DNA and then to ds DNA by a virion-associated, RNA-dependent DNA polymerase (reverse transcriptase [RT]). The viral DNA is subsequently integrated into cellular DNA and mRNA synthesized by cellular RNA polymerase II.
   f. The **genome replication strategy** of DNA and RNA viruses is summarized in Figure 10–2.
   g. All DNA viruses, with the exception of poxviruses, replicate their genome in the nucleus.
   h. Small nuclear ds DNA viruses such as papillomaviruses, utilize host cell DNA polymerase for synthesis of new viral DNA, whereas more complex adenoviruses and herpesviruses encode their own DNA polymerase and other enzymes important in DNA synthesis.
   i. Large cytoplasmic ds DNA viruses, such as poxviruses, encode DNA polymerase and other proteins necessary for viral DNA replication.
   j. The nuclear DNA virus, hepatitis B, is unique in that its genome is partially ds with 2 ss regions. The ss regions are converted to ds DNA by a virus-associated enzyme. Viral RNA synthesized from the DNA genome serves as a template for reverse transcription into progeny DNA.
   k. All RNA viruses except influenza virus and retroviruses replicate in the cytoplasm.
   l. Genome replication by all RNA viruses, except retroviruses, requires an RNA-dependent RNA polymerase.

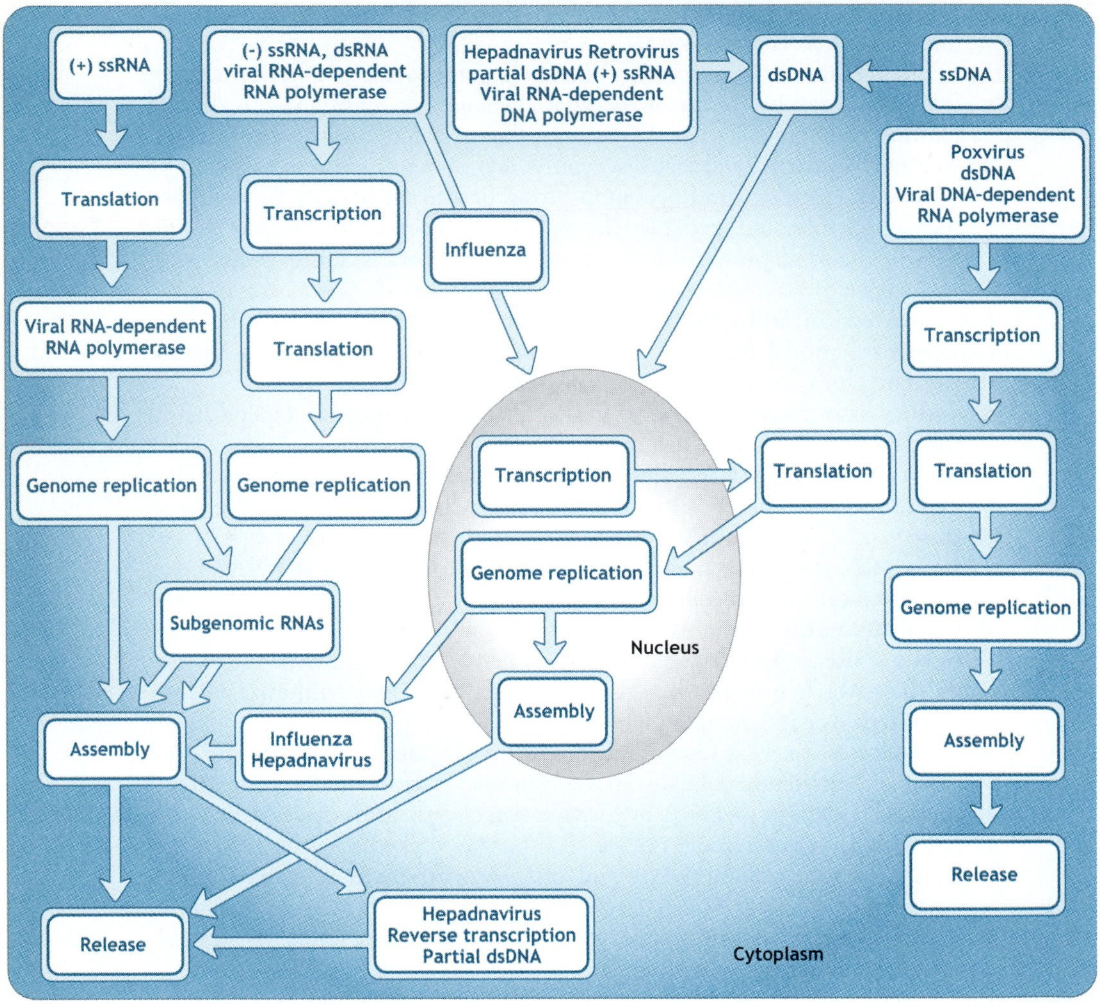

Figure 10–2. Replication strategies of DNA and RNA viruses. Diagram courtesy of Dr. Julie A. Kerry.

m. In (+) strand RNA viruses, such as picornaviruses, the viral genome acts as mRNA and is translated into a large, single protein that is subsequently cleaved into individual proteins, including an RNA polymerase. The RNA-dependent RNA polymerase produces a complementary (–) sense RNA from the (+) sense template. This (–) sense intermediate serves as a template for the production of the (+) strand genome.

n. In (–) strand RNA viruses, such as paramyxoviruses and rhabdoviruses, the virion-associated, RNA-dependent RNA polymerase produces (+) strands that may be subgenomic and function as mRNA or genome length (+) RNA that acts as a template for the production of the (–) strand genome.

o. In ds RNA viruses, such as reoviruses, a virion-associated, RNA-dependent RNA polymerase transcribes each segment into (+) mRNA. The (+) mRNAs are utilized for protein synthesis and as a template for complementary (–) RNA strand synthesis in a subviral particle to generate the formation of ds RNA genomes.
p. Retroviruses have a (+) strand RNA genome that does not function as mRNA. The virion-associated RT synthesizes a (–) strand DNA copy of the viral RNA that is subsequently converted to ds DNA by the same RT. ds DNA is integrated into the host cell chromosomal DNA, where cell DNA-dependent RNA polymerase transcribes subgenomic mRNAs for viral protein synthesis as well as genome length RNA for production of the (+) strand genome.

4. Virion **assembly and release** generally take place at the site of viral nucleic acid replication.
   a. Newly synthesized capsid proteins self-assemble and package or encapsidate the viral nucleic acid.
   b. Enveloped viruses acquire their envelope by budding through the plasma membrane or nuclear membrane (herpesviruses).
   c. Virions are released by cell lysis (nonenveloped viruses) or by budding from cell membranes (enveloped viruses).
   d. Release of enveloped viruses often occurs without cell death with virions shed extracellularly.

B. Virus Cell Interactions

1. **Lytic infections** are characterized by virion production and death of the permissive host cell. Examples of lytic infections are rhinovirus and influenza virus infection.
2. **Abortive infections** are characterized by no virion production and host cell survival. They may result from viral infection of a nonpermissive cell either lacking cell receptors or factors required for complete viral replication.
3. **Persistent infections** are characterized generally by cell survival with or without production of infectious viruses.
   a. Persistent infections can be chronic, latent, or transforming.
   b. **Chronic infections,** exemplified by hepatitis B, are characterized by the nonlytic continuous shedding of virus from the infected cell.
   c. **Latent infections,** typified by herpesviruses, are characterized by no production of progeny virus, but the viral genome remains quiescent in the cell for months or years; virus can later be produced by reactivation.
   d. **Transforming infections,** exemplified by papillomaviruses and human T-cell leukemia virus (HTLV-1), are characterized by the acquisition of growth, morphologic, and behavioral properties of tumor cells.
   e. Integration of viral DNA and continuous expression of specific viral genes are a common theme in cell transformation.
4. **Slow infections,** such as prion diseases, are characterized by the slow (years to decades) clinical course, accumulation of misfolded prion protein in the brain resulting in neuronal degeneration, and spongiform encephalopathy (see Chapter 16).

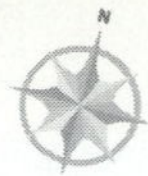

VI. Viral Genetics

A. Types of Viral Mutations

1. **Spontaneous mutations** occur randomly in viruses with low rates among DNA viruses (10^{-8}–10^{-11} per incorporated nucleotide), comparable to mutation rates in cellular DNA, and generally higher rates in RNA viruses (10^{-3}–10^{-4}) due primarily to high error rates in RNA-dependent RNA polymerases.
   a. Spontaneous mutations may have no effect, be lethal to virus production, or result in altered virus phenotype with a selective advantage.
   b. Spontaneous mutants may acquire phenotypes that enable the virus to evade host immunity (eg, **antigenic drift** due to point mutations in influenza virus envelope proteins, hemagglutinin, and neuraminidase) or acquire antiviral drug resistance (eg, HIV).
   c. Live, attenuated viral vaccines are derived from the selection of spontaneous mutants that have lost the capacity to cause disease while retaining antigenicity.
2. **Induced mutations** can be generated in the laboratory using chemical mutagens that modify viral nucleic acids. Specific induced mutations can be engineered into viruses by recombinant DNA techniques to construct deletion, insertion, or substitution mutations in viral genes.

B. Genetic Interactions between Viruses

1. Intramolecular homologous **recombination** between 2 strains of the same DNA virus (eg, herpes simplex virus [HSV] types 1 and 2) results in a hybrid virus with genes from both parents (Figure 10–3). Homologous recombination is common among DNA viruses.
2. Random **reassortment** of gene segments is common in RNA viruses with segmented genomes (eg, influenza A virus, reoviruses).
   a. When a cell is coinfected with 2 different viral strains, gene segments are exchanged and progeny viruses are produced with RNA segments from either parental virus (Figure 10–4).
   b. Reassortment of RNA segments occurring during infection of a cell with a human and animal influenza virus can result in major antigenic changes in the virus, termed **antigenic shift** (see Chapter 13, IV. Orthomyxoviridae Family).

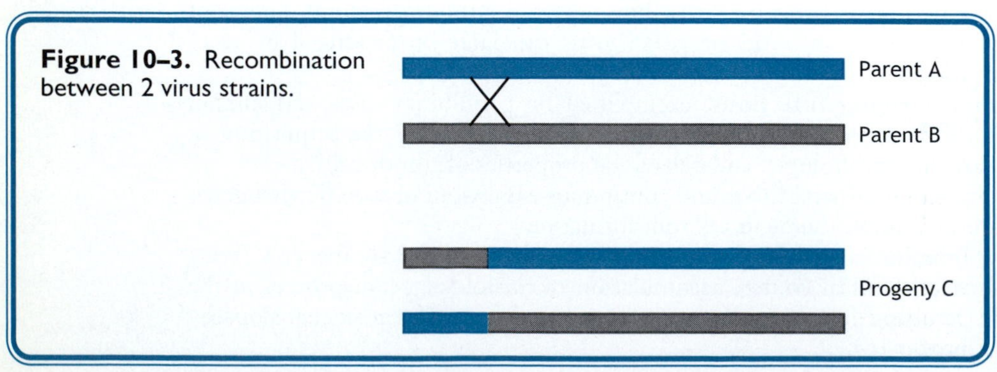

Figure 10–3. Recombination between 2 virus strains.

Figure 10–4. Gene reassortment between 2 segmented RNA viruses.

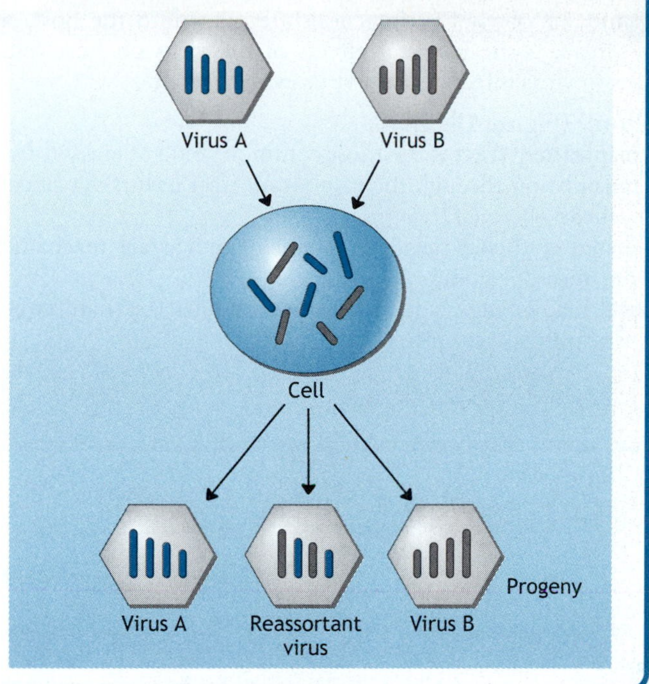

3. **Complementation** is the interaction between viral proteins in a mixedly infected cell that results in increased production of 1 or both parental types.
   a. Complementation usually consists of one virus providing the functional gene product that is defective in the other virus.
   b. In complementation, viral proteins provide the missing or defective function, but the genotypes of parental and progeny viruses are unchanged.

INFLUENZA A VIRUS ANTIGENIC SHIFT

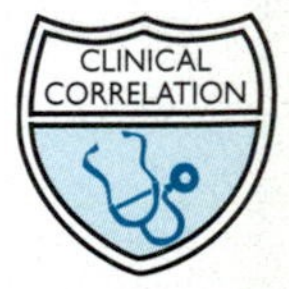

- *The 1918 "Spanish" flu pandemic that killed more than 20 million people worldwide is a sober reminder of the devastating consequences of influenza A virus antigenic shift.*
- *Influenza A virus has a genome composed of multiple RNA segments.*
- *The virus can infect birds and pigs as well as humans. RNA segments from bird or pig influenza can be exchanged with human influenza A virus by genetic reassortment in a dually infected cell and can lead to the emergence of a hybrid virus capable of pandemic disease in nonimmune humans.*

VII. Viral Pathogenesis

A. Key Concepts

1. Viral pathogenesis is a delicate and dynamic balance between virus offense and host defense.
2. Pathogenesis is a multifactorial process by which viruses cause disease.
3. Most virus infections are subclinical or inapparent.
4. Viral pathogenesis is an unintended consequence of the way the virus has chosen to reproduce, spread, and evade host defenses.

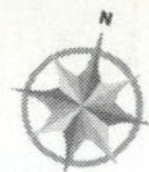

5. **Virulence** is the capacity of a virus to cause disease.
6. Determinants of viral pathogenesis are entry into the host, mechanisms of virus spread, tissue tropism, effects of the virus on host cells, the host responses to virus infection, and virus evasion tactics.

B. Site of Entry (Figure 10–5)

1. The **respiratory tract** is the most common route of entry for viruses.
   a. Transmission through the respiratory tract occurs via aerosol or exchange of saliva.
   b. Ciliated epithelial cells and a layer of mucus are mechanical barriers the virus must overcome.
   c. Local macrophages and secretory antibodies (IgA) are important host defenses against virus infection.

Figure 10–5. Sites of virus entry.

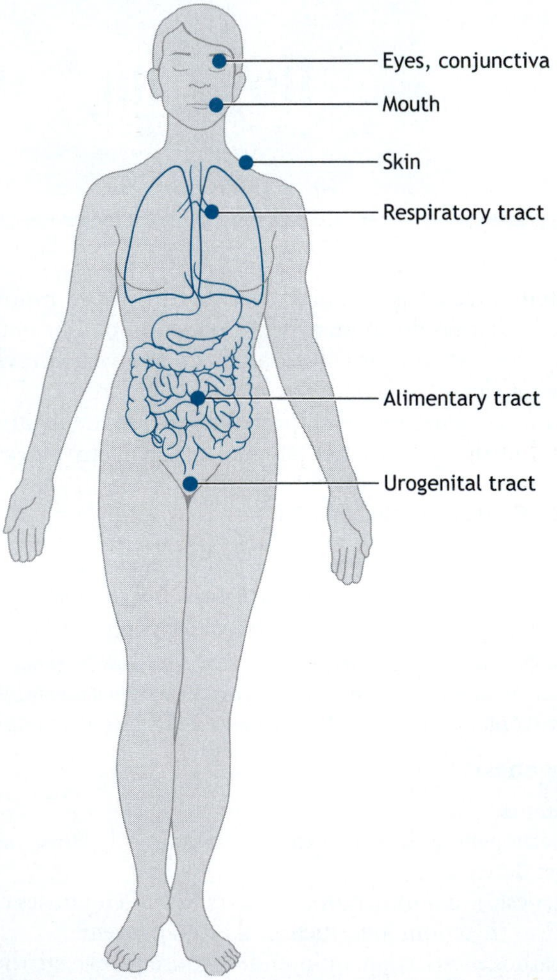

d. Viruses that breach the host defenses and infect the respiratory tract include rhinoviruses, paramyxoviruses, influenza viruses, coronaviruses, arenaviruses, hantavirus, adenoviruses, HSV, and Epstein-Barr virus.

2. Viruses that infect the **alimentary/digestive tract** must survive acid pH of the stomach, alkaline pH of the intestine, digestive enzymes, and bile detergents.
   a. Mucosal IgA, local macrophages, and lymphocytes are important host defenses of the alimentary tract.
   b. Most viruses that infect the digestive tract are naked. Enveloped viruses are readily destroyed by bile detergents and enzymes in the digestive tract.
   c. Viruses that survive the hostile environment of the digestive tract include enteroviruses, hepatitis A virus, rotaviruses, caliciviruses, astroviruses, and adenoviruses.
3. The **urogenital tract** is the route of entry for sexually transmitted viruses.
   a. Barrier defenses of the urogenital tract are the stratified epithelium of the vagina, acid pH, and a layer of mucus that contains IgA.
   b. Viruses may gain entry into the urogenital tract through small tears or breaks in the mucosal epithelium during sexual activity.
   c. Viruses that infect the urogenital tract include HSV, human papillomavirus, and HIV.
4. The **skin** represents the largest target for entry but is the most difficult barrier to penetrate.
   a. The outer layer of skin consists of an impermeable barrier of dead keratinocytes that do no support virus growth.
   b. Viruses gain entry to the underlying vascular dermis when skin is torn by cuts or abrasions or through the bite of an arthropod vector, animal bites, or needle inoculation.
   c. Viruses that gain entry via the skin include papillomaviruses, poxviruses, and HSV following mechanical abrasion; rabies virus by an animal bite; togaviruses, flaviviruses, bunyaviruses, and reoviruses transmitted by mosquito or tick bites; and HIV, hepatitis B, and C viruses transmitted by intravenous drug use.
5. The **eyes and conjunctiva** are an exposed and relatively unprotected site for virus entry.
   a. The flow of secretions and the eyelid act as a barrier to wash away foreign particles from the eye.
   b. Eye infections often are associated with an eye injury, an ophthalmologic procedure, or environmental contamination (eg, swimming in an unsanitized pool).
   c. Viruses that gain entry through the eye are adenovirus types, HSV, and enterovirus 70.

C. Mechanisms of Virus Spread

1. **Some virus infections remain localized** to the site of entry after primary replication.
   a. The virus spreads locally to infect adjacent cells and is prevented from spreading systemically by the host response.
   b. Examples of localized virus infections are rhinovirus and influenza virus replication restricted to the respiratory tract, rotavirus and norovirus replication restricted to the digestive tract, and papillomavirus and molluscum contagiosum virus replication restricted to the skin.

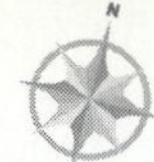

2. Virus spread beyond the primary site of entry to multiple organs is termed **systemic infection.**
   a. Physical and immune barriers are breached in systemic infections.
   b. Measles is an example of a systemic infection in which measles virus initiates infection in the upper respiratory tract and spreads to the lymphatic system and then to the blood, which disseminates the virus to multiple organs, including capillary endothelium, and causes a skin rash.
   c. Viruses spread systemically either via the bloodstream (hematogenous spread) or the nervous system (neural spread).
   d. In hematogenous spread, the virus is either inoculated directly by an insect bite or released into the lymphatic or vascular capillaries at the site of local multiplication.
   e. Primary **viremia** (ie, virus in the blood) allows spread to distant organs, further replication (secondary viremia), and spread to target organs where disease is manifested.
   f. Viruses spread by blood may be either free in plasma (eg, poliovirus) or as infected cell-associated virus (eg, monocyte and macrophage: Dengue virus, HIV; B lymphocyte: Epstein-Barr virus; T lymphocytes: HIV, HTLV-1; erythrocytes: Colorado tick fever virus).
   g. In neural spread, virus spread occurs either by contact with neurons at the site of local multiplication or by the hematogenous route.
   h. Virus invades the CNS by axonal transport along neurons.

D. Determinants of Tissue Tropism

1. **Cell receptors** determine the susceptibility of cells and tissues to virus infection.
   a. Viruses attach to and enter cells via cell receptors.
   b. Cell receptors are normal cell surface proteins that have important cellular functions (ie, they are not solely for virus attachment).
   c. Examples of cell receptors for viruses are the complement protein CR2 on B lymphocytes for Epstein-Barr virus and intercellular adhesion molecule-1 (ICAM-1) on epithelial cells for rhinoviruses. (See also p. 80 for additional examples.)
2. Viruses use VAP to attach and adsorb to cell receptors. Examples of **virus receptors** are the hemagglutinin of measles virus and influenza virus; the G protein of respiratory syncytial virus; and the VP1, VP2, and VP3 capsid protein complex of rhinovirus and poliovirus.
3. **Other cellular proteins:** Cellular transcription factors that control transcription of viral genes are active in specific cell types or tissues that are permissive for virus infection. Cell proteases in the lung are important determinants of influenza virus tropism and act by specifically cleaving the hemagglutinin precursor into 2 subunits essential for infectivity.

E. Host Response to Virus Infection

1. **Cellular level:** Virus infections cause phenotypic changes in cells.
   a. Cytocidal infections are characterized by cytopathic effects (CPEs) typified by morphologic changes, such as inclusion bodies, multinucleated giant cells, and cell lysis.
   b. Persistent infections are characterized by the coexistence of the virus and the host cell. The host cell retains viability and function.

c. Transforming infections caused by oncogenic viruses result in altered morphologic and growth properties of the transformed cell and a risk of malignant potential.

2. **Host response:** Host defense against virus infections consists of nonspecific (innate) immune defense mechanisms and specific (adaptive) immune defense mechanisms.
   a. The nonspecific (innate) immune response is the front line of defense activated early in infection and includes interferon (IFN), natural killer (NK) cells, complement, and phagocytosis.
   b. IFNs are produced by virus-infected cells that produce an "antiviral state" in uninfected cells, thereby protecting them from infection.
   c. IFNs are generally host species specific but virus nonspecific.
   d. There are three groups of IFN proteins: IFN-alpha produced by leukocytes, IFN-beta produced by fibroblasts and epithelial cells, and IFN-gamma produced by NK cells and activated T lymphocytes.
   e. IFNs are induced by most viruses with ds RNA (a product of RNA and DNA virus replication) acting as a potent IFN inducer.
   f. IFNs bind to an IFN receptor found on most cells and activate 2 IFN-responsive genes: a ds RNA-activated protein kinase (PKR) and 2′-5′-oligoadenylate (oligo A) synthetase.
   g. PKR phosphorylates and inactivates eIF2, which is required to initiate protein synthesis; thus, protein synthesis is blocked.
   h. 2′-5′-oligo A synthetase produces short 2′-5′ oligomers of adenylic acid that then activate a latent endoribonuclease (RNase L) that, in turn, degrades viral mRNA, thereby blocking viral protein synthesis.
   i. NK cells produce IFN-gamma that activates macrophages and the inflammatory response.
   j. NK cells act to control the viral infection until acquired immunity is induced.
   k. NK cells kill virus-infected cells.
   l. Macrophages phagocytize virions, and both macrophages and NK cells have antibody receptors on their surface that bind to antibodies on infected cells and target them for elimination in a process known as **antibody-dependent cellular cytotoxicity (ADCC).**
   m. Complement component C3b binds to virions that then become a target for digestion by macrophages with surface C3b receptors in a process known as **opsonization.**
   n. The specific (adaptive) immune response consists of acquired humoral and cell-mediated immunity essential for clearing the viral infection.
   o. Neutralizing antibody to viral surface proteins prevents infection or targets the virus for destruction by phagocytosis, ADCC, or the complement system.
   p. Cytotoxic T lymphocytes target viral antigens expressed in infected cells and destroy them.
   q. In some virus infections, the pathology is a consequence of the host immune response.
   r. Examples of virus-induced immunopathology include noncytolytic hepatitis A and B viruses, in which damage to infected hepatocytes is mediated by cytotoxic T lymphocytes, and severe respiratory syncytial virus infections, in which helper T lymphocytes produce inflammatory cy-

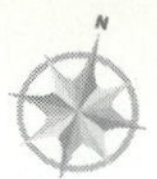

tokines that cause injury by recruiting a massive inflammatory cell infiltrate in the bronchioles and alveoli.

F. Virus Immune Evasion Strategies

1. **Antigenic variation:** HIV, hepatitis C virus (HCV), influenza virus, and rotavirus are examples of antigenic hypermutation or variation.
2. **Establish an immunologically silent latent phase:** The herpesvirus is an example of this strategy involving restricted viral gene expression.
3. **Hide in immunologically privileged sites:** Herpesviruses, JC polyoma virus, and papillomaviruses are examples of viruses that establish persistent infections with reduced immune surveillance.
4. **Infect immune cells and suppress their function:** HIV is the most powerful example of this strategy; measles virus is another.
5. **Inhibit viral antigen presentation:** Adenoviruses and herpesviruses are examples of viruses that interfere with the presentation of viral antigens by MHC class I proteins for recognition by cytotoxic T lymphocytes.
6. **Express extracellular immunomodulatory proteins:** Poxviruses and herpesviruses are examples of viruses that express secreted cytokines or soluble cytokine receptors that sabotage host defenses.
7. **Counteract the antiviral action of IFNs:** Adenovirus, herpesviruses, poliovirus, and influenza virus interfere with the antiviral activity of IFN.

HCV CHRONIC INFECTION

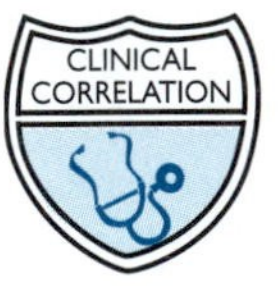

- *HCV infects some 170 million people worldwide, frequently leading to cirrhosis and liver cancer.*
- *HCV is a (+) RNA virus and takes advantage of its error-prone RNA polymerase to produce mutant viruses that evade host immune defenses and establish lifelong, chronic infection.*
- *Chronic infection by HCV is a cycle of immune killing of virus and infected liver cells, and HCV escape by a high rate of mutation.*

VIII. Laboratory Diagnosis of Viral Infections

A. Noncculture Methods

1. **Cytology:** The presence of virus in clinical specimens can sometimes be detected by characteristic cytologic changes in infected cells.
   a. Cytologic alterations are often typified by the presence of **inclusion bodies.**
   b. The presence of inclusion bodies can be pathognomonic for a specific viral infection (eg, intracytoplasmic **Negri bodies** caused by **rabies virus** in brain tissue).
   c. In most cases, cytologic changes are nonspecific and require confirmation by more sensitive and specific immunochemical techniques.
2. **Electron microscopy (EM):** EM is a rapid technique to detect viruses but lacks sensitivity and specificity.
   a. Detection of viral particles by EM requires $\geq 10^6$ virions in the original specimen; most clinical specimens have low quantities of virus.
   b. EM can be used to identify virus groups based on size and shape, but morphologically similar viruses (eg, herpesviruses) cannot be differentiated.
3. **Immunofluorescence (IF) and enzyme immunoassay (EIA) for viral antigen detection:** Monoclonal antibodies specific for unique viral epitopes and labeled with fluorescent molecules or enzymes are available

commercially and can be used as diagnostic tools to detect viral antigens in clinical specimens.

   a. IF is used routinely to detect viral antigens in direct cell smears and requires intact cells for interpretation.
   b. EIA is used to detect viral antigen in cell lysates and tissue sections by immunocytochemistry.
   c. Both IF and EIA methods are sensitive, specific, relatively inexpensive, and rapid (1–4 hours).

4. **Detection of viral nucleic acid:** DNA probes complementary to specific viral sequences are used to detect the presence of virus in clinical specimens.
   a. Viral nucleic acid can be detected in whole cells or tissues fixed to microscope slides by **in situ hybridization.**
   b. The **polymerase chain reaction (PCR)** has revolutionized the detection and identification of viruses in clinical specimens.
   c. PCR is used directly to amplify viruses with DNA genomes.
   d. For RNA viruses, viral RNA is converted to complementary DNA by RT before PCR (RT-PCR).

B. Cell Culture Methods

1. **Cytopathic viruses** can be detected and presumptively identified by characteristic CPEs produced when grown in cell cultures.
   a. CPEs are characterized by microscopic changes in cells after inoculation of the clinical specimen and may include cell rounding, cell clumping, cell degeneration, cell detachment, or cell fusion resulting in multinucleated giant cells.
   b. Definitive identification of the CPE-inducing virus is determined routinely by immunologic detection of viral antigens (eg, IF).
2. **Noncytopathic viruses** do not produce CPEs in cultured cells. Noncytopathic viruses can be detected with assays that measure viral antigen expression in cultured cells (eg, immunocytochemistry).

C. Serologic Methods

1. **Detection of antiviral antibody:** Serology is used to detect a rise in antibody titer to a specific virus in serum collected during the acute and convalescent phase of the infection.
   a. A rise greater than fourfold between acute and convalescent serum is diagnostic evidence of a recent viral infection.
   b. Detection of virus-specific IgM antibody by serology is indicative of a recent infection.
   c. Commonly used serologic assays are EIAs to detect IgG or IgM antibody and the immunoblot assay.
   d. The immunoblot assay uses immobilized viral antigens to detect antibodies to specific viral proteins.
   e. The Western blot is an immunoblot assay that is used to confirm a positive HIV antibody result reported by EIA.
2. **Detection of viral antigen:** Serologic assays (EIAs) are used to detect viral antigen in blood, particularly for those viruses that cannot be detected in any other way. Hepatitis B virus surface antigen and HIV p24 core antigen are examples of viral antigens detected in this way.

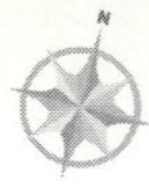

LABORATORY DIAGNOSIS OF SEVERE ACUTE RESPIRATORY SYNDROME (SARS)-CORONAVIRUS

- *In a remarkable tour de force, international collaboration of 13 laboratories from 10 countries identified a virus associated with SARS in 2 weeks and in 2 more weeks had sequenced the entire virus genome.*
- *Identification of a novel coronavirus as the causative agent of SARS was accomplished using traditional virus isolation in cell culture and sophisticated molecular biology techniques.*
- *Availability of the SARS-coronavirus genome aids in the development of diagnostic tests, specific therapies, and vaccines.*

IX. Antiviral Therapy

A. Approaches to Specific Control of Viral Infections (Figure 10–6)

1. **Immunologic control:** Virus infections can be controlled immunologically with vaccines that have a narrow specificity (virus specific) but generally induce long-term effects. Passive immunity in the form of immune serum globulin is virus specific but with relatively short-term effects because of the short half-life of IgG.
2. **Chemotherapy:** Virus infections can be controlled by antiviral drugs that are relatively virus specific (narrow specificity) and provide relatively short-term effects.
3. **IFN therapy:** Virus infections can be controlled by IFN that has broad specificity (virus nonspecific) and provides relatively short-term effects.

B. Rationale for Antiviral Therapy

1. Antiviral drugs are under development for prophylaxis of rhinovirus infections in which vaccination is impractical because of numerous serotypes.
2. Antiviral drugs are being developed for influenza A virus, which undergoes antigenic variation and thus requires annual vaccination.
3. Antiviral drugs are being developed to find life-saving therapies for HIV and AIDS and to overcome viral drug resistance.
4. Antiviral drugs are being developed for use by immunodeficient patients who are unable to mount an immune response.

C. Antiviral Drug Targets

1. Viruses have complex life cycles that are susceptible to attack by drugs at several stages.
2. Examples of targets for antiviral therapy include virus attachment and entry, transcription of viral nucleic acid, translation of viral mRNA into protein, replication of viral nucleic acid, and virus assembly and release.

D. Antiviral Therapies that Block Attachment or Entry

1. Antiviral antibody and receptor analogues or decoys, such as the ICAM-1 receptor used by rhinoviruses and the CD4 or CCR5 receptor used by HIV, are examples of antiviral therapies that **block attachment of the virus to the cell receptor.**
2. Amantadine and rimantadine (an analogue of amantadine with fewer side effects) inhibit influenza A virus infections by **blocking penetration and uncoating.**
   a. They are lipophilic amines that act as weak bases to buffer the acidic environment of the endosome and block fusion of the viral envelope with the endosomal membrane, an acid pH-mediated event.
   b. They are active only against influenza A virus, not influenza B.

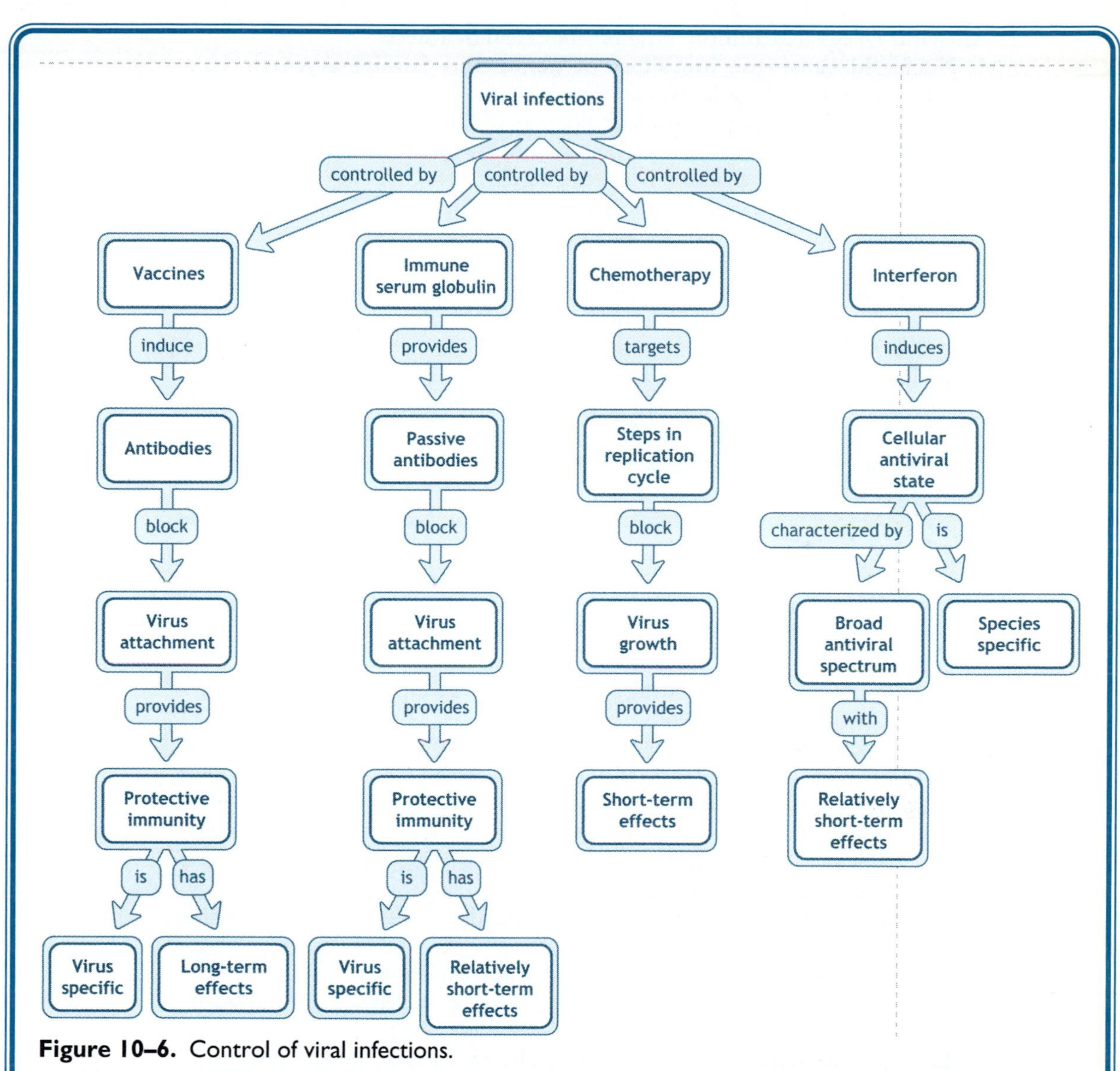

Figure 10–6. Control of viral infections.

   c. They bind to and block the ion channel formed by the viral M2 protein, preventing viral uncoating.

3. Enfuvirtide (T-20) **blocks HIV-1 entry** by inhibiting the fusion of HIV-1 with CD4+ cells.
   a. It is a synthetic peptide that binds to HIV-1 transmembrane gp41 glycoprotein and prevents fusion with the CD4 receptor of T lymphocytes.
   b. It is used with a cocktail of other antiretroviral drugs to treat HIV-1 in patients in whom multiple resistance mutations against other antiretroviral drugs have developed.

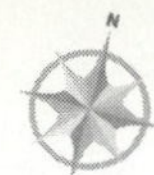

E. Antiviral Drugs that Inhibit Viral Nucleic Acid Synthesis

1. Nucleoside analogue inhibitors of herpesvirus family: acyclovir (acycloguanosine), valacyclovir, and famciclovir

a. All three drugs are nucleoside analogues of guanosine.
b. Valacyclovir and famciclovir are prodrugs (precursor forms) with improved oral bioavailability relative to acyclovir.
c. The drugs are selectively phosphorylated in herpesvirus-infected cells by viral-encoded thymidine kinase (TK).
d. Acyclovir is phosphorylated by herpesvirus TK to form acyclovir monophosphate, which is converted to acyclovir triphosphate (by cellular enzymes) that preferentially inhibits viral DNA polymerase and leads to DNA chain termination.
e. The drugs are approved to treat most HSV and varicella zoster virus infections, including primary and recurrent genital herpes, herpes encephalitis, and varicella or zoster (shingles) in immunocompromised patients.
f. Resistance to these drugs occurs most commonly by mutation of the viral TK and less commonly by mutation of viral DNA polymerase.

2. Nucleoside analogue inhibitors of herpesvirus family: ganciclovir and valganciclovir

a. Ganciclovir and valganciclovir are nucleoside analogues of guanosine.
b. The drugs are approved to treat cytomegalovirus (CMV) disease and CMV retinitis and to prevent CMV disease in patients who receive organ transplants.
c. Valganciclovir is the prodrug of ganciclovir, is administered orally, and is metabolized to ganciclovir.
d. Ganciclovir's mechanism of action is similar to that of acyclovir.
   (1) The drug is preferentially phosphorylated by CMV-encoded protein kinase (UL 97), further phosphorylated by cellular kinases to produce ganciclovir triphosphate that inhibits viral DNA synthesis by inhibiting viral DNA polymerase and by incorporation into viral DNA leading to chain termination.
   (2) Resistance to ganciclovir is due to mutation of the viral protein kinase (UL 97) and, less frequently, mutation of the viral DNA polymerase.

3. Nonnucleoside analogue inhibitor of herpesvirus family: foscarnet

a. Foscarnet (phosphonoformic acid) is not a nucleoside or nucleotide analogue.
b. It does not require intracellular metabolism for activation.
c. It is a pyrophosphate analogue that binds directly to the pyrophosphate binding site of DNA polymerase to inhibit viral DNA polymerase.
d. It has a broad spectrum of activity against herpesviruses. It also has activity against HIV.
e. It is used in the treatment of HSV and VZV resistant to acyclovir and CMV resistant to ganciclovir.

4. Nucleotide analogue inhibitor of CMV: cidofovir

a. Cidofovir is an acyclic phosphonate nucleotide analogue of deoxycytidine monophosphate.
b. It does not require viral kinases to be converted to an active form.
c. It is converted by cellular kinases to its active diphosphorylated form, which acts as a competitive inhibitor of viral DNA polymerase.

d. It is used for treatment of CMV retinitis in patients with HIV and AIDS and has also been used for treatment of acyclovir- and foscarnet-resistant HSV or CMV infections.

e. Cidofovir has activity against a wide range of DNA viruses.

(1) It may have efficacy in the topical treatment of human papillomavirus infections, the treatment of JC polyomavirus-induced progressive multifocal leukoencephalopathy in patients with HIV and AIDS, and the topical treatment of immunocompromised patients with molluscum contagiosum.

(2) It may have use in human smallpox infection.

5. Antisense oligonucleotide inhibitor of CMV: fomivirsen

a. Fomivirsen is an antisense oligonucleotide that binds to CMV mRNA, inducing its degradation and preventing synthesis of essential CMV proteins.

b. It is highly specific against CMV.

c. It is approved for the intraocular treatment of CMV retinitis.

6. Nucleoside analogue RT inhibitors of retroviruses: zidovudine, didanosine, zalcitabine, lamivudine, stavudine

a. Zidovudine (azidothymidine) is a nucleoside analogue of thymidine that is phosphorylated by cellular kinases, acts as a competitive inhibitor of RT, and is incorporated into growing DNA chains resulting in chain termination.

(1) It is used to treat HIV infections in adults, usually in combination with other antiretroviral agents.

(2) It is used as monotherapy for prevention of maternal-fetal transmission of HIV and is given to pregnant HIV-positive women and neonates born to HIV-positive women.

(3) Zidovudine resistance is caused by mutations in the HIV RT gene.

b. Didanosine (dideoxyinosine; ddI) and zalcitabine (dideoxycytidine; ddC) are nucleoside analogues of deoxyadenosine (dATP) and deoxycytidine (dCTP), respectively.

(1) Both drugs are converted intracellularly by cellular kinases to dATP and dCTP, respectively, which competitively inhibit HIV RT and act as chain terminators of viral DNA synthesis.

(2) They are used to treat HIV infections in combination with other antiretroviral drugs.

c. Lamivudine (3TC) and stavudine (d4T) are nucleoside analogues of cytidine and thymidine, respectively, and act as competitive inhibitors of HIV RT and chain terminators of viral DNA synthesis.

(1) They are used to treat HIV infections in combination with other antiretroviral drugs.

(2) Lamivudine is also used to treat hepatitis B virus, which uses RT to convert RNA copies of its genome into DNA.

7. Nonnucleoside RT inhibitors of retroviruses: nevirapine, delavirdine, efavirenz

a. These drugs bind to specific sites on HIV RT that are different from the substrate-binding site.

b. They are used to treat HIV infections in combination with other antiretroviral drugs.

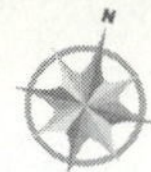

8. **Inhibitors of other viruses: ribavirin**
   a. Ribavirin is a nucleoside analogue of guanosine, phosphorylated by cellular enzymes to the triphosphate form (RTP), which is incorporated into newly synthesized viral genomes by viral RNA-dependent RNA polymerase.
   b. It exerts its antiviral effect by lethally mutating the viral RNA genome.
   c. In an alternate mechanism, ribavirin acts by inhibiting the biosynthesis of guanosine triphosphate, resulting in depleted cellular guanosine triphosphate pools required for viral transcription and replication.
   d. Aerosolized ribavirin is used to treat hospitalized infants and young children with severe lower respiratory tract disease caused by respiratory syncytial virus, but its use is controversial.
   e. In combination with IFN-alpha, ribavarin is used to treat chronic hepatitis C infection.
   f. It has been used to treat hemorrhagic fever viruses (eg, Lassa fever virus).

F. Antiviral Therapies That Inhibit Viral Protein Processing and Assembly and Viral Protein Synthesis

1. **Protease inhibitors of retroviruses: indinavir, ritonavir, saquinavir, nelfinavir, amprenavir**
   a. HIV-1–encoded protease functions to cleave precursor retroviral structural proteins necessary for correct assembly and production of infectious virus.
   b. Protease inhibitors bind to the active site of HIV-1 protease to inhibit its action.
   c. A combination of protease inhibitors plus nucleoside and nonnucleoside analogue RT inhibitors is the standard therapy for HIV-1 infection.
2. **IFNs:** IFNs are host cell proteins with significant antiviral and immunomodulatory effects.
   a. The 2 major types of human IFN are IFN-alpha and IFN-beta.
   b. Antiviral activity induced by IFN results in the generation of at least 2 types of enzymatic activity (a PKR and 2′-5′-oligo A synthetase) that inhibit viral protein synthesis.
   c. The mechanism of IFN-induced antiviral activity is described in Section VII.E.2.
   d. Recombinant IFN-alpha-2b is used to treat chronic hepatitis B virus infection.
   e. Recombinant IFN-alpha-2b in combination with ribavirin is used to treat chronic hepatitis C infection.

G. Antiviral Drugs That Inhibit Virus Release

1. **Neuraminidase inhibitors** (**zanamivir** and **oseltamivir**) are selective inhibitors of influenza virus neuraminidase.
2. Neuraminidase inhibitors are sialic acid analogues that block the active site of the viral neuraminidase responsible for cleaving sialic acid on the cell surface and releasing the virus.
3. They are active against both influenza A and B viruses.
4. These drugs block release of influenza virus from infected cells and reduce virus spread to adjacent cells.
5. Zanamivir and oseltamivir are used for treatment of influenza A and B virus infections.

ANTIRETROVIRAL DRUG RESISTANCE

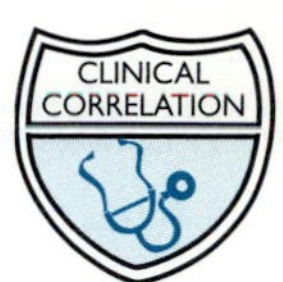

- *The success of current HIV-1 therapy is limited by the emergence of drug-resistant mutants.*
- *This antiviral drug resistance stems from the error-prone HIV-1 RT that permits the virus to mutate rapidly.*
- *Highly active antiretroviral therapy that uses 3 or more drugs directed against 2 targets, RT and protease, is aimed to keep resistance at bay.*

CLINICAL PROBLEMS

1. Negative-strand (–) RNA viruses transcribe functional mRNA by using:

A. RNA-dependent RNA polymerase

B. RNA-dependent DNA polymerase

C. DNA-dependent RNA polymerase

D. DNA-dependent DNA polymerase

2. HIV-1 with a deletion mutation in the protease gene would be blocked in which step of virus replication?

A. Attachment

B. Entry

C. Genome expression and replication

D. Assembly

E. Release

3. Acute infection followed by a quiescent phase in which the cell survives, no infectious virus is detectable, and then repeated episodes of virus reactivation occur best describes:

A. Lytic infection

B. Abortive infection

C. Chronic infection

D. Latent infection

E. Transforming infection

4. Resistance to the antiviral drug acyclovir is due to a mutation in the gene for:

A. RT

B. Protease

C. TK

D. RNA polymerase

E. Neuraminidase

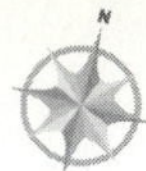

5. A major cellular determinant of virus tropism is the presence of:
   A. The complement system
   B. Cell surface receptors
   C. The cell lipid bilayer
   D. Viral attachment protein
   E. Hemagglutinin

ANSWERS

1. The answer is A. (–) RNA viruses express their genome by using virion-associated, RNA-dependent RNA polymerase to synthesize viral mRNA. Choices B and D are incorrect because the polymerase synthesizes DNA, not mRNA. Choice C is the mechanism used by DNA viruses and retroviruses (but not [–] RNA viruses) to synthesize viral mRNA.

2. The answer is D. A functional HIV-1 protease is required to cleave precursor proteins necessary for proper virion assembly. The other steps in the virus replication cycle are unaffected by the protease gene mutation.

3. The answer is D. Latent infections are typical of the herpesviruses. Lytic infections result in cell death and infectious virus production. Abortive infections result in neither cell death nor virus production. Chronic infections are characterized by cell survival and continuous production of progeny viruses. Transforming infections result in acquisition of the tumor cell phenotype.

4. The answer is C. Acyclovir is selectively phosphorylated by viral encoded TK. TK mutants do not phosphorylate and activate acyclovir. None of the other choices activate acyclovir.

5. The answer is B. Cell surface receptors are the major determinant of cell susceptibility to virus infection. The complement system is part of the host innate defense mechanism against virus infections. The cell lipid bilayer is present in all cells and does not dictate virus tropism. Viral attachment proteins and hemagglutinin are viral, not cellular determinants of virus tropism.

CHAPTER 11
DNA VIRUSES

I. Key Concepts

A. Most DNA viruses contain double-stranded (ds) DNA genomes; the one human virus exception is the Parvoviridae family, whose members have a single-stranded DNA genome.

B. All DNA viruses, except poxviruses, have icosahedral nucleocapsid symmetry; poxviruses have complex symmetry.

C. Medically important DNA viruses comprise 7 virus families (Parvoviridae, Polyomaviridae, Papillomaviridae, Adenoviridae, Herpesviridae, Poxviridae, and Hepadnaviridae) and share similar properties of nucleic acid composition, shape, and site of replication (Table 11–1).

II. Parvoviridae Family

A. Parvoviruses

1. Parvoviruses (*parvo* = small) are very small, icosahedral viruses lacking an envelope and contain linear single-stranded DNA.
2. Parvovirus DNA replication occurs in the nucleus of actively dividing cells.
3. Two genera in the Parvoviridae family, *Dependovirus* and *Erythrovirus,* infect humans.
4. Members of the *Dependovirus* genus include adeno-associated viruses (AAVs), which require helper adenovirus for replication.
5. AAVs have not been associated with any human disease but are being evaluated as vectors for gene therapy because they can integrate into chromosomal DNA.

B. Parvovirus B19

1. Human parvovirus B19 replicates autonomously and is the only known human pathogen in the *Erythrovirus* genus.
2. **Clinical manifestations:** B19 causes **erythema infectiosum,** or fifth disease, a childhood rash characterized by a generalized erythema and a rash of the face, giving a "slapped-cheek" appearance.
   a. A prodromal period with a mild systemic illness is followed by the characteristic rash that usually appears a week or 2 later and then resolves over the course of a few weeks.
   b. B19 infection of erythroid precursors in patients with hemolytic anemia or sickle cell disease can lead to suppression of erythropoiesis and **aplastic crisis.**

 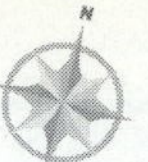

Table 11–1. Properties of DNA viruses.

Virus Family	DNA Structure	Shape	Envelope	Virion Polymerase	Site of Replication	Human Viruses
Parvoviridae	Linear ss	Icosahedral	No	No	Nucleus	B19 virus
Polyomaviridae	Circular ds	Icosahedral	No	No	Nucleus	JC & BK viruses
Papillomaviridae	Circular ds	Icosahedral	No	No	Nucleus	Papillomavirus
Adenoviridae	Linear ds	Icosahedral	No	No	Nucleus	Adenovirus
Herpesviridae	Linear ds	Icosahedral	Yes	No	Nucleus	HSV, CMV, EBV, VZV
Poxviridae	Linear ds	Complex	Yes	Yes	Cytoplasm	Smallpox, MCV
Hepadnaviridae	Circular, partially ds	Icosahedral	Yes	Yes	Nucleus	Hepatitis B virus

HSV, herpes simplex virus; CMV, cytomegalovirus; EBV, Epstein-Barr virus; VZV, varicella-zoster virus, MCV, molluscum contagiosum virus.

   c. B19 infection of pregnant women can lead to fetal anemia and death or a generalized fetal anemia and congestive heart failure called **hydrops fetalis.**
   d. B19 infection in immunodeficient patients can result in persistent anemia.
3. **Transmission/epidemiology:** B19 virus is transmitted by the **respiratory route** with high transmission rates among household members.
   a. B19 is also transmitted **transplacentally** from infected mother to fetus.
   b. B19 infections occur worldwide with seroconversion rates of 75–90% in persons over 50 years of age.
4. **Pathogenesis:** B19 virus initiates infection in the respiratory tract followed by viremia about a week after infection.
   a. B19 infects erythroid precursors in bone marrow, replicating preferentially in proliferating hematopoietic cells.
   b. B19 is cytolytic to immature erythroid cells, resulting in suppression of erythropoiesis and anemia.
   c. In immunocompetent persons, recovery is associated with an antibody response that clears the virus and confers long-term protection.
5. **Virulence factors:** No virulence factors have been identified.
6. **Laboratory diagnosis:** B19 virus infection is diagnosed by the detection of B19-specific IgM antibody or polymerase chain reaction (PCR) detection of viral DNA.

7. **Treatment:** There is no specific antiviral therapy for B19 virus. Immunodeficient patients in whom a chronic B19 infection develops are treated with intravenous immune globulin.
8. **Prevention:** There is no vaccine to prevent B19 virus infection.

III. Polyomaviridae Family

A. Polyomaviruses

1. Polyomaviruses (*poly* = many, *omas* = tumors), so named because they cause numerous tumors in mice, are icosahedral, nonenveloped viruses that contain circular ds DNA and replicate in the nucleus.
2. Polyomaviruses cause oncogenic transformation in cell cultures and tumors in laboratory animals.
3. Some polyomaviruses have been associated with human tumors, but their precise role remains controversial.
4. BK and JC viruses (BKV and JCV) are polyomaviruses that infect humans.

B. BK and JC Viruses

1. **Clinical manifestations:** JCV causes **progressive multifocal leukoencephalopathy (PML),** a demyelinating disease of the brain, in immunocompromised patients.
   a. PML is an AIDS-defining illness.
   b. BKV causes kidney/urinary tract infections and **hemorrhagic cystitis,** especially in immunocompromised patients.
   c. Most infections with JCV or BKV are subclinical.
2. **Transmission/epidemiology:** JCV and BKV are transmitted by **respiratory droplets.** The viruses are ubiquitous, with 70–80% of adults demonstrating antibody to them.
3. **Pathogenesis:** JCV and BKV initiate infection in the respiratory tract and spread by viremia to localize in the kidney as a latent asymptomatic infection. They are opportunistic viruses reactivated in immunodeficient patients to cause kidney/urinary tract infections (BKV) and central nervous system infection of oligodendrocytes and PML (JCV).
4. **Virulence factors:** BKV and JCV have the capacity to establish latent infections and reactivate in the immunodeficient host.
5. **Laboratory diagnosis:** BKV and JCV are detected by PCR or in situ DNA hybridization.
6. **Treatment:** There is no specific antiviral therapy for BKV or JCV.
7. **Prevention:** There are no vaccines to prevent BKV or JCV infection.

IV. Papillomaviridae Family

A. Papillomaviruses

1. Papillomaviruses are icosahedral, nonenveloped viruses that contain circular ds DNA and that replicate in the nucleus.
2. Papillomaviruses cause papillomas (ie, benign growths often called warts) in various mammalian species and are species specific.
3. Papillomaviruses are epitheliotropic, and different types induce hyperplastic epithelial lesions of the skin and mucous membranes.

B. Human Papillomavirus

1. **Clinical manifestations:** Human papillomavirus (HPV) causes **common warts** on the hands and feet (HPV types 1, 2, and 4), and **anogenital warts** (**condyloma acuminata**) are associated with HPV types 6 and 11.
   a. Genital HPV (types 6 and 11) is the cause of **laryngeal papillomas** in children infected in the birth canal of a mother with genital warts.
   b. **Epidermodysplasia verruciformis (EV),** a rare skin condition in patients with cell-mediated immune deficiency, is characterized by widespread, chronic cutaneous HPV lesions.
   c. Patients with EV and skin warts associated with specific HPV types may progress to skin carcinomas after many years of exposure to sunlight.
   d. HPV types 16 and 18 are oncogenic and strongly associated with **anogenital cancer** and some sites of **head and neck cancer.**
   e. Most HPV infections are clinically unapparent.
2. **Transmission/epidemiology:** HPV is transmitted by direct physical contact with an infected individual or indirectly by contact with fomites on which the virus has been deposited.
   a. Direct skin-to-skin contact transmits cutaneous HPV infections.
   b. Anogenital HPV infections are transmitted **sexually.**
   c. HPV is second only to chlamydia infection as the most commonly acquired sexually transmitted disease.
   d. HPV infections are common, with cervical HPV detected in 10–40% of sexually active females. Most infections are transitory.
   e. Risk factors for HPV infection include multiple sex partners, a history of sexually transmitted diseases, and the age at first intercourse.
   f. More than 100 different genotypes of HPV have been identified based on DNA sequencing of their cloned genomes.
   g. Genital HPV types are classified as **low-risk** and **high-risk oncogenic types** and have distinctive properties (Table 11–2).
      (1) High-risk oncogenic HPV types (HPV 16 and 18) are closely linked with cervical cancer.
         (a) Cervical cancer is the second most common cancer in women.
         (b) HPV DNA is detected in over 99% of cervical cancer cases.
      (2) Low-risk oncogenic types (HPV 6 and 11) are the cause of benign genital warts.
3. **Pathogenesis:** HPV targets basal epithelial cells and gains entry through cracks in the skin or tears or lacerations in mucosal surfaces during sexual intercourse.
   a. The infection remains localized and may resolve spontaneously, remain latent, or (depending on the HPV type) progress to dysplasia and carcinoma.
   b. HPV replication and virus production are tied to squamous epithelial cell differentiation.
   c. HPV DNA replicates in synchrony with basal stem cell DNA, but no capsid proteins are produced.
   d. As the epithelial cells mature as part of the differentiation program, they become permissive for viral reproduction, resulting in capsid protein synthesis, virion assembly, and viral particle production in the terminally differentiated cells.
   e. HPV encodes two proteins, E6 and E7, that inactivate tumor suppressor proteins p53 and Rb, respectively, and stimulate cell proliferation.

Table 11–2. Comparison of low-risk and high-risk human papillomavirus (HPV) types.

Property	HPV-6 & 11	HPV-16 & 18
Clinical association	Benign wart	Cervical cancer
Risk of malignant progression	Low	High
Immortalization of keratinocytes in vitro	No	Yes
Integration into cellular DNA	No	Yes
Affinity of E7 protein to bind Rb tumor suppressor protein	Low	High
E6 protein binds to & degrades tumor suppressor protein p53	No	Yes

f. High-risk HPV types integrate into cellular DNA, leaving the E6 and E7 genes intact, thus allowing continuous and increased expression of E6 and E7 proteins that facilitate cell cycle dysregulation and the evolution of the malignant tumor cell phenotype.
g. HPV infections are eradicated and controlled by cell-mediated immunity.

4. **Virulence factors:** HPV has the capacity to establish latent infections. High-risk HPV types integrate into chromosomal DNA.
5. **Laboratory diagnosis:** Cervical cytology in the form of the Papanicolaou (Pap) smear is the gold standard in cervical cancer diagnosis.
   a. The Pap smear detects cellular atypia and a characteristic perinuclear clearing known as koilocytosis, a hallmark of cervical HPV infection; however, the test has a high rate of false-negatives.
   b. HPV cannot be isolated in cell culture.
   c. Detection of HPV is based on molecular techniques using PCR to detect viral DNA or by in situ or liquid hybridization using HPV type-specific probes.
6. **Treatment:** Warts are treated surgically (cryotherapy, laser therapy) or with topical chemical agents (podophyllin, trichloroacetic acid) to remove the wart, but these methods do not remove adjacent HPV-infected tissue, and recurrences are common.
   a. Intralesional injection of interferon-alpha has shown some efficacy in the treatment of genital warts.
   b. Imiquimod, an inducer of interferon and other cytokines, is used for the topical treatment of genital warts and skin warts.
   c. The antiviral drug cidofovir has shown some efficacy in the treatment of genital warts and laryngeal papillomatosis.
7. **Prevention:** No vaccine is available for HPV. Prophylactic and therapeutic HPV vaccines are in development.

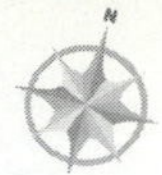

CERVICAL CANCER AS A SEXUALLY TRANSMITTED DISEASE

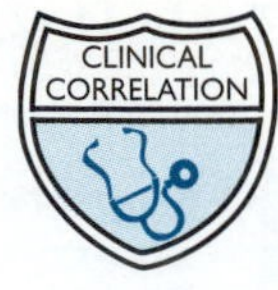

- *The link between HPV infection and cervical cancer is overwhelming.*
  —Cervical cancer is the second most common cancer and one of the leading causes of cancer-related death in women.
  —It is estimated that 25 million Americans are infected with HPV.
  —These epidemiologic data emphasize the need to develop vaccination strategies for HPV.
- *Two types of HPV vaccine trials are under way.*
  —One is a prophylactic vaccine aimed to prevent HPV infection and subsequent HPV-associated disease.
  —The other is a therapeutic vaccine aimed to induce regression of precursor lesions or remission of advanced cervical cancer.

V. Adenoviridae Family

A. Adenoviruses

1. Adenoviruses are icosahedral, nonenveloped viruses that contain linear ds DNA and that replicate in the nucleus.
2. Adenoviruses were originally isolated from the adenoids, from which the name is derived.
3. There are about 50 different human adenovirus serotypes that are species specific and that share a common group-specific antigen.
4. Certain human adenovirus types are oncogenic in rodent hosts, but there is no evidence that adenoviruses are associated with tumors in humans.

B. Adenovirus

1. **Clinical manifestations:** Adenovirus types 1–7 cause upper respiratory tract illness such as the common cold, **pharyngitis,** and tonsillitis in infants and young children, characterized by coryza, fever, cough, and lymphadenopathy.
   a. Adenoviruses cause approximately 20% of childhood **pneumonias** characterized by bronchitis and bronchiolitis.
   b. Adenovirus types 4 and 7 cause epidemics, primarily in military recruits, of **acute respiratory disease (ARD),** characterized by pharyngitis, cough, fever, and malaise.
   c. Certain adenoviruses are associated with eye infections.
      (1) **Pharyngoconjunctival fever** is caused by adenovirus types 3 and 7, occurs primarily in children, and is characterized by fever, pharyngitis, conjunctivitis, and cervical adenopathy.
      (2) **Keratoconjunctivitis** is associated with adenovirus types 8, 19, and 37, and usually occurs in adults.
   d. Enteric adenovirus types 40 and 41 are second only to rotaviruses as the cause of **acute gastroenteritis** in infants and young children.
   e. Adenovirus type 11 causes hemorrhagic cystitis, which is characterized by fever and hematuria.
2. **Transmission/epidemiology:** Depending on the syndrome, adenoviruses are transmitted by the **respiratory route,** by the **fecal-oral route,** or through **direct inoculation** of the eyes by fingers. Adenovirus infections are endemic worldwide and are more prevalent in young children.
3. **Pathogenesis:** Adenoviruses infect epithelial cells of the respiratory tract and intestinal tract and cause direct cytotoxic damage.
   a. The virus may spread to involve lymphoid tissues and can persist as a latent infection in tonsils and adenoids.

   b. Adenoviral infections are cleared by cell-mediated immunity, and type-specific, serum-neutralizing antibody provides long-term protection.
4. **Virulence factors:** Adenoviruses have the capacity to establish latent infections.
   a. Adenoviruses encode a protein, E3-19K, that combines with MHC class I molecules and prevents antigen presentation and recognition of infected cells by cytotoxic T lymphocytes.
   b. Adenoviruses encode a specific RNA that interferes with the antiviral action of interferon.
5. **Laboratory diagnosis:** Adenovirus infections can be diagnosed by virus isolation and detection in cell culture, antigen detection, PCR, and serology.
6. **Treatment:** There is no specific antiviral therapy for adenovirus.
7. **Prevention:** There is no vaccine available for adenovirus.
   a. A vaccine developed for the prevention of adenovirus type 4– and 7–associated ARD in military recruits is no longer produced commercially.
   b. Handwashing and good infection-control practices are effective in preventing adenovirus infections.

ENTERIC ADENOVIRUSES

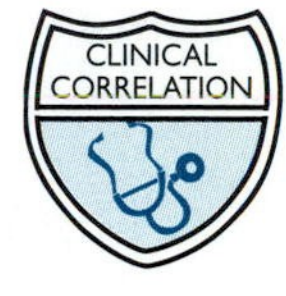

- *Enteric adenovirus serotypes 40 and 41 account for up to 15% of the cases of watery, nonbloody infantile diarrhea.*
- *Most enteric adenovirus infections are asymptomatic.*
- *When symptomatic, adenovirus diarrhea is clinically indistinguishable from diarrhea induced by other viruses.*
- *Relative to rotavirus diarrhea, the adenovirus incubation period of infection is longer, and adenovirus diarrhea is more prolonged.*

VI. Herpesviridae Family

A. Herpesviruses

1. Herpesviruses are icosahedral, enveloped viruses that contain linear ds DNA and that replicate in the nucleus.
2. Herpesviruses have the ability to establish a **latent infection** that persists for life after primary infection and that can be **reactivated** at a later time.
3. In the latent phase, viral DNA is maintained as an episome (not integrated) in the cell nucleus with restricted transcription of viral genes required for the maintenance of latency.
4. Reactivation of latent virus can be triggered by a variety of factors that result in production of progeny virus in permissive cells.
5. The 8 medically important members of the Herpesviridae family are divided into 3 subfamilies.
   a. Alphaherpesvirinae (or alphaherpesviruses) include herpes simplex types 1 and 2 (HSV-1 and HSV-2) and varicella-zoster virus (VZV).
   b. Betaherpesvirinae (or betaherpesviruses) include cytomegalovirus (CMV) and human herpesvirus types 6 and 7 (HHV-6 and HHV-7).
   c. Gammaherpesvirinae (or gammaherpesviruses) include Epstein-Barr virus (EBV) and Kaposi sarcoma herpesvirus (KSHV), also called human herpesvirus type 8 (HHV-8).

 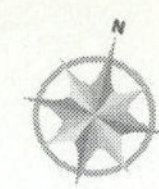

B. Herpes Simplex Types 1 and 2 (a.k.a. Human Herpesvirus Types 1 and 2)

1. **Clinical manifestations:** Most HSV-1 and HSV-2 infections are asymptomatic.
   a. Primary infections by HSV-1 are generally in the facial area, whereas HSV-2 infects the genital area, but there is considerable clinical overlap.
   b. Primary infection by HSV-1 causes **gingivostomatitis,** which is characterized by painful vesicular and ulcerative lesions in the facial area and oral mucosa accompanied by fever, sore throat, localized lymphadenopathy, and malaise lasting 1–2 weeks.
   c. HSV-1 infection of the eye causes **herpetic keratoconjunctivitis,** the second leading cause of corneal blindness in the United States.
   d. HSV-1 or HSV-2 infection of the fingers, termed **herpetic whitlow,** is caused by inoculation of infected secretions through small cuts in the skin.
   e. Primary infection by HSV-2 causes **herpes genitalis,** characterized by painful vesicular and ulcerative lesions of the penis, cervix, vulva, vagina, or perineum and accompanied by fever, dysuria, localized lymphadenopathy, and malaise lasting 1–2 weeks.
   f. **Herpes encephalitis** is a rare complication of HSV-1 infection in adults and HSV-2 infection in neonates, and is associated with a high fatality rate.
   g. **Herpes meningitis** is a complication of HSV-2 herpes genitalis.
   h. HSV-1 or HSV-2 primary infection is followed by latent infection of the **trigeminal ganglia** in the case of herpetic gingivostomatitis and the **sacral or lumbar ganglia** in the case of herpes genitalis.
   i. Reactivation of latent HSV infections results in recurrent disease, with the eruption of vesicles containing infectious virus in the same region as the primary infection, such as around the lips (fever blisters, cold sores), or the eruption of genital vesicular lesions.
2. **Transmission/epidemiology:** HSV-1 and HSV-2 are transmitted by direct contact with virus-containing secretions and body fluids, such as saliva and genital secretions during sexual contact.
   a. Neonatal HSV infections are transmitted from the infected maternal genital secretions to the newborn during delivery.
   b. HSV infections occur worldwide, and there is no animal reservoir.
   c. Seroepidemiologic surveys indicate that 80% of the US population have antibodies to HSV-1 and HSV-2 by age 50.
   d. More than 1 in 5 Americans are infected with genital herpes.
   e. Infected individuals can shed infectious virus in the absence of clinical symptoms.
3. **Pathogenesis:** HSV-1 and HSV-2 cause a localized, lytic infection of mucosal epithelial cells.
   a. The virus spreads to innervating neurons and is transported to dorsal root ganglia, where latency is established.
   b. Reactivation of latency is triggered by external factors (eg, fever, sunlight, stress, immune suppression) that induce the virus to travel down the axon with infection of epithelial cells innervated by the sensory nerve, resulting in recurrent vesicular lesions.
   c. HSV infections are controlled by cytotoxic T lymphocytes. Immunosuppressed individuals exhibit disseminated disease.

4. **Virulence factors:** HSV evades the immune system by establishing a latent infection in neurons. HSV-encoded protein (ICP47) downregulates MHC class I antigen presentation and cytotoxic T-cell recognition.
5. **Laboratory diagnosis:** HSV can be detected by the demonstration of multinucleated giant cells in a Tzanck smear of cells from vesicular fluid.
   a. HSV-1 or HSV-2 can be detected by cell culture cytopathic effects and identified by HSV type-specific fluorescent antibody staining.
   b. PCR of HSV DNA in cerebrospinal fluid is used to diagnose patients with HSV encephalitis.
6. **Treatment:** HSV infections are treated with acyclovir or the acyclovir prodrugs valacyclovir and famciclovir. Acyclovir-resistant HSV infections are treated with foscarnet.
7. **Prevention:** There is no vaccine to prevent HSV infection. Barrier contraceptives and safe sex are important preventive measures.

GENITAL HERPES

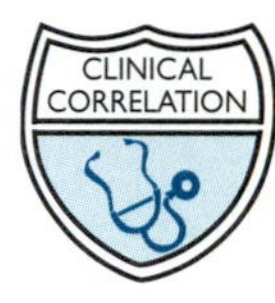

- *Genital herpes is one of the most common sexually transmitted diseases in the United States and is increasing in prevalence.*
- *It has a high morbidity in adults and can cause potentially fatal encephalitis in infants whose mothers are shedding the virus during vaginal delivery.*
- *Genital HSV infections can facilitate the spread of HIV and AIDS by allowing HIV access to dendritic cells, macrophages, and lymphocytes in the herpes lesion.*

C. Varicella-Zoster Virus (a.k.a. Human Herpesvirus Type 3)

1. **Clinical manifestations:** Primary infection by VZV causes **varicella (chickenpox),** usually in childhood, which reactivates as **zoster (shingles),** usually in adults.
   a. Primary infection by VZV has an incubation period of 10–21 days followed by a prodrome consisting of fever and malaise and then a generalized vesicular rash that progresses to pustules and scabs (chickenpox) lasting 5–7 days.
   b. Varicella-chickenpox lesions generally begin on the head and face and progress to the trunk and extremities.
   c. Reactivation of latent VZV results in herpes zoster or shingles and is characterized by unilateral, localized, painful, vesicular lesions in skin along a dermatome innervated by a particular sensory ganglion.
   d. Maternal infection with VZV during pregnancy can cause congenital varicella syndrome characterized by birth defects.
   e. Complications of varicella include bacterial superinfections of skin lesions, varicella pneumonia, varicella encephalitis, and disseminated varicella, most commonly in immunosuppressed patients.
   f. **Postherpetic neuralgia,** a debilitating pain in the dermatome, is a common complication of herpes zoster that may persist for months to years.
   g. Disseminated varicella may occur in immunosuppressed zoster patients.
2. **Transmission/epidemiology:** VZV is transmitted by **respiratory droplets.**
   a. Vesicular lesions of zoster contain infectious VZV that can be transmitted via the respiratory route to cause a primary varicella-chickenpox infection.
   b. VZV infections occur worldwide and are highly contagious.
   c. Herpes zoster occurs only in individuals who had a previous primary varicella-chickenpox infection.

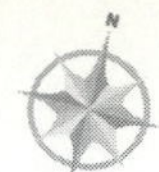

3. **Pathogenesis:** VZV initially infects respiratory epithelial cells, spreads to and multiplies in lymph nodes, enters the bloodstream and spreads to the liver and spleen, and then is disseminated back to the respiratory tract and skin, where the vesicular rash occurs.
   a. VZV spreads to innervating neurons and is transported to dorsal root ganglia to establish the latent state.
   b. Reactivation of latency can be triggered by increasing age, immunocompromise due to cancer, AIDS, or immunosuppressive therapy for organ transplantation or cancer.
   c. Reactivation results in virus travel down the axon with recurrent infection of epithelial cells innervated by the sensory nerve and resultant vesicular lesions on skin, usually involving a dermatome (shingles).
   d. Humoral immunity is important in preventing respiratory infection, and cell-mediated immunity is paramount for clearing primary and recurrent VZV infections.
4. **Virulence factors:** VZV evades the immune system by establishing a latent infection in neurons.
5. **Laboratory diagnosis:** Varicella or zoster is usually diagnosed clinically based on the appearance and distribution of vesicular lesions.
   a. Multinucleated giant cells detected cytologically in scrapings of lesions by the Tzanck test are characteristic of herpesvirus infection but not specific for VZV.
   b. VZV can be detected by isolation in cell culture and identified with VZV-specific fluorescent antibody staining.
6. **Treatment:** Acyclovir or the prodrugs valacyclovir and famciclovir are used to treat varicella and zoster, particularly in immunosuppressed patients. VZV infections resistant to acyclovir are treated with foscarnet.
7. **Prevention:** A live, attenuated VZV vaccine is effective in preventing varicella and is recommended for vaccination of healthy children after 1 year of age and susceptible adults.
   a. Passive administration of varicella-zoster immune globulin (VZIG) is used to prevent disease in immunocompromised patients exposed to VZV.
   b. Isolation of hospitalized patients is critical to prevention of nosocomial spread.
   c. The live, attenuated varicella vaccine is highly effective in preventing chickenpox and induces long-term protective immunity.
   d. Ninety percent of immunized, healthy children are protected after only one dose of vaccine.
   e. Transmission of the vaccine strain to susceptible contacts is rare and much less common than the transmission rate after exposure to wild-type VZV.

D. Cytomegalovirus (a.k.a. Human Herpesvirus Type 5)

1. **Clinical manifestations:** Most primary infections by CMV are clinically unapparent.
   a. CMV causes a **mononucleosislike syndrome** in older children and adults characterized by persistent fever, pharyngitis, fatigue, malaise, and lymphadenopathy that is clinically similar to EBV mononucleosis.
   b. CMV is the common cause of **pneumonia** in immunosuppressed patients who have received organ transplants.

c. CMV is a common opportunistic pathogen in patients with HIV or AIDS and can cause retinitis, encephalitis, and colitis.

d. **Congenital infection** by CMV causes **cytomegalic inclusion disease,** with severity ranging from relatively mild disease in seropositive mothers to severe disease in seronegative mothers that is characterized by hepatosplenomegaly, jaundice, petechiae, microcephaly, growth retardation, and neurologic complications such as deafness, chorioretinitis, and mental retardation.

2. **Transmission/epidemiology:** CMV is transmitted by direct contact with bodily fluids such as saliva, urine, semen, cervical secretions, breast milk, and blood.
   a. CMV has a worldwide distribution and is acquired in early childhood, with approximately 70–90% of adults seropositive for CMV depending on socioeconomic status.
   b. It is frequently shed in saliva, urine, semen, and cervical secretions from asymptomatic individuals.
   c. It is transmitted efficiently in daycare centers from a child excreting CMV to other children and, in turn, to seronegative parents.
   d. Latent CMV infection of leukocytes accounts for blood transfusion–associated and organ transplant transmission of CMV.
3. **Pathogenesis:** CMV initiates infection in the oropharynx and usually causes a subclinical, asymptomatic infection.
   a. The virus spreads locally to lymphoid tissues—replicating in monocytes, macrophages, and endothelial cells—and produces a viremia.
   b. Viremia disseminates CMV systemically to involve multiple organs (liver, spleen, kidney, lungs).
   c. CMV remains latent in mononuclear cells and is reactivated in immunosuppressed patients.
   d. Congenital infection derived from a maternal primary CMV infection or a reactivated infection results in cytomegalic inclusion disease, which is characterized by multiorgan involvement and congenital abnormalities.
   e. CMV infections are controlled by cell-mediated immunity.
   f. Disseminated CMV disease occurs in immunosuppressed patients.
4. **Virulence factors:** CMV evades host immune defense by establishing a latent infection in mononuclear cells. CMV-encoded protein downregulates MHC class I expression and cytotoxic T-cell recognition.
5. **Laboratory diagnosis:** CMV can be isolated by cytopathic effects in cell culture and identified by CMV-specific fluorescent antibody staining of infected cells.
   a. Rapid diagnosis of CMV infection is accomplished by detection of CMV early antigens before cytopathic effects occur by immunocytochemical staining of infected cells in culture.
   b. CMV can be detected in body fluids by PCR.
6. **Treatment:** Ganciclovir and the prodrug valganciclovir are the antiviral drugs of choice for treatment of CMV infection.
   a. Foscarnet is used to treat CMV infections resistant to ganciclovir.
   b. Cidofovir is used to treat CMV retinitis in patients with HIV and AIDS and those with foscarnet-resistant CMV infections.
   c. Fomivirsen, an antisense oligonucleotide inhibitor, is used for the specific treatment of CMV retinitis.

 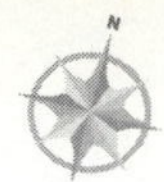

7. **Prevention:** There is no vaccine available to prevent CMV infections. Barrier contraception and safe sex practices are important preventive measures.

E. Human Herpesvirus Types 6 and 7

1. **Clinical manifestations:** Primary infection by HHV-6 or HHV-7 causes **exanthem subitum (roseola)** in children and is characterized by high fever for 2–5 days, followed by a generalized, maculopapular rash.
   - a. More severe forms of HHV-6 or HHV-7 infection with or without rash can result in febrile seizures.
   - b. HHV-6 infections in adults are uncommon but can cause severe disease characterized by a mononucleosislike syndrome, protracted lymphadenopathy, and fulminant hepatitis.
   - c. Reactivation of latent HHV-6 or HHV-7 can occur in immunocompromised individuals such as transplant recipients and patients with AIDS, with CMV potentiating transplant rejection or pneumonitis and encephalitis.
2. **Transmission/epidemiology:** HHV-6 and HHV-7 are transmitted by **saliva.**
   - a. HHV-6 and HHV-7 account for 30% and 5–10% of the cases of roseola, respectively.
   - b. HHV-6 and HHV-7 infections are acquired in childhood, with 60–90% of adults seropositive for viral antibody.
3. **Pathogenesis:** HHV-6 and HHV-7 infect T cells infiltrating the site of infection and establish a latent infection in T lymphocytes.
   - a. HHV-6 and HHV-7 infections are controlled by cell-mediated immunity.
   - b. HHV-6 and HHV-7 are opportunistic viruses usually not associated with disease in the immunocompetent host but reactivated in patients with AIDS, transplant recipients, and others with lymphoproliferative and immunosuppressive disorders.
   - c. HHV-6 may be a cofactor in the pathogenesis of AIDS by transactivating the HIV-1 promoter and inducing CD4 expression in T lymphocytes.
4. **Virulence factors:** HHV-6 and HHV-7 have the capacity to establish latent infections in T lymphocytes.
5. **Laboratory diagnosis:** HHV-6 and HHV-7 can be detected by PCR, and serologic tests are useful to detect virus-specific IgM and IgG antibodies.
6. **Treatment:** There is no specific antiviral therapy of HHV-6 or HHV-7 infection.
7. **Prevention:** There is no vaccine for the prevention of HHV-6 or HHV-7 infection.

F. Epstein-Barr Virus (a.k.a. Human Herpesvirus Type 4)

1. **Clinical manifestations:** EBV causes **infectious mononucleosis** in young adults characterized by fever, pharyngitis, fatigue, headache, malaise, lymphadenopathy, splenomegaly, and elevated liver enzymes.
   - a. Infectious mononucleosis is usually self-limiting, with symptoms resolving in 1–2 weeks, but fatigue may persist for months.
   - b. Primary EBV infections in children are usually asymptomatic.
   - c. EBV is associated with **lymphoproliferative disorders,** particularly in posttransplant patients, often seen as a benign polyclonal B-cell proliferation or malignant lymphoma.
   - d. EBV is closely linked with **Burkitt lymphoma, nasopharyngeal carcinoma,** and **Hodgkin disease.**

2. **Transmission/epidemiology:** EBV is transmitted by **saliva.**
   a. EBV is distributed worldwide, with over 90% of adults seropositive.
   b. Burkitt lymphoma is a B-cell lymphoma of African children linked to EBV.
   c. Nasopharyngeal carcinoma is an epithelial cell malignancy endemic in southeast Asia that is linked to EBV infection and other environmental cofactors.
3. **Pathogenesis:** EBV initiates infection of oropharyngeal epithelial cells (causing pharyngitis) and spreads to infiltrating B lymphocytes by binding to the cellular complement receptor C3d, causing a latent infection that persists for life.
   a. EBV stimulates B-cell mitogenesis and immortalizes B cells.
   b. Cytotoxic T lymphocytes control B-cell infection and limit B-cell outgrowth.
   c. Latent infection and immortalization of a small proportion of B cells may result in EBV-associated tumors years later.
   d. EBV DNA and proteins are commonly found in Burkitt lymphoma and nasopharyngeal carcinoma.
4. **Virulence factors:** EBV has the capacity to cause latent infection of B lymphocytes.
   a. EBV encodes an interleukin-10 mimic that inhibits helper T-cell functions required for cytotoxic T cells.
   b. EBV evades cytotoxic T-cell recognition by EBNA1-mediated downregulation of EBV genes.
5. **Laboratory diagnosis:** EBV mononucleosis is diagnosed by the demonstration of atypical lymphocytosis (Downey cells) in a blood smear.
   a. A **heterophile antibody**–positive test result (Monospot test) is diagnostic for EBV infectious mononucleosis.
   b. EBV-specific serologic tests can be used to diagnose EBV infection.
   c. EBV DNA can be detected by PCR.
6. **Treatment:** There is no specific antiviral therapy for EBV.
7. **Prevention:** There is no vaccine to prevent EBV infection.

G. Kaposi's Sarcoma Herpesvirus (a.k.a. Human Herpesvirus Type 8)

1. **Clinical manifestations:** KSHV causes **Kaposi sarcoma (KS),** a spindle cell tumor of endothelial origin, characterized by lesions on the skin, face, or oral cavity that appear as bruised or discolored spots and that progress to ulcerated nodules, primarily in patients with AIDS.
   a. KSHV also causes **primary effusion lymphoma,** an AIDS-associated malignancy, characterized as effusions of B-cell lymphoma in body cavities, with the pleural cavity the most common site.
   b. KSHV also is the cause of **multicentric Castleman disease,** a multicentric angiofollicular B-cell lymphoproliferative disorder.
2. **Transmission/epidemiology:** KSHV is transmitted by **saliva** and **semen.**
   a. KS is the most common AIDS-associated malignancy
   b. In the United States, KS is found almost exclusively in patients with AIDS, particularly homosexual men infected with HIV.
   c. Seropositivity to HHV-8 is high (30–50%) in HIV-infected gay and bisexual men but low in HIV-infected women and noninfected men or women.

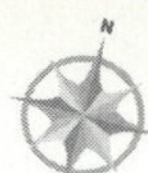

3. **Pathogenesis:** HHV-8 preferentially infects B lymphocytes and endothelial cells and establishes a latent infection in B cells.
   a. HHV-8 encodes a number of viral homologues of cell growth regulatory genes that promote angiogenesis, stimulate cell proliferation, and inhibit apoptosis.
   b. Uncontrolled expression of these HHV-8 latency genes leads to cell transformation of endothelial cells and B-cell proliferation, culminating in vascular tumors and B-cell lymphomas.
4. **Virulence factors:** HHV-8 has the capacity to establish latent infection in B lymphocytes. HHV-8 encodes many potentially oncogenic products: cellular homologues of cytokines (IL-6), cell regulatory proteins (cyclin D, bcl-2), and survival and proliferation factors (G protein–coupled receptor).
5. **Laboratory diagnosis:** HHV-8 infection is detected by PCR and hybridization with HHV-8–specific probes or by in situ immunohistochemistry or hybridization.
6. **Treatment:** There is no specific antiviral therapy for HHV-8 infection.
7. **Prevention:** There is no vaccine to prevent HHV-8 infection. Safe sex practices should reduce the risk of transmission.

KAPOSI SARCOMA

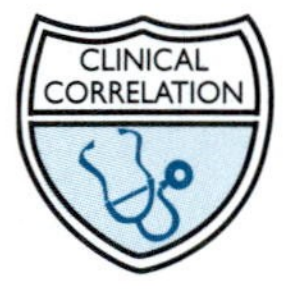

- *KS was originally described as a rare tumor in elderly men of Mediterranean descent.*
  —In the early 1980s, a cluster of KS cases was reported among homosexual men in New York City and California.
  —Thereafter, the prevalence of KS increased dramatically in parallel with the AIDS epidemic and is now an AIDS-defining malignancy.
- *HHV-8 or viral DNA is found in nearly all KS cases.*
  —Antibodies to HHV-8 are detected in groups at risk for KS, and KS seroconversion precedes KS development.
  —Several HHV-8 genes have transforming and angiogenic potential; other HHV-8 genes encode inflammatory cytokines.
  —Taken together, the evidence implicates HHV-8 as a necessary factor, in combination with immunosuppression, in the cause of KS.

VII. Poxviridae Family

A. Poxviruses

1. Poxviruses are large, brick-shaped viruses with complex symmetry; they are enveloped, contain ds DNA, and replicate in the cytoplasm.
2. Poxviruses carry many virion-associated enzymes and encode enzymes needed for DNA genome replication in the cytoplasm.
3. Three medically important members of the Poxviridae family are in 2 genera: *Orthopoxvirus* (variola virus [smallpox virus], monkeypox virus) and *Molluscipoxvirus* (molluscum contagiosum virus [MCV]).
4. Naturally occurring smallpox was eradicated from the world in 1977 and represents one of the great success stories of virus eradication by vaccination.

5. Heightened interest in smallpox virus is fueled by its use as a potential bioterrorist weapon.

B. Variola Virus

1. **Clinical manifestations:** Variola virus causes **smallpox,** which has a case fatality rate of 30% in unvaccinated persons.
   a. Smallpox has an incubation period of 10–14 days with abrupt onset of fever, chills, headache, backache, and myalgia followed by a characteristic rash 3–4 days later.
   b. The smallpox rash begins as macular and progresses to papular, vesicular, and pustular before encrusting and sloughing off, sometimes leaving pocklike scars on survivors.
   c. Smallpox lesions characteristically are all in the same stage of development.
   d. The smallpox lesions have a characteristic centrifugal distribution, being more prominent on the extremities and face than on the trunk.
   e. Death results from overwhelming toxemia and systemic shock.
2. **Transmission/epidemiology:** Variola virus is highly contagious and is transmitted from person to person by **respiratory droplets.**
   a. The greatest risk for infection occurs among household members and close contacts of persons with smallpox.
   b. The virus survives in the environment and can be transmitted by fomites (eg, clothes or bedding) and less commonly by aerosol.
   c. Variola virus only infects humans and has no animal reservoir.
3. **Pathogenesis:** Variola virus is acquired by inhalation and infects respiratory epithelial cells and macrophages.
   a. The virus multiplies in regional lymph nodes and spreads via the blood to the spleen and liver, where further multiplication occurs.
   b. The virus is disseminated by a secondary viremia to the skin, where lesions develop.
   c. Cell-mediated immunity is important in clearing the infection. Humoral immunity protects against reinfection.
   d. Recovery from disease confers lifelong immunity.
4. **Virulence factors:** Variola virus encodes a variety of anti-immune proteins, such as a secreted glycoprotein that inhibits the complement pathway. Poxviruses express secreted cytokine mimics or soluble cytokine receptors that inhibit host defenses.
5. **Laboratory diagnosis:** Specimen collection and laboratory diagnosis of variola should be performed only by the state health department, the Centers for Disease Control and Prevention, or both. Laboratory testing to evaluate rash illnesses includes PCR for viral DNA, electron microscopy, histopathology, and culture.
6. **Treatment:** Vaccinia immune globulin is given for certain adverse reactions to smallpox vaccine. The antiviral drug cidofovir is used for therapy.
7. **Prevention:** A live, attenuated vaccine made from vaccinia virus confers solid immunity against the disease smallpox.
   a. Vaccinia virus is a poxvirus related to smallpox.
   b. Strategies to control a smallpox outbreak are containment and isolation of smallpox cases and vaccination of household and other close contacts of the infected person.

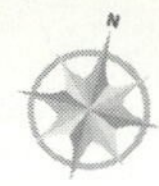

C. Monkeypox Virus

1. **Clinical manifestations:** Monkeypox virus causes a vesicular and pustular rash clinically similar to smallpox with a case fatality rate of 1–10% in Africa. Monkeypox is differentiated from smallpox by the pronounced lymphadenopathy in most patients with monkeypox.
2. **Transmission/epidemiology:** Transmission of monkeypox virus to humans in the United States is by close contact with infected mammalian pets.
   a. Person-to-person transmission is inefficient and uncommon.
   b. Human monkeypox is a rare, sporadic **viral zoonosis** that occurs mostly in the rain forests in central and west Africa.
   c. Monkeypox virus has a broad host range capable of infecting nonhuman primates, rabbits, squirrels, and some rodents.
   d. A multistate outbreak of monkeypox in persons exposed to infected pet prairie dogs and a giant Gambian rat occurred in the United States in 2003. The source was traced to an Illinois pet distributor.
3. **Pathogenesis:** Monkeypox pathogenesis is probably similar to smallpox.
4. **Virulence factors:** Like other poxviruses, monkeypox encodes a variety of anti-immune proteins.
5. **Treatment:** There are no specific treatment recommendations for monkeypox.
6. **Prevention:** Vaccination with smallpox vaccine (vaccinia) provides protective immunity against monkeypox but is not recommended for general use.
   a. If monkeypox infection is suspected, appropriate contact, isolation, and infection control guidelines should be instituted.
   b. The Centers for Disease Control and Prevention has placed an embargo on the importation of rodents from Africa.

D. Molluscum Contagiosum Virus

1. **Clinical manifestations:** MCV causes **benign nodular skin lesions** that appear as pearly, flesh-colored, raised, umbilicated nodules without systemic symptoms.
   a. The lesions are painless and resolve over time.
   b. MCV is an opportunistic pathogen in immunosuppressed patients, resulting in widespread and recurrent lesions.
2. **Transmission/epidemiology:** MCV is transmitted by **direct bodily contact** with the skin lesions.
   a. Genital MCV lesions can be transmitted **sexually.**
   b. MCV is distributed worldwide, and infection occurs mainly in children and young adults.
3. **Pathogenesis:** MCV infects epidermal cells to form a localized, fleshy lesion with an umbilicated center. Because of its epidermal localization, MCV provokes a minimal inflammatory or immune response.
4. **Virulence factors:** No virulence factors have been identified.
5. **Laboratory diagnosis:** A diagnosis of MCV can be made by the histologic detection of eosinophilic cytoplasmic inclusions (molluscum bodies) in biopsy specimens of skin lesions. Characteristic pox virions can be detected by electron microscopy.
6. **Treatment:** There is no specific antiviral therapy for MCV.
7. **Prevention:** There is no vaccine to prevent MCV infection.

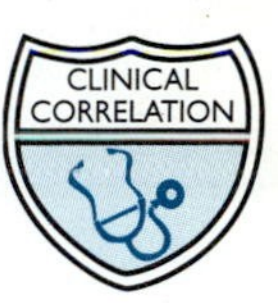

SMALLPOX

- *Smallpox is a contagious, infectious disease with a high fatality rate.*
- *There is no specific treatment, and routine vaccination was discontinued after the disease was eradicated in 1977.*
- *The terrorist attacks in 2001 raised the possibility and fear that variola virus might be used as an agent of bioterrorism.*
- *To respond to a possible terrorist attack, smallpox vaccination is recommended for persons designated by public health authorities to conduct investigation and follow-up of initial smallpox cases that might necessitate direct patient contact.*

VIII. Hepadnaviridae Family

A. Hepadnaviruses

1. Hepadnaviruses (*hepa*totropic *DNA* viruses) are icosahedral, enveloped viruses that contain circular partially ds DNA and that replicate in the nucleus.
2. Hepadnaviruses have a reverse transcriptase–DNA polymerase that replicates the DNA genome by reverse transcription of an RNA intermediate.
3. Hepatitis B virus (HBV) is the one medically important member of the Hepadnaviridae family.

B. Hepatitis B Virus

1. **Clinical manifestations:** HBV causes hepatitis in humans with a highly variable clinical outcome and with symptoms that range from mild and self-limited to severe and chronic.
   a. Most HBV primary infections are subclinical; 60–70% of infected individuals have no symptoms.
   b. **Acute hepatitis** occurs in 25–35% of infected individuals after an incubation period of 60–180 days.
   c. Acute hepatitis is characterized by the onset of fever, fatigue, anorexia, nausea, and pain associated with hepatomegaly.
   d. Symptoms indicative of more liver involvement include elevated liver enzymes, jaundice, pale stools, and dark urine.
   e. Markers of HBV infection, hepatitis B surface antigen (HBsAg), hepatitis B e antigen (HBeAg associated with the core antigen), and hepatitis B DNA, are detected in serum and disappear with acute disease resolution and the appearance of anti-HBs and anti-HBe antibodies.
   f. Extrahepatic manifestations such as arthralgias and rashes occur in 25% of acute HBV infections.
   g. Fulminant hepatitis resulting in liver failure and death is an uncommon complication (< 1% of cases) of acute HBV infection.
   h. **Chronic hepatitis** occurs in about 10% of HBV infections and is defined as the detection of HBsAg, HBV DNA, and HBeAg for 6 months or more.
   i. Patients with chronic HBV infection are at risk for liver cirrhosis, liver failure, and **hepatocellular carcinoma.**
   j. Risk of chronic infection is high (90%) in neonates born to chronically HBV-infected mothers and is increased in immunocompromised patients.

 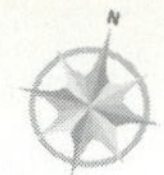

2. **Transmission/epidemiology:** HBV is transmitted **sexually,** by **blood and other bodily fluids,** by **intravenous drug use**, and **perinatally** from infected mother to child.
   a. Perinatal infection is acquired at the time of birth.
   b. Sexual transmission of HBV (heterosexual or homosexual) is associated with duration of sexual activity, number of sex partners, and a history of other sexually transmitted disease.
   c. Intravenous drug use is a common mode of HBV transmission in the United States.
   d. Occupational exposure to contaminated blood products (eg, needle stick injury) is a risk factor for HBV transmission.
   e. HBV can also be transmitted horizontally via saliva or skin lesions, particularly by children under conditions of crowding in some daycare centers.
3. **Pathogenesis:** HBV infects hepatocytes but does not cause direct cytopathology.
   a. Hepatocellular injury is due to immune attack by cytotoxic T cells.
   b. Individuals who fail to clear the virus from the body (eg, neonates who have an impaired ability to make antibody to HBsAg because of an immature immune system or patients who are endogenously or exogenously immunosuppressed) become virus carriers and chronic hepatitis and cirrhosis result.
   c. Hepatocellular carcinoma, linked with chronic HBV infection, may result from HBV DNA integration into hepatocyte DNA.
   d. Chronic hepatitis associated with active viral replication leads to a cycle of liver cell damage and regeneration, providing a pool of proliferating hepatocytes susceptible to mutations and contributing to loss of cell growth control and malignant transformation.
   e. Antibody to HBsAg is protective and leads to disease resolution.
   f. Cell-mediated immunity is important in clearing the infection.
4. **Virulence factors:** Overproduction of excess HBsAg during viral replication acts as a decoy, binding neutralizing antibodies and evading the immune response.
5. **Laboratory diagnosis:** Diagnosis of HBV infection is made by biochemical tests (liver enzymes, bilirubin) and serologic assays.
   a. EIA assays that detect HBV-specific antigens and antibodies are sensitive, and specific tests used routinely in HBV diagnosis.
   b. IgM antibody to hepatitis B core antigen (HBcAg) is an indicator of acute HBV infection.
   c. The presence of antibody to HBsAg is associated with immunity to HBV infection.
6. **Treatment:** There is no specific treatment for acute hepatitis B.
   a. Chronic hepatitis B is treated with interferon-alpha, lamivudine, or adefovir.
   b. Lamivudine is a nucleoside reverse transcriptase inhibitor.
   c. Adefovir is a nucleotide analogue of adenine with anti-HBV activity used in the treatment of lamivudine-resistant HBV mutants.
7. **Prevention:** Active immunization against HBV is achieved with a recombinant **HBsAg vaccine.**
   a. Passive immunization with **HBV immune globulin** is given to neonates born to HBsAg (+) mothers and after needlestick exposures.
   b. Avoidance of high-risk behavior is an important preventive measure.

HBV INFECTION

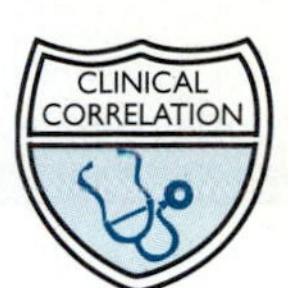

- *HBV infection is a global public health problem.*
  —Chronic HBV infection can cause chronic hepatitis and cirrhosis and is a risk factor for primary liver cancer.
  —It is estimated that nearly 500 million people worldwide are chronic HBV carriers with more than a million deaths annually.
- *HBV vaccination is the most effective way to prevent chronic HBV infection and its associated sequelae.*
  —In parts of the world where HBV infection is endemic, active immunization has dramatically reduced the chronic infection rate and decreased the incidence of hepatocellular carcinoma in children.
  —Recommended universal immunization of infants against HBV is aimed at preventing chronic HBV infection and eliminating the excess mortality associated with cirrhosis and hepatocellular carcinoma.

CLINICAL PROBLEMS

A 6-year-old child is seen with a prominent bright red rash that appeared 2 days earlier on the cheeks. The child has a sore throat and a low-grade fever.

1. The DNA virus most likely responsible for this illness is:

A. VZV
B. Adenovirus
C. Parvovirus B19
D. Measles virus
E. Rubella virus

A 20-year-old woman is admitted to the university health clinic with painful vesicular lesions on the vulva and perineum. She reports not feeling well the past week and having pain on urination. On physical examination, she has a low-grade fever and inguinal lymphadenopathy.

2. Electron microscopy of lesion cells would be expected to show:

A. Naked intranuclear virions
B. Enveloped intranuclear virions
C. Naked cytoplasmic virions
D. Enveloped cytoplasmic virions
E. No virions

3. Appropriate therapy for this patient is:

A. Acyclovir
B. Ganciclovir
C. Foscarnet
D. Zidovudine
E. Zanamivir

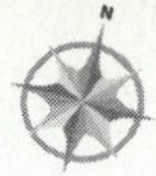

A 19-year-old college student presents to the student health clinic complaining of fever, fatigue, and sore throat that developed about a month after spring break. Physical examination shows pharyngitis, cervical and axillary lymphadenopathy, and splenomegaly. Laboratory tests show atypical lymphocytes and are positive for heterophile antibody.

4. The virus most likely responsible for this disease is:
   A. HSV
   B. CMV
   C. HHV-7
   D. EBV
   E. HHV-8

5. The patient is at risk for development of:
   A. Anogenital carcinoma
   B. T-cell lymphoma
   C. Hodgkin disease
   D. KS
   E. Hepatocellular carcinoma

A 30-year-old homosexual man is seen in the sexually transmitted disease clinic with numerous skin-colored, umbilicated, nodular lesions in the groin and perineum. He has a history of multiple sex partners and infection with HSV. Histologic examination of the lesions shows cells with eosinophilic cytoplasmic inclusions.

6. This infection is most likely caused by:
   A. HSV
   B. VZV
   C. CMV
   D. EBV
   E. MCV

ANSWERS

1. The answer is C. Parvovirus B19 is a DNA virus that causes erythema infectiosum, a common childhood exanthem. The characteristic clinical feature of B19 infection is a "slapped cheek" appearance. VZV is incorrect because the lesions of chickenpox are characteristically vesicular and pustular. Adenoviruses cause childhood upper respiratory tract infections not noted for rash. Measles virus and rubella virus cause childhood exanthems, but both are RNA viruses.

2. The answer is B. The clinical case is descriptive of a genital infection by HSV. HSV is an enveloped DNA virus that replicates in the nucleus. Although choice E could be

correct based on sampling error, it is highly unlikely because infectious virus can be recovered routinely from HSV vesicles.

3. The answer is A. Acyclovir is the antiviral drug of choice for the treatment of primary HSV infection. Ganciclovir is used to treat CMV. Foscarnet is used to treat acyclovir-resistant HSV. Zidovudine is a reverse transcriptase inhibitor without effect on HSV. Zanamivir is an influenza neuraminidase inhibitor without effect on HSV.

4. The answer is D. The clinical case, typical of infectious mononucleosis, coupled with a positive heterophile antibody test (Monospot test) is indicative of EBV infection. HSV can cause sore throat but is not associated with mononucleosislike syndrome. CMV can cause a mononucleosislike syndrome clinically similar to EBV with a negative Monospot test. HHV-7 causes roseola characterized by a generalized rash in young children. HHV-8 is the causative agent of KS.

5. The answer is C. EBV infectious mononucleosis is a risk factor for Hodgkin disease. Infectious mononucleosis is not a risk factor for the other malignancies.

6. The answer is E. MCV is a poxvirus that is transmitted sexually and that causes benign, nodular skin lesions. Cytoplasmic inclusion bodies in the skin lesions are characteristic of MCV and its replication in the cytoplasm. The other choices are herpesviruses, which replicate in the nucleus.

CHAPTER 12

POSITIVE-STRAND RNA VIRUSES

I. Key Concepts

A. Positive-strand (+) RNA viruses have single-stranded RNA genomes of the same polarity or sense as mRNA.

B. The **(+) strand RNA virus genome functions as mRNA,** and the naked RNA is infectious.

C. All (+) RNA viruses encode an RNA-dependent RNA polymerase used in genome replication. Unlike other RNA viruses, (+) RNA viruses do not carry the polymerase as part of the virion structure.

D. Medically important (+) RNA viruses encompass 6 virus families (Picornaviridae, Caliciviridae, Astroviridae, Togaviridae, Flaviviridae, and Coronaviridae) and share similar features in terms of nucleic acid composition, lack of a virion polymerase, and site of replication (Table 12–1).

II. Picornaviridae Family

A. Picornaviruses

1. Picornaviruses (*pico* = small, *RNA*-containing viruses) are small, nonenveloped, (+) RNA viruses with icosahedral symmetry.
2. Picornavirus (+) RNA is translated into a single polyprotein that is subsequently processed by virion and cellular proteases into nonstructural and structural proteins.
3. Enteroviruses, Rhinoviruses, and Hepatoviruses are representative genera within the picornavirus family.
4. Members of the *Enterovirus* genus infect the gastrointestinal tract and include polioviruses, coxsackieviruses, and echoviruses.
5. Enteroviruses are acid stable and resistant to the low pH of the stomach.
6. Rhinoviruses are acid labile and replicate optimally at about 33 °C, a temperature maintained in the nasopharynx.

B. Poliovirus

1. **Clinical manifestations:** Poliovirus is the etiologic agent of **poliomyelitis.**
   a. Most (90–95%) poliovirus infections are asymptomatic, with no disease manifestations.
   b. Abortive poliomyelitis is the most common clinical form and is characterized by a flulike illness, with fever, headache, sore throat, and nausea followed by spontaneous recovery without central nervous system (CNS) sequelae.

Table 12–1. Properties of positive-strand RNA viruses.

Virus Family	RNA Structure	Virion Polymerase	Shape	Envelope	Site of Replication	Human Viruses
Picornaviridae	Linear, ss, (+), non-segmented	No	Icosahedral	No	Cytoplasm	Poliovirus Coxsackievirus Echovirus Rhinovirus Hepatitis A virus
Caliciviridae	Linear, ss, (+), non-segmented	No	Icosahedral	No	Cytoplasm	Norovirus Hepatitis E virus
Astroviridae	Linear, ss, (+), non-segmented	No	Icosahedral	No	Cytoplasm	Astrovirus
Togaviridae	Linear, ss, (+), non-segmented	No	Icosahedral	Yes	Cytoplasm	Alphaviruses (EEE, WEE, VEE viruses) Rubella virus
Flaviviridae	Linear, ss, (+), non-segmented	No	Icosahedral	Yes	Cytoplasm	Yellow fever virus Dengue virus JE, MVE, SLE, WN viruses Hepatitis C & G viruses
Coronaviridae	Linear, ss, (+), non-segmented	No	Helical	Yes	Cytoplasm	Coronavirus

ss, single-stranded; EEE, eastern equine encephalitis; WEE, western equine encephalitis; VEE, Venezuelan equine encephalitis; JE, Japanese encephalitis; MVE, Murray Valley encephalitis; SLE, St. Louis encephalitis; WN, West Nile.

c. A minority (~1%) of poliovirus infections result in either nonparalytic or paralytic poliomyelitis.

d. Nonparalytic poliomyelitis is characterized by symptoms of aseptic meningitis with fever, headache, and stiff neck followed by spontaneous recovery.

e. Paralytic poliomyelitis is characterized by asymmetric **flaccid paralysis,** most often affecting the legs. Respiratory paralysis can occur if the brainstem is infected. Overall paralytic poliomyelitis mortality is about 5%.

f. A postpolio syndrome is observed in about 25% of persons who survived paralytic poliomyelitis. The syndrome appears 30–40 years after acute polio infection and is characterized by fatigue, pain, muscle weakness, and atrophy.

2. **Transmission/epidemiology:** Poliovirus is transmitted by the **fecal-oral** route.
   a. Humans are the only natural hosts.
   b. Poliovirus has 3 serotypes: poliovirus types 1–3.
   c. Poliomyelitis has been largely eradicated from the western hemisphere because of the successful vaccination program.
   d. The rare cases of paralytic polio in the United States are caused by live, attenuated vaccine strains that have reverted to virulence.
   e. Paralytic polio remains high in developing countries, with global eradication of polio targeted for the next decade.
3. **Pathogenesis:** Poliovirus initiates infection in the pharynx and gastrointestinal tract after ingestion.
   a. The virus spreads to draining lymph nodes followed by viremic dissemination to other sites with particular tropism for the CNS.
   b. Invasion of the CNS results in direct killing of motor neurons located in the anterior horn of the spinal cord.
   c. Destruction of motor neurons results in paralysis.
   d. Clearance of poliovirus and recovery from infection are primarily due to IgA and IgG antibody response. Acquired immunity is permanent.
4. **Virulence factors:** Poliovirus is stable under the acid conditions (pH 3–5) found in the gastric tract. Poliovirus encodes proteins that interfere with the antiviral action of interferon.
5. **Laboratory diagnosis:** Poliovirus is detected by cytopathic effects (CPEs) induced in cell culture and identified by neutralization with type-specific antiserum or immunocytochemical staining of infected cells with poliovirus-specific antibody. A reverse transcriptase–polymerase chain reaction (RT-PCR) assay can be used to discriminate between polioviruses and nonpolio enteroviruses.
6. **Treatment:** No specific antiviral therapy is available for poliovirus.
7. **Prevention:** Poliomyelitis can be prevented by either the live, attenuated (Sabin) or killed (Salk) vaccine. Because of the rare cases of live vaccine–associated paralytic poliomyelitis, the killed, inactivated polio vaccine is recommended in the United States.

C. Coxsackievirus Groups A and B and Echoviruses

1. **Clinical manifestations:** Coxsackieviruses and echoviruses cause a variety of diseases but are the most frequently recognized cause of **aseptic meningitis.**
   a. No clinical syndrome is specifically associated with a given coxsackievirus or echovirus type, but serotypes most commonly associated with disease syndromes are noted below.
   b. Enteric disease is an uncommon manifestation of coxsackievirus or echovirus infection, even though the viruses are classified as enteroviruses.
   c. Respiratory syndromes associated with coxsackievirus and echovirus infection include the common cold, herpangina (coxsackie A and echoviruses), hand-foot-and-mouth disease (coxsackie A), and pleurodynia and myalgia (coxsackie B).
   d. Cardiovascular syndromes associated with coxsackievirus and echovirus infection include pericarditis and myocarditis (coxsackie B).

e. Aseptic meningitis is characterized by acute onset of fever, headache, and stiff neck. Most patients recover in about a week with no CNS sequelae.

2. **Transmission/epidemiology:** Coxsackieviruses and echoviruses are transmitted horizontally, primarily by the **fecal-oral** route and less commonly by respiratory droplets.
   a. Human enteroviruses are classified into groups A–D and include 6 coxsackie B, 24 coxsackie A, and 34 echovirus serotypes.
   b. Coxsackievirus and echoviruses are distributed worldwide.
   c. Coxsackieviruses are named after Coxsackie, New York, where the first virus was isolated.
   d. Echovirus is an acronym for *e*nteric *c*ytopathic *h*uman *o*rphan viruses, originally isolated during a search for the cause of polio and not associated initially with any disease (ie, orphan viruses).
   e. Coxsackievirus and echovirus infections are more common in the summer and fall in temperate climates.
3. **Pathogenesis:** Coxsackievirus and echovirus pathogenesis is similar to that of poliovirus. However, these viruses differ from poliovirus by commonly infecting the meninges rather than the motor neurons.
   a. Virus is shed from the nasopharynx (weeks) and in the feces (weeks to months) after infection.
   b. Virus directly damages and kills target cells.
   c. Clearance of the virus is antibody mediated.
4. **Virulence factors:** No virulence factors have been identified.
5. **Laboratory diagnosis:** Laboratory diagnosis of coxsackievirus and echovirus infections is similar to that described for polioviruses.
6. **Treatment:** No specific antiviral therapy is available for coxsackievirus or echovirus infection.
7. **Prevention:** No vaccines are available to prevent coxsackievirus or echovirus disease.

D. Rhinovirus

1. **Clinical manifestations:** Rhinoviruses cause the **common cold,** characterized by an incubation period of 2–3 days followed by rhinorrhea, nasal congestion, sneezing, headache, mild sore throat, and cough, with little or no fever. Symptoms resolve after a week generally without complications.
2. **Transmission/epidemiology:** Rhinovirus is transmitted by **hand-to-nose** or **hand-to-eye contact** with contaminated respiratory tract secretions or **respiratory droplets.**
   a. Rhinoviruses are distributed worldwide and cause about 50% of cases of the common cold in older children and adults.
   b. Rhinovirus infections are seasonal with peak prevalence in the fall and spring in temperate climates.
   c. More than 100 rhinovirus serotypes are known, making vaccine development unrealistic.
3. **Pathogenesis:** Rhinoviruses gain entry to cells in the nasopharynx and nasal passages by attachment to the intercellular cell adhesion molecule-1 (ICAM-1) receptor.
   a. Virus replication is localized to nasal epithelial cells and is shed into respiratory secretions.

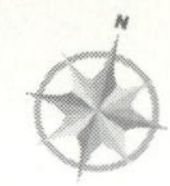

b. Rhinovirus grows optimally at 33 °C, the temperature of the upper airway.
c. The virus causes minimal pathology to respiratory epithelial cells with subsequent rapid repair of involved areas.
d. The major pathogenesis of rhinovirus infection is associated with chemical mediators of inflammation (eg, bradykinin, prostaglandins).
e. The inflammatory mediators cause vasodilation, mucus secretion, and stimulation of the sneeze and cough reflexes, consistent with clinical symptoms of the common cold.
f. Immunity is serotype specific, transient, and correlates with secretory IgA response.

4. **Virulence factors:** No virulence factors have been identified.
5. **Laboratory diagnosis:** Laboratory diagnosis is rarely performed. The common cold is usually self-diagnosed.
6. **Treatment:** There is no specific antiviral therapy for rhinovirus colds. A variety of anti-inflammatory treatments (antihistamines, decongestants) provide symptomatic relief.
7. **Prevention:** No vaccine is available to prevent rhinovirus colds given the plurality of rhinovirus serotypes. Hand washing is an effective method of prevention.

E. Hepatitis A Virus (HAV)

1. **Clinical manifestations:** HAV is the cause of **infectious hepatitis,** characterized by an incubation period ranging from 15–50 days followed by the onset of fever, anorexia, nausea, vomiting, dark urine due to bilirubinuria, and jaundice.
   a. The duration of illness varies but is usually self-limiting with recovery in 3–4 weeks.
   b. Fulminant hepatitis leading to total liver failure and death is a rare complication.
2. **Transmission/epidemiology:** HAV is transmitted horizontally by the **fecal-oral** route.
   a. Epidemics of HAV are usually due to food- or water-borne infections associated with poor sanitary conditions and personal hygiene.
   b. HAV infections in children under the age of 5 years are often clinically unapparent. Symptomatic infections increase with age.
   c. Overall mortality from HAV in the United States is below 0.5%.
   d. HAV is the single serotype in the genus *Hepatovirus.*
   e. It is heat stable and resistant to the stomach's acidic pH.
3. **Pathogenesis:** HAV is ingested from contaminated food or water and initially infects cells in the oropharynx and gastrointestinal tract.
   a. HAV spreads to the liver by viremia and infects hepatocytes without producing marked cytopathology.
   b. Hepatic cell injury is mediated by immune attack by cytotoxic T cells.
   c. Virus from infected liver cells is shed into the intestine and excreted in the feces.
   d. HAV does not establish a chronic infection or carrier state.
   e. Serum IgG is important in recovery from infection and in long-term protection.
4. **Virulence factors:** No HAV virulence factors have been identified.

5. **Laboratory diagnosis:** HAV-specific IgM antibody detected by enzyme immunoassay (EIA) is the most common laboratory method to diagnose HAV infection.
6. **Treatment:** There is no specific antiviral therapy for HAV infection.
7. **Prevention:** A formalin-inactivated **HAV vaccine** is available for use in individuals at risk for HAV infection and for travelers to areas of high HAV prevalence.
   a. HAV vaccine is highly effective and confers long-term protection.
   b. Passive immunization with **HAV immune globulin** is recommended for postexposure prophylaxis in individuals exposed to infection but not previously immunized.
   c. Hand washing is an effective means of prevention.

HEPATITIS A

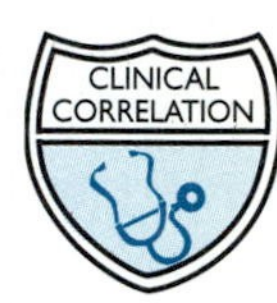

- *HAV outbreaks are usually spread by eating food contaminated with infected feces, often traced to an infected food handler.*
- *HAV is spread by lax hygiene and the capacity of the virus to resist the pH of the stomach en route to the infection of intestinal cells.*
- *HAV immune globulin can prevent infection or diminish the severity of illness but only if given within 2 weeks of exposure.*

III. Caliciviridae Family

A. Caliciviruses

1. Caliciviruses are small, nonenveloped, (+) RNA viruses with icosahedral symmetry.
2. Caliciviruses have characteristic cuplike depressions (*calyx* is Latin for cup) on the surface of the virion that are readily visualized by electron microscopy.
3. Caliciviruses are acid stable and resistant to the low pH in the stomach.
4. Human caliciviruses have been classified into 2 genera: Norwalk-like viruses, also called Noroviruses, and Sapporo-like viruses. Hepatitis E virus (HEV) is provisionally classified as a calicivirus.
5. Noroviruses are the prototypical caliciviruses.

B. Norovirus (Norwalk-like Virus)

1. **Clinical manifestations:** Noroviruses cause **acute gastroenteritis** in older children and adults, characterized by acute onset of vomiting, diarrhea, nausea, abdominal cramps, and fever.
   a. The constellation of symptoms is indistinguishable from those associated with rotavirus or with bacterial or parasitic agents.
   b. Norovirus incubation is short (mean, 24 hours), and the duration of illness is 1–2 days.
   c. Diarrhea is generally watery without blood or mucus.
2. **Transmission/epidemiology:** Noroviruses are transmitted horizontally by the **fecal-oral** route.
   a. Noroviruses are the most common cause of gastroenteritis in the United States and cause an estimated 23 million cases annually.
   b. Noroviruses have a worldwide distribution and affect older children and adults, whereas acute gastroenteritis caused by rotaviruses is a disease of infants and young children.

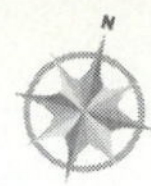

c. Norovirus outbreaks have occurred in schools, camps, cruise ships, restaurants, and families.
d. Norovirus outbreaks are associated with the ingestion of contaminated food or water, direct person-to-person contact, and contact with contaminated environmental surfaces.

3. **Pathogenesis:** Norovirus infects the small bowel and directly damages enterocytes.
   a. Intestinal microvilli are broadened and blunted as damaged enterocytes slough off.
   b. Norovirus-induced pathology leads to transient malabsorption of water and nutrients and reduced gastric motility, culminating in vomiting and diarrhea.
   c. Norovirus antibody is detected after infection and confers short-term protection.
   d. Knowledge about the role of immunity in norovirus infections is incomplete.
4. **Virulence factors:** No norovirus virulence factors have been identified.
5. **Laboratory diagnosis:** RT-PCR assays have been developed to detect norovirus in stools and other clinical or environmental samples. EIAs are also available to detect norovirus-specific IgM antibody in serum.
6. **Treatment:** There is no specific antiviral therapy for norovirus infections.
7. **Prevention:** No vaccine is available to prevent norovirus infection.
   a. Frequent hand washing is an effective means of prevention.
   b. Disposal of contaminated food and disinfection of contaminated materials will prevent transmission.

NOROVIRUS: A HIT-AND-RUN VIRUS

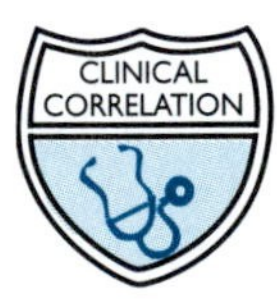

- *Noroviruses have gained notoriety for causing outbreaks of acute gastroenteritis on cruise ships sailing into US ports. However, 60–80% of all such outbreaks occur on land.*
- *Noroviruses have evolved an efficient strategy to infect cells of the intestinal tract.*
  —They are resistant to the acid pH in the digestive tract.
  —They reproduce quickly.
  —They leave the host before the immune system can become fully activated.

C. Hepatitis E Virus

1. **Clinical manifestations:** HEV is the cause of enterically transmitted, waterborne epidemics of hepatitis.
   a. Hepatitis caused by HEV is clinically indistinguishable from other forms of acute viral hepatitis.
   b. Most HEV infections are subclinical.
   c. In symptomatic cases, onset of illness is abrupt, is generally self-limiting, and has a mortality rate of about 1% in the general population.
   d. Fulminant hepatitis is a major complication of HEV infections among pregnant females, with a mortality rate of up to 40% during the third trimester of pregnancy.
2. **Transmission/epidemiology:** HEV is transmitted by the **fecal-oral** route, usually by contaminated water. It is endemic and the most common cause of acute hepatitis in developing countries with poor sanitation.
3. **Pathogenesis:** HEV pathogenesis is similar to that of HAV. HEV does not establish a chronic infection or carrier state.
4. **Virulence factors:** No virulence factors have been identified.

5. **Laboratory diagnosis:** Diagnosis of HEV is made by the detection of HEV-specific IgM or IgG antibody by EIA.
6. **Treatment:** There is no specific antiviral therapy for HEV.
7. **Prevention:** There is no vaccine for HEV.
   a. Improved sanitary conditions should lower the rate of transmission.
   b. Travelers to HEV-endemic areas should be cautioned about drinking potentially contaminated water.

IV. Astroviridae Family

A. Astroviruses

1. Astroviruses are small, nonenveloped, (+) RNA viruses with icosahedral symmetry.
2. Astroviruses are so named because they have a characteristic 5- or 6-point star on the virion surface that can be visualized by electron microscopy.
3. Human astrovirus 1 is the prototypical human virus member of the family Astroviridae.

B. Human Astrovirus 1

1. **Clinical manifestations:** Astroviruses cause **acute gastroenteritis,** primarily in infants and young children, characterized by vomiting, abdominal pain, fever, and watery diarrhea that is self-limiting.
2. **Transmission/epidemiology:** Astroviruses are transmitted by the **fecal-oral** route, usually by person-to-person contact or by contaminated food or water.
   a. Astroviruses are distributed worldwide with peak incidence of infections reported in the winter months in temperate climates.
   b. Astrovirus is second only to rotavirus as the cause of diarrhea in children.
3. **Pathogenesis:** Astrovirus infects intestinal epithelial cells and directly damages enterocytes. Viral clearance and protective immunity are correlated with serum IgG antibody.
4. **Virulence factors:** No virulence factors have been identified.
5. **Laboratory diagnosis:** Astroviruses can be detected by EIA for viral antigen and RT-PCR for genomic RNA.
6. **Treatment:** There is no specific antiviral therapy for astrovirus infections.
7. **Prevention:** There is no astrovirus vaccine. Good hygienic practices in hospitals, daycare centers, and families are effective means to prevent transmission.

V. Togaviridae Family

A. Togaviruses

1. Togaviruses are enveloped, (+) RNA viruses with icosahedral symmetry.
2. Togaviruses are named for the cloak (*toga* is Latin for cloak) that denotes the virion envelope.
3. The Togaviridae family consists of 2 genera: *Alphaviruses* with 26 members and *Rubivirus.*
4. Major human pathogens in the *Alphavirus* genus are eastern and western equine encephalitis (EEE and WEE) viruses and Venezuelan equine encephalitis (VEE) virus.
5. Rubella virus is the only member in the *Rubivirus* genus.

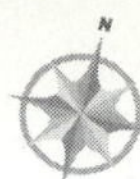

B. Alphaviruses (EEE, WEE, and VEE)

1. **Clinical manifestations:** EEE and WEE viruses cause encephalitis characterized by fever, headache, myalgia that may progress to dizziness, vomiting, confusion, convulsions, coma, and death.
   a. VEE viruses cause encephalitis and pneumonitis that may be complicated by secondary bacterial infections.
   b. WEE tends to be less severe clinically than EEE.
   c. Mortality from EEE is 35% with neurologic deficits in 35% of EEE survivors.
   d. Mortality from WEE is 4% and 1% from VEE with milder neurologic deficits.
2. **Transmission/epidemiology:** Alphaviruses are **arboviruses** transmitted by the bite of infected **mosquitoes.**
   a. They are maintained and amplified in nature in wild birds (EEE and WEE) or small mammals (VEE).
   b. Humans and horses are dead-end hosts.
   c. EEE viruses are found in the western hemisphere and concentrated in the eastern part of the United States.
   d. WEE viruses are found in North and South America and concentrated in the western part of the United States.
   e. VEE viruses are found in Central and South America.
   f. Persons over 50 years of age and young children are at greatest risk for development of severe disease.
3. **Pathogenesis:** Infection by alphaviruses is initiated by the bite of an infected mosquito.
   a. The mosquito regurgitates virus-containing saliva into the bloodstream.
   b. Virus is spread by viremia and invades the CNS via capillary endothelial cells or the choroid plexus.
   c. Serum IgG antibody confers protective immunity to alphavirus infections.
4. **Virulence factors:** No virulence factors have been identified.
5. **Laboratory diagnosis:** EEE, WEE, and VEE infections are diagnosed serologically by a rise in virus-specific antibody titer.
6. **Treatment:** There is no specific antiviral therapy for alphavirus infections.
7. **Prevention:** There are no vaccines available for human EEE, WEE, or VEE infections.
   a. A killed vaccine is available to protect horses.
   b. Mosquito vector control is an important means of prevention.
   c. People should avoid mosquito bites by wearing protective clothing and using insect repellant containing DEET.

EASTERN EQUINE ENCEPHALITIS

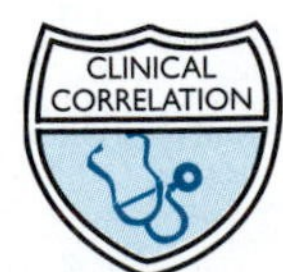

- *EEE is the most deadly of the mosquito-borne diseases but relatively rare (average of 4 cases per year in the United States).*
- *Human cases of EEE are often preceded by cases in horses, signifying that mosquitoes in the area are a risk to human health.*
- *Personal and household protection from mosquitoes is the best preventive method.*

C. Rubella Virus

1. **Clinical manifestations:** Rubella virus causes a mild illness (commonly called rubella or German measles) in children and adults characterized by an incubation period of 14–21 days followed by a generalized maculopapular rash, low-grade fever, and lymphadenopathy.
   a. Common complications of postnatal rubella are arthritis and arthralgia, most frequently in adults.
   b. Rubella virus infection of women in the first trimester of pregnancy causes **congenital rubella syndrome** in the child, which is characterized by cataracts, cardiac abnormalities, deafness, and mental retardation.
2. **Transmission/epidemiology:** Rubella virus is recognized as one of the most potent infectious teratogenic agents.
   a. Congenital infections occur by **transplacental transmission** from infected mother to the fetus.
   b. Risk of congenital rubella syndrome is greatest during the first trimester of pregnancy but can occur throughout pregnancy.
   c. Infants with congenital rubella syndrome excrete virus for many months and are capable of transmitting the virus to susceptible individuals.
   d. The rubella vaccine was licensed to protect against future fetal infections and birth defects.
   e. Rubella virus is transmitted postnatally by **respiratory droplets** of infected individuals.
   f. Rubella outbreaks in the United States are rare, and the source is usually traced to infected individuals from countries where rubella vaccination is not routine, undervaccinated populations in the United States, or religious communities that shun vaccination programs.
   g. Rubella remains endemic in some developing countries.
3. **Pathogenesis:** In postnatal infections, rubella virus enters through the respiratory tract and spreads to local lymph nodes, coinciding with lymphadenopathy.
   a. The virus spreads to spleen and regional lymph nodes and disseminates by viremia to skin, kidney, joints, and respiratory tract.
   b. In congenital rubella syndrome, the virus infects the placenta and spreads to the fetus with multiple organ involvement and teratogenic effects.
   c. Antibody response limits viral spread, but cell-mediated immunity is required to resolve infection.
4. **Virulence factors:** No virulence factors have been identified.
5. **Laboratory diagnosis:** Rubella virus–specific IgM and IgG antibody detection by EIA is the most common diagnostic test for rubella virus infection.
6. **Treatment:** There is no specific antiviral therapy for rubella virus infection.
7. **Prevention: Live, attenuated rubella virus vaccine** is highly effective in preventing rubella. The vaccine is usually given in combination with the measles, mumps, and rubella (MMR) vaccine.

VI. Flaviviridae Family

A. Flaviviruses

1. Flaviviruses are enveloped, (+) RNA viruses with icosahedral symmetry.

 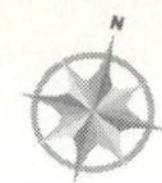

2. The Flaviviridae family has 2 genera with several human pathogens: the *Flavivirus* genus, with more than 70 antigenically related members, and the *Hepacivirus* genus, with 2 members (hepatitis C virus [HCV] and hepatitis G virus [HGV]).
3. Major pathogens in the *Flavivirus* genus are **arboviruses,** which are transmitted by mosquitoes and which include yellow fever virus, dengue virus, St. Louis encephalitis virus, Japanese encephalitis virus, Murray Valley encephalitis virus, and West Nile virus.
4. Medically important members of the *Flavivirus* genus are associated with several clinical syndromes, including febrile illness with rash, hemorrhagic fever, and encephalitis.

B. Yellow Fever Virus

1. **Clinical manifestations:** Yellow fever virus causes **hemorrhagic fever,** which is characterized by jaundice, fever, headache, myalgia, black vomit, other hemorrhages, and shock. The mortality rate is 20–50%.
2. **Transmission/epidemiology:** Yellow fever virus is transmitted by the bite of infected **mosquitoes.**
   a. It is endemic in Africa and South America but is not present in the United States.
   b. In the jungle cycle, mosquitoes acquire the virus from viremic monkeys that act as a permanent reservoir. Humans encroaching on the jungle environment are accidental hosts.
   c. In the urban cycle, infected viremic humans act as the reservoir for mosquitoes that then transmit the virus to other humans.
3. **Pathogenesis:** Yellow fever virus infects mosquitoes and establishes a persistent infection.
   a. The virus is inoculated directly into the blood stream of the host by the biting mosquito.
   b. It spreads via the blood to cells of the monocyte-macrophage lineage with liver as the target organ.
   c. Antibody and cell-mediated immunity are important in controlling infection.
4. **Virulence factors:** No yellow fever virus virulence factors are known.
5. **Laboratory diagnosis:** Yellow fever virus–specific IgM detected by EIA is the laboratory method to diagnose infections. Less often, a rise in virus-specific antibody titer between paired acute and convalescent serum samples is used diagnostically.
6. **Treatment:** There is no specific antiviral therapy for yellow fever virus infections.
7. **Prevention:** A highly effective live, attenuated yellow fever virus **vaccine** is available for prevention of urban yellow fever.
   a. The vaccine is given to those traveling to areas where yellow fever is endemic.
   b. Mosquito vector control is an important means of preventing yellow fever.

C. Dengue Virus

1. **Clinical manifestations:** Dengue virus causes **dengue fever,** an acute febrile disease with headache, retroocular pain, rash, myalgia, and deep bone pain ("breakbone fever").
   a. Dengue fever may be mild or severe but rarely fatal.
   b. Dengue virus can also cause **dengue hemorrhagic fever** or **dengue shock syndrome,** characterized by symptoms of dengue fever that progress to prostration, gastrointestinal and skin hemorrhages, shock, coma, and death in up to 10% of victims.

2. **Transmission/epidemiology:** Dengue virus is transmitted by the bite of infected **mosquitoes.**
   a. Dengue viruses are endemic in southeast Asia, Central and South America, and the Caribbean Islands but are not present in the United States, except for imported cases in travelers returning to the United States from endemic areas.
   b. Dengue viruses are transmitted primarily in urban environments where humans serve as both hosts and viremic reservoirs of infection.
3. **Pathogenesis:** Dengue virus pathogenesis is similar to that of yellow fever virus, with the vasculature as the target organ.
   a. Serum antibody and cell-mediated immune responses limit the outcome and severity of dengue fever and confer long-term protection.
   b. Dengue hemorrhagic fever–shock syndrome has an immunopathologic basis characterized by dengue virus antibody–mediated enhancement of monocyte-macrophage infection and activation of dengue virus–specific lymphocytes, with release of cytokines, activation of complement, and subsequent tissue damage.
4. **Virulence factors:** No dengue virus virulence factors are known.
5. **Laboratory diagnosis:** Dengue virus–specific IgM antibody detected by EIA is commonly used to diagnose dengue virus infections. Serologic diagnosis that shows a rise in dengue antibody titer between acute and convalescent serum and RT-PCR for genomic RNA are adjunctive diagnostic tests.
6. **Treatment:** There is no specific antiviral therapy for dengue virus infections.
7. **Prevention:** There are no vaccines available to prevent dengue virus infections. Mosquito vector control is an important preventive measure.

D. Japanese Encephalitis Virus and Related Viruses (Murray Valley Encephalitis Virus, St. Louis Encephalitis Virus, and West Nile Virus)

1. **Clinical manifestations:** Japanese encephalitis and related viruses cause clinical illness ranging from a nonspecific flulike febrile illness to **encephalitis.**
   a. Symptoms in more severe infections include headache, nausea, high fever, malaise, myalgia, backache, neck stiffness, and disorientation.
   b. Japanese encephalitis and related viruses cause significant mortality, ranging from 10–40% with young children and the elderly at increased risk.
2. **Transmission/epidemiology:** Japanese encephalitis and related viruses are transmitted by the bite of infected **mosquitoes.**
   a. Transmission of West Nile virus has also been documented via blood transfusions, organ transplants, breast milk from an infected mother to her infant, and transplacentally.
   b. Japanese encephalitis virus is present throughout Asia, and Murray Valley encephalitis virus is endemic in Australia. St. Louis encephalitis virus is widely distributed in North America. West Nile virus is present in Africa, Europe, the Middle East, India, Australia, and since 1999 in the United States.
   c. All these viruses are maintained in a mosquito-bird-mosquito cycle.
   d. Domestic pigs also act as a reservoir for Japanese encephalitis virus.
   e. Humans are considered dead-end hosts for Japanese encephalitis virus and related viruses.
   f. Japanese encephalitis and related virus infections usually occur in the late summer and early fall.

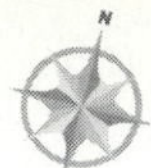

3. **Pathogenesis:** Japanese encephalitis virus and related viruses infect mosquitoes and establish a persistent infection.
   a. The virus is inoculated directly into the blood stream of the host by the infected mosquito.
   b. Virus spreads through the blood to cells of the monocyte-macrophage lineage, with the brain as the target organ; it spreads to the CNS via capillary endothelial cells or the choroid plexus.
   c. Antibody and cell-mediated immunity are important in controlling infections.
4. **Laboratory diagnosis:** Detection of virus-specific IgM by EIA in serum or cerebrospinal fluid is the laboratory method of choice.
5. **Treatment:** There is no effective treatment for Japanese encephalitis virus and related viruses.
6. **Prevention:** There are no vaccines available to prevent St. Louis encephalitis, Murray Valley encephalitis, or West Nile virus infections in humans.
   a. Killed and live, attenuated vaccines to prevent Japanese encephalitis virus infection are available for routine immunization of infants and children in Japan and China.
   b. Mosquito vector control is a key means of prevention.
   c. Wearing protective clothing and applying mosquito repellant containing DEET are important preventive steps to avoid mosquito bites.

WEST NILE VIRUS

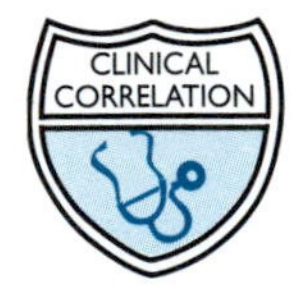

- *In 1999, a cluster of encephalitis cases occurred in New York City.*
- *In 4 years, West Nile virus infections evolved from an initial localized epidemic to a disease endemic in North America.*
- *The mosquito-borne disease is more common but less fatal than EEE. Infection in birds often precedes appearance of the human disease.*
- *Like other mosquito-borne viral diseases, personal and household protection from mosquitoes is the best means of prevention.*

E. Hepatitis C and Hepatitis G Viruses

1. **Clinical manifestations:** HCV causes **acute and chronic hepatitis,** and HCV infection predisposes individuals to the development of **hepatocellular carcinoma.**
   a. Primary HCV infections are asymptomatic or result in a mild illness with nonspecific symptoms and rare jaundice.
   b. Chronic hepatitis develops in 75% of HCV infections.
   c. About half of the patients with chronic hepatitis are asymptomatic for 20–30 years. The other half experience chronic liver disease characterized by fatigue and elevated liver enzymes.
   d. Approximately 25% of patients have moderate to severe chronic hepatitis that progresses to liver cirrhosis and are at increased risk for hepatocellular carcinoma (1–4% per year).
   e. HGV is related to HCV, is not a major cause of hepatitis, and is of uncertain clinical significance.
2. **Transmission/epidemiology:** HCV is transmitted **parenterally** by exposure to **blood** and blood products.
   a. Intravenous drug users and organ transplant recipients are at high risk for HCV infection.

b. Sexual and maternal-fetal routes of transmission are less common for HCV.
c. HCV is distributed worldwide. Before routine screening of blood for HCV, HCV infection was the major cause of posttransfusion hepatitis.
d. HCV-associated cirrhosis is the most common indication for a liver transplant.
e. HGV is transmitted predominately by the parental route but can also be transmitted sexually.
f. HGV is distributed worldwide and is estimated to cause 0.3% of posttransfusion hepatitis in the United States.
g. Coinfections of HCV and HGV are common, and HGV does not increase the severity of HCV infection.

3. **Pathogenesis:** HCV infects hepatocytes, causing acute and chronic hepatitis.
   a. Liver injury is mediated by cytotoxic T cells that contribute both to inflammation and viral clearance.
   b. Hepatocellular carcinoma linked to HCV infections is indirect (ie, the virus does not encode an oncogene) and is likely due to compensatory hepatocyte proliferation as a consequence of liver injury, thus providing a pool of dividing cells susceptible to genetic mutations.
   c. HGV pathogenesis is poorly understood.
4. **Virulence factors:** HCV can mutate at high frequency, creating significant variations in the major envelope protein and allowing escape from virus-neutralizing antibodies. HCV NS3/4A serine protease blocks cellular interferon activation and synthesis to circumvent a major host immune response mechanism.
5. **Laboratory diagnosis:** HCV is diagnosed most commonly by EIA for HCV antibody and by RT-PCR for virion RNA. HGV can be detected in serum by RT-PCR, but routine testing for HGV is not recommended because its clinical significance is unknown.
6. **Treatment:** A combination of interferon-alpha and ribavirin is recommended for treatment of chronic HCV hepatitis. There is no specific antiviral therapy for HGV.
7. **Prevention:** There are no vaccines available for HCV or HGV. Screening blood products and avoiding intravenous drug use are important steps in preventing HCV infection.

HEPATITIS C

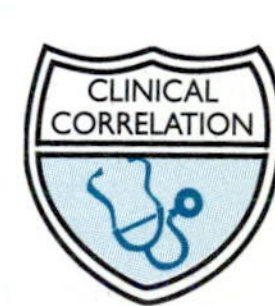

- *Some 170 million people worldwide and 4 million people in the United States are estimated to be infected with HCV and at risk for chronic hepatitis and its associated morbidity.*
- *The development of a serologic assay to detect HCV antibody in blood donors dramatically reduced the incidence of hepatitis contracted by blood transfusions.*
- *HCV remains highly prevalent in intravenous drug users.*

VII. Coronaviridae Family

A. Coronaviruses

1. Coronaviruses are enveloped, (+) RNA viruses with helical symmetry.
2. Coronaviruses were so named (*corona* = crown in Latin) to depict the crown-like spikes seen under electron microscopy and that adorn the virion envelope.
3. Coronaviruses have the largest known RNA genome.

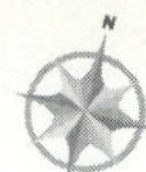

4. The error-prone, RNA-dependent RNA polymerase of coronaviruses results in a high frequency of recombination and the generation of mutant progeny viruses.
5. Coronaviruses consist of four serologically unrelated groups and cause disease in a range of birds and mammals, including humans.

B. Human Coronavirus

1. **Clinical manifestations:** A novel coronavirus causes **severe acute respiratory syndrome (SARS),** an emerging infectious disease with high morbidity and a mortality rate of 10%.
   a. Previously known coronaviruses cause about 30% of cases of the **common cold.**
   b. SARS is characterized by an incubation period of 2–7 days followed by the onset of high fever, usually accompanied by headache, generalized discomfort, body aches, and diarrhea in 10–20% of cases.
   c. Two to 7 days later, patients with SARS experience a dry, nonproductive cough, hypoxia requiring mechanical ventilation, and pneumonia.
2. **Transmission/epidemiology:** SARS coronavirus transmission is by **respiratory droplets** produced by coughing or sneezing and requires close person-to-person contact.
   a. Infection may also be spread by contaminated fomites and by the fecal-oral route.
   b. SARS was first reported in Hong Kong in 2003. Within months, the SARS outbreak spread to North America, South America, Europe, and Asia and accounted for more than 8000 cases worldwide and approximately 800 deaths.
   c. There were no SARS-associated deaths in the United States, and all cases were attributed to travelers returning from areas with documented SARS.
   d. SARS is an emerging infectious disease that may have jumped from an animal reservoir to humans.
3. **Pathogenesis:** Information as to the full extent of SARS coronavirus pathogenesis is limited.
   a. Lymphopenia (decreased CD4 and CD8 T lymphocytes) and low-grade disseminated intravascular coagulation (thrombocytopenia) are seen in patients with SARS.
   b. Pathologic studies in patients who died of SARS show diffuse alveolar damage.
   c. Severe pulmonary damage may be due to coronavirus directly or may represent secondary effects of cytokines or other host factors induced by coronavirus infection.
4. **Virulence factors:** The capacity of coronavirus to undergo high-frequency recombination provides an immune evasion strategy.
5. **Laboratory diagnosis:** The SARS coronavirus can be identified by RT-PCR, by serologic tests to detect coronavirus-specific antibody, or by viral isolation in cell culture.
6. **Treatment:** There is no specific antiviral therapy for SARS coronavirus infection.
7. **Prevention:** There are no vaccines available to prevent SARS coronavirus infection.
   a. Preventive measures to contain the spread of the SARS coronavirus are to isolate persons who are ill and to quarantine persons who have been exposed to the SARS coronavirus.

b. Measures to prevent the spread and exposure of the SARS coronavirus include washing hands frequently, imposing travel restrictions to areas with SARS, and health care workers' wearing masks, gloves, and eye protection.

SARS

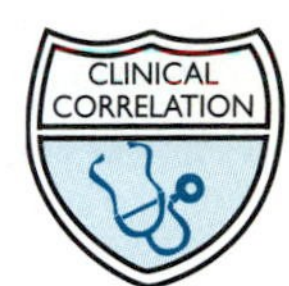

- *SARS represents an emerging infectious disease.*
- *Within months after the outbreak, the virus was isolated, identified, and contained because of strict isolation and quarantine procedures.*
- *Genome sequencing determined that the SARS coronavirus was different from all known coronaviruses.*
- *The identification of the natural host for the SARS coronavirus and the development of antiviral drugs and vaccines for it are urgently needed research and public health objectives.*

CLINICAL PROBLEMS

During 2002, the state health department reported 60 outbreaks of acute gastroenteritis affecting more than 1500 persons from a community hospital, the county jail, 3 restaurants, and 6 nursing homes. Illness was characterized by diarrhea, nausea, and vomiting, with an average duration of 48 hours and an incubation period of 24–48 hours.

1. The virus most likely responsible for the outbreaks of acute gastroenteritis is:

A. Rotavirus

B. HAV

C. HEV

D. Norovirus

E. Astrovirus

A 25-year-old man is seen in an outpatient clinic with a chief complaint of fatigue, nausea, and vomiting for the past several days. He had noticed that morning that his urine was dark yellow. On physical examination, the patient has a low-grade fever and mild abdominal pain and is jaundiced. He denies intravenous drug use or multiple sexual partners. He had attended a 5-day outdoor rock concert in North Carolina 3 weeks earlier. He is a cook at the local university dining hall.

2. The picornavirus most likely responsible for this case of viral hepatitis is:

A. HAV

B. HBV

C. HCV

D. HEV

E. HGV

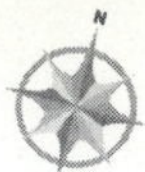

3. The recommended prophylaxis of exposed contacts to prevent spread of the disease is:
   A. Interferon-alpha
   B. Interferon-alpha with ribavirin
   C. Lamivudine
   D. Virus-specific immune globulin
   E. Acyclovir

A 50-year-old woman was admitted to the hospital with symptoms of high fever, headache, neck stiffness, and disorientation. She received medical treatment and recovered. Serum results sent to the state public health laboratory were positive for St. Louis encephalitis virus IgM antibody.

4. How is St. Louis encephalitis virus transmitted?
   A. By the fecal-oral route
   B. Sexually
   C. By respiratory droplets
   D. By infected mosquitoes
   E. By infected ticks

5. St. Louis encephalitis virus and West Nile virus are closely related flaviviruses that produce similar clinical symptoms in humans. One difference that distinguishes them is:
   A. The insect vector
   B. The mode of transmission
   C. A preventive vaccine for St. Louis encephalitis
   D. Effective antiviral therapy for West Nile virus
   E. The vector control measure

ANSWERS

1. The answer is D. Noroviruses cause acute gastroenteritis primarily in adults and characterized by a short incubation period (1–2 days) and brief, self-limited illness (1–2 days). Rotaviruses and astroviruses cause acute gastroenteritis primarily in infants and young children. HAV and HEV cause hepatitis after a longer incubation period (15–50 days).

2. The answer is A. This is a typical case of HAV infection with clinical and epidemiologic clues to support the presumptive diagnosis. None of the other hepatitis viruses are picornaviruses. HBV, HCV, and HGV are transmitted parenterally. HEV is a calicivirus transmitted by the fecal-oral route.

3. The answer is D, virus-specific immune globulin, specifically HAV immune globulin. Postexposure prophylaxis with HAV immune globulin is recommended for those ex-

posed to the index case within 2 weeks of exposure. Interferon-alpha with ribavirin is effective in treatment (not prophylaxis) of HCV infection. Interferon alone is not effective. Lamivudine is an RT inhibitor used to treat HBV infection. Acyclovir, an inhibitor of thymidine kinase, is used to treat herpesvirus infections.

4. The answer is D. St. Louis encephalitis is a mosquito-borne viral encephalitis. It is not spread from person to person.

5. The answer is B, modes of transmission. West Nile virus can be transmitted by the bite of infected mosquitoes and through blood transfusion, organ transplants, breast milk, and transplacentally. St. Louis encephalitis is known to be transmitted only by mosquitoes. The mosquito is the insect vector for both viruses. There are no vaccines or antiviral drugs for either virus, and vector control measures are the same to prevent both.

CHAPTER 13
NEGATIVE-STRAND RNA VIRUSES

I. Key Concepts

A. Negative-strand (–) RNA viruses have single-stranded (ss) RNA genomes complementary to mRNA (ie, they are of negative polarity and are incapable of acting as mRNA).

B. All (–) RNA viruses carry a virion-associated, RNA-dependent-RNA polymerase that transcribes genomic RNA into mRNA. (The same polymerase synthesizes a full-length, positive-strand copy of the viral RNA genome that acts as a template for new (–) RNA genomes.)

C. Medically important (–) RNA viruses are a diverse collection of 6 virus families (Paramyxoviridae, Rhabdoviridae, Orthomyxoviridae, Filoviridae, Bunyaviridae, Arenaviridae) that share similar characteristics in terms of nucleic acid composition, shape, virion polymerase, and replication site (Table 13–1).

II. Paramyxoviridae Family

A. Paramyxoviruses

1. Members of the Paramyxoviridae family include parainfluenza virus (PIV), respiratory syncytial virus (RSV), measles virus, and mumps virus.
2. All paramyxoviruses initiate infection via the respiratory tract.
3. PIV and RSV cause localized infections of the respiratory tract, whereas measles virus and mumps virus cause systemic infections and produce generalized disease.
4. Paramyxovirus envelope has 2 important viral proteins (Table 13–2): the hemagglutinin and neuraminidase (HN) protein and the fusion (F) protein.
   - **a.** A viral attachment protein is the HN protein, with both *h*emagglutinating and *n*euraminidase activities, typical of PIV and mumps, the H protein of measles virus, and the G protein of RSV.
   - **b.** The fusion (F) protein mediates fusion of the viral envelope with the plasma membrane of the susceptible cell, facilitating entry.

B. Parainfluenza Virus

1. **Clinical manifestations:** There are four known serotypes (PIV types 1, 2, 3, and 4).
   - **a.** **PIV types 1 and 2** are the major cause of **croup** (ie, laryngotracheobronchitis) in infants and young children.
   - **b.** **Croup** is characterized by a fever, hoarseness, a barking cough, and inspiratory stridor.
   - **c.** **PIV type 3** is associated with **bronchiolitis** and **pneumonia** in infants and young children.

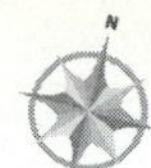

Table 13–1. Common properties of negative-strand RNA viruses.

Virus family	RNA Structure	Virion Polymerase	Shape	Envelope	Site of Replication	Human Viruses
Paramyxoviridae	Linear, ss, (–), non-segmented	Yes	Helical	Yes	Cytoplasm	Parainfluenza virus Respiratory syncytial virus Measles virus Mumps virus
Rhabdoviridae	Linear, ss, (–), non-segmented	Yes	Helical, bullet shaped	Yes	Cytoplasm	Rabies virus
Orthomyxoviridae	Linear, ss, (–), segmented	Yes	Helical	Yes	Nucleus	Influenza virus
Filoviridae	Linear, ss, (–), non-segmented	Yes	Helical, filamentous	Yes	Cytoplasm	Ebola virus Marburg virus
Bunyaviridae	Circular, ss, (–), segmented	Yes	Helical	Yes	Cytoplasm	LaCrosse virus California encephalitis virus Hantavirus
Arenaviridae	Circular, ss, (–), segmented	Yes	Helical	Yes	Cytoplasm	Lassa fever virus Lymphocytic choriomeningitis virus

ss, single-stranded.

d. PIV type 4 is infrequently detected and causes a mild upper respiratory infection in children and adults.
e. PIVs cause mild, nonspecific upper respiratory infections in immunocompetent adults but may have serious consequences in immunocompromised patients.
f. Reinfections with PIVs are common in children and adults.

2. **Transmission/epidemiology:** PIV infections are transmitted by **respiratory droplets** or by direct contact with secretions or fomites.
   a. Infection occurs when virus contacts mucous membranes of the eyes, nose, or mouth or via inhalation of respiratory droplets.
   b. Reinfections are common and immunity transient.

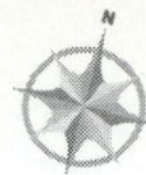

Table 13–2. Envelope glycoproteins of paramyxoviruses.

Envelope Protein	Parainfluenza Virus	Respiratory Syncytial Virus	Measles Virus	Mumps Virus	Functions
Hemagglutinin (H)	–	–	+	-	Viral attachment
Hemagglutinin neuraminidase (HN)[a]	+	–	–	+	Viral attachment & release
Attachment (G)	–	+	-	–	Viral attachment
Fusion (F)	+	+	+	+	Penetration & entry

[a]Hemagglutinin and neuraminidase activity on the same protein

3. **Pathogenesis:** PIV infects and damages respiratory epithelial cells without systemic spread. Histopathologic changes include the presence of multinucleated giant cells caused by the viral F protein.
4. **Virulence factors:** PIV evades host antibody by direct cell-to-cell spread mediated by the F protein.
5. **Laboratory diagnosis:** PIV can be isolated and detected in cell culture by hemadsorption.
   a. PIV can be identified by immunocytochemistry with PIV-specific antibodies.
   b. Rapid, direct detection of PIV antigen in epithelial cells of nasal aspirates is achieved by immunofluorescence.
6. **Treatment:** There is no specific therapy for PIV infections.
7. **Prevention:** No vaccine is available to protect against PIV infection. Strict attention to infection control practices reduces nosocomial PIV infection.

CROUP

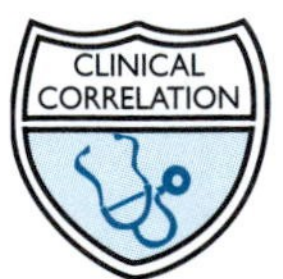

- *Croup is an acute viral infection caused by PIVs.*
- *PIVs are second to RSVs as the most important cause of lower respiratory disease in young children.*

C. Respiratory Syncytial Virus

1. **Clinical manifestations:** RSV is the most common cause of **bronchiolitis** and **pneumonia** in infants and children under age 1.
   a. Bronchiolitis in infants is characterized by a pronounced cough, expiratory wheezing, and cyanosis.
   b. Otitis media is the most common complication of RSV infection in infants.
   c. RSV causes nonspecific upper respiratory tract disease symptoms in healthy adults.
   d. RSV causes an influenzalike syndrome in elderly patients.

2. **Transmission/epidemiology:** RSV infections are transmitted by **respiratory droplets** and by direct contact of contagious secretions from contaminated hands.
    a. RSV has 2 serotypes (A and B). Subgroup A infections are more prevalent and severe than subgroup B.
    b. Community outbreaks of RSV infection occur annually in late fall to early spring.
    c. Infants at high risk of mortality from RSV infection include neonates, premature infants, and infants with underlying cardiopulmonary disease or those who are immunologically compromised.
    d. Reinfections with RSV are common in children and adults.
3. **Pathogenesis:** RSV infection is localized primarily to the lower respiratory tract in infants without viremia or systemic spread.
    a. Multinucleated giant cells are a common histopathologic finding in pulmonary specimens.
    b. The narrow airways of infants are readily obstructed by virus-induced pathology.
    c. Severe disease in infants may have an immunologic basis (eg, tissue injury from inflammatory cytokines).
4. **Virulence factors:** RSV evades host antibody by direct cell-to-cell spread mediated by the F protein.
5. **Laboratory diagnosis:** RSV can be isolated in cell culture and detected by characteristic formation of syncytia (ie, multinucleated giant cells).
    a. RSV identity can be confirmed by immunocytochemistry with virus-specific antibody.
    b. Rapid diagnosis of RSV infection can be made by direct detection of RSV antigen in nasal aspirates by EIA.
6. **Treatment:** Ribavirin aerosol is approved for treatment of infants hospitalized with severe RSV infection.
7. **Prevention:** No vaccine is available to prevent RSV infection.
    a. Passive immunization with a monoclonal antibody directed against RSV F protein (palivizumab) or hyperimmune globulin is available for high-risk infants.
    b. Nosocomial infection is reduced by strict attention to infection control practices.

RSV

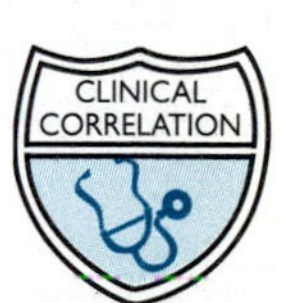

- *The characteristic syncytia formation in cell culture mediated by RSV F protein enabled the development of a rapid and sensitive method to detect RSV in clinical specimens and to diagnose RSV disease.*

D. Measles Virus

1. **Clinical manifestations:** Measles infections are marked by a prodromal phase characterized by fever, cough, coryza, and conjunctivitis.
    a. One to 2 days later, **Koplik's spots** (ie, small white spots on inflamed buccal mucosa) appear inside the cheek, followed a day later by a maculopapular rash, appearing first on the head and spreading to the trunk and extremities and lasting 3–5 days.
    b. The complications of measles, particularly in developing countries, in malnourished children, and in immunocompromised individuals, include
        (1) Encephalitis.
        (2) Virus-induced giant cell pneumonia.

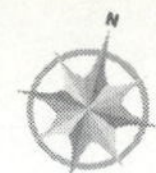

(3) Opportunistic bacterial superinfections (otitis media, pneumonia).

(4) **Subacute sclerosing panencephalitis,** a rare late progressive neurologic disease that occurs months or years after clinical measles.

2. **Transmission/epidemiology:** Measles virus is transmitted by **respiratory droplets.**
   - **a.** Measles virus has a single serotype.
   - **b.** Measles virus is highly contagious with an 85–95% infection rate.
3. **Pathogenesis:** Measles virus initially infects respiratory epithelial cells and then spreads and multiplies in the lymph nodes.
   - **a.** The virus then enters the blood (viremia) and is disseminated to distant sites throughout the body, including the skin and mucosa.
   - **b.** Formation of multinucleated giant cells, resulting from fusion of infected cells with neighboring uninfected cells, is a characteristic pathologic feature of measles virus infection.
   - **c.** The maculopapular rash is due to a cell-mediated immune attack by cytotoxic T cells on virus-infected vascular endothelial cells in the skin.
   - **d.** General temporary suppression of cell-mediated immunity associated with measles is a consequence of infection of T and B cells, which results in a depressed immune response and is the major cause of secondary infections responsible for morbidity and mortality.
   - **e.** Cell-mediated immunity is essential to recovery from measles.
4. **Virulence factors:** Measles virus evades host antibody by direct cell-to-cell spread mediated by the F protein. The ability to induce a temporary general immunosuppression either directly or indirectly enables the virus to evade immune recognition.
5. **Laboratory diagnosis:** Cell culture isolation of the virus is uncommon. Serologic diagnosis by enzyme immunoassay (EIA) of measles virus-specific antibody is the most common diagnostic approach.
6. **Treatment:** There is no specific therapy for measles virus infection.
7. **Prevention:** Live, attenuated measles virus vaccine is highly effective in preventing measles. The vaccine is usually given in combination with mumps and rubella vaccines.

EFFECTIVE MEASLES VACCINE

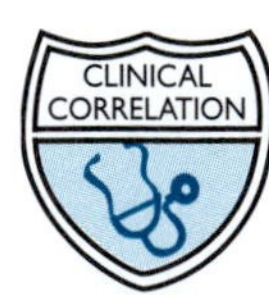

- *Measles virus is highly contagious.*
- *Widespread use of the live, attenuated measles vaccine has dramatically reduced the incidence of measles from the prevaccine level of 7–8 million deaths worldwide to 1 million deaths annually, mostly in developing countries.*

E. Mumps Virus

1. **Clinical manifestations:** Mumps, a common disease of school-age children, is rare in the United States because of an effective vaccine.
   - **a.** Classic symptoms of mumps virus infection include a prodromal phase characterized by fever, malaise, and headache followed by **parotitis** (ie, parotid gland pain and inflammation and swelling).
   - **b.** Parotitis occurs in less than 50% of infections.
   - **c.** Aseptic meningitis is a common manifestation of mumps; encephalitis is rare.
   - **d.** Complications of mumps include **orchitis** (ie, inflammation/swelling of the testis) in adult males. Sterility is uncommon.

2. **Transmission/epidemiology:** Mumps virus is highly contagious.
   a. The virus is spread by respiratory droplets, salivary secretions, or urine.
   b. Mumps virus has a single serotype.
3. **Pathogenesis:** Mumps virus initially infects the respiratory epithelial cells and spreads to regional lymph nodes.
   a. After a transient viremia, the virus is disseminated to the salivary glands, central nervous system (CNS), and other sites.
   b. Parotid gland swelling is due to inflammation, lymphocyte infiltration, and edema.
   c. Viruria (ie, virus in the urine) is common.
   d. Cell-mediated immunity is essential to recovery from disease.
4. **Virulence factors:** Mumps virus evades host antibody by direct cell-to-cell spread that is mediated by the F protein.
5. **Laboratory diagnosis:** Mumps virus isolation in cell culture is not a routinely available test. Serologic diagnosis by EIA of mumps virus-specific antibody is the most common diagnostic approach.
6. **Treatment:** There is no specific therapy for mumps virus infection.
7. **Prevention:** A live, attenuated mumps virus vaccine is highly effective in preventing mumps. The vaccine is usually given in combination with measles and rubella vaccines.

MUMPS VACCINE

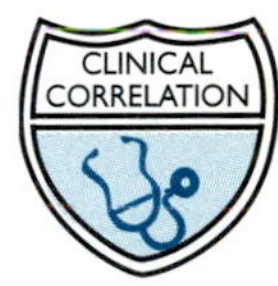

- *Isolation and propagation of mumps virus in cell culture led to the development of a safe, effective mumps virus vaccine.*
- *Widespread mumps vaccination resulted in a 98% reduction in the incidence of mumps and its CNS sequelae.*

III. Rhabdoviridae Family

A. Rhabdoviruses

1. Rhabdoviruses have a distinctive bullet-shaped morphology.
2. Rabies virus is the most important human pathogen.
3. Rabies is a **viral zoonotic infection,** an infection in which viruses are transmitted between animals and humans.

B. Rabies Virus

1. **Clinical manifestations:** The incubation period is variable, averaging 30–60 days after a bite exposure.
   a. A prodromal phase is characterized by fever, malaise, nausea, vomiting, and pain or itching at the site of the bite wound.
   b. The neurologic phase is characterized by hyperactivity, agitation, hydrophobia, encephalitis, and coma.
   c. The disease is almost always fatal.
2. **Transmission/epidemiology:** Rabies virus is transmitted by infectious saliva from the bite of a rabid animal or aerosol contact with mucous membranes. Raccoons, skunks, bats, coyotes, and foxes are natural reservoirs of infection in the United States.
3. **Pathogenesis:** Rabies virus multiplies at the site of the bite, then infects sensory neurons by attaching to the acetylcholine receptor.
   a. The virus ascends axons to the CNS and replicates in gray matter.
   b. Virus then descends down peripheral nerves to skin and salivary glands.

 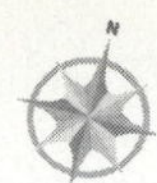

c. **Negri bodies** (ie, cytoplasmic eosinophilic inclusions of rabies virus nucleocapsids) detected in neurons are pathognomonic of rabies.
d. Cell-mediated immunity is insufficient to prevent disease.

4. **Virulence factors:** The neurotropic virus evades immune surveillance by sequestration in neurons, an immunologically privileged site.
5. **Laboratory diagnosis:** Rabies is diagnosed by cytologic detection of Negri bodies or by immunocytochemical detection of viral antigen in brain tissue at autopsy.
   a. In live patients, rabies virus antigens can be detected by immunocytochemistry in biopsy specimens from corneal scrapings or skin from the nape of the neck.
   b. Rabies virus RNA in saliva can be detected by reverse transcriptase–polymerase chain reaction.
6. **Treatment:** There is no specific treatment for rabies once clinical symptoms have developed.
7. **Prevention:** Postexposure prophylaxis (ie, treatment after exposure to a bite of a rabid animal) and preexposure prophylaxis are available.
   a. Postexposure prophylaxis consists of
      (1) Thorough washing of the wound.
      (2) Passive immunization with human rabies immune globulin into the wound.
      (3) Active immunization with rabies vaccine.
   b. Pre-exposure prophylaxis by active immunization with rabies vaccine is recommended for high-risk individuals (eg, veterinarians and animal handlers).

RABIES INCUBATION PERIOD

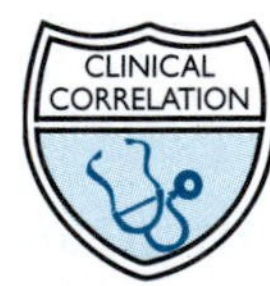

- *Rabies is one of the rare examples in medicine in which active immunization against infection can be initiated after a bite exposure because of the long incubation period.*

IV. Orthomyxoviridae Family

A. Orthomyxoviruses

1. Influenza viruses are members of the Orthomyxoviridae family.
2. Three types are known: influenza A, B, and C.
3. Influenza A and B contain ss (–) RNA in 8 segments. Influenza C has 7 discrete RNA segments.
4. Influenza A causes epidemic disease with significant mortality. Influenza B causes sporadic and epidemic disease, usually milder than influenza A. Influenza C causes infrequent, subclinical disease (Table 13–3).

B. Influenza A and B Viruses

1. **Clinical manifestations:** Influenza has an abrupt onset characterized by fever, chills, prostration, myalgia, and headache.
   a. This is followed by respiratory symptoms of rhinitis and dry cough.
   b. Recovery is often slow with fatigue, weakness, and cough persisting for 2–4 weeks.
   c. Complications of influenza virus include
      (1) Secondary bacterial pneumonia (common), usually caused by *Streptococcus pneumoniae, Staphylococcus aureus,* or *Haemophilus influenzae.*
      (2) Primary viral pneumonia (uncommon).
   d. Individuals at greater risk for complications include the elderly and individuals with chronic cardiac or pulmonary disease.

Table 13–3. Comparison of influenza A, B, and C viruses.

Property	Influenza A	Influenza B	Influenza C
RNA segments	8	8	7
Antigenic variation	Frequent	Less frequent	Less frequent
Host range	Humans, pigs, birds, horses	Humans only	Humans only
Human disease	Influenza epidemics & pandemics	Influenza; occasional epidemics	Subclinical infections

2. **Transmission/epidemiology:** Influenza is spread directly by **respiratory droplets.**
   - **a.** Influenza A has a broad host range capable of infecting humans, swine, horses, and birds.
   - **b.** Influenza B host range is limited to humans.
   - **c.** Antigen variation of influenza virus envelope protein **hemagglutinin (H)** or **neuraminidase (N)** is responsible for epidemic and pandemic diseases.
   - **d.** Two types of antigenic variation are known.
     - *(1)* **Antigenic shift** (influenza A only) entails a major change in H or N antigens or both as a result of **genetic reassortment** of RNA gene segments between 2 influenza A subtypes. For example, coinfection of a cell with a human influenza A virus and a swine influenza A virus yields a hybrid virus with antigens derived from either of the parental viruses (Figure 13–1).
     - *(2)* **Antigenic drift** (influenza A and B) involves minor changes affecting H or N antigens due to point mutations in RNA segments coding for H or N.
   - **e.** Antigenic shifts are responsible for influenza **pandemics** because the new virus variant is introduced into a population with no preexisting immunity.
   - **f.** Antigenic drift favors the emergence of new viruses that account for yearly outbreaks of influenza.
3. **Pathogenesis:** Virus attaches via the envelope H protein to sialic acid–containing cell receptors.
   - **a.** Infection is limited primarily to ciliated epithelial cells of the respiratory tract, leading to cell death.
   - **b.** Denudation of the respiratory epithelium causes an acute inflammatory response and renders the individual susceptible to bacterial superinfection.
   - **c.** The systemic complaints common with influenza are caused by host production of various cytokines.
   - **d.** Interferon, virus-specific secretory IgA, and cytotoxic T-cell responses are associated with recovery from infection.
4. **Virulence factors:** The segmented genome facilitates genetic reassortment and antigenic shift in influenza A. Mutability of viral envelope proteins H and N permits escape from immune recognition.

Figure 13–1. Mechanism of antigenic shift in influenza A virus.

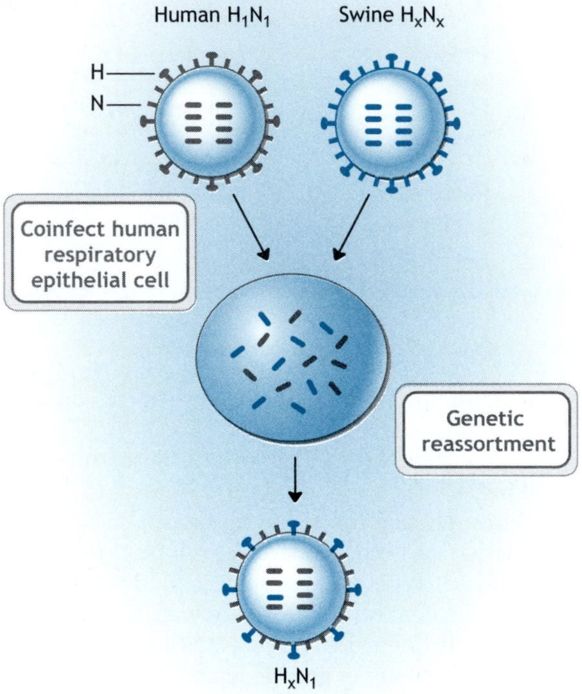

Human H_1N_1

Swine H_xN_x

H

N

Coinfect human respiratory epithelial cell

Genetic reassortment

H_xN_1

5. **Laboratory diagnosis:** Virus can be detected in clinical specimens by EIA or immunocytochemistry. Virus can be isolated in cell culture and identified by immunocytochemistry with virus-specific antibody.
6. **Treatment:** Antiviral drugs are an adjunct but not a substitute for influenza vaccine.
   a. Amantadine and rimantadine are approved for treatment of influenza A (neither is effective for influenza B).
   b. Neuraminidase inhibitors (zanamivir and oseltamivir) are approved for treatment of both influenza A and B viruses.
7. **Prevention:** Vaccination with a killed vaccine containing current influenza A and B strains is the single most effective method to prevent influenza and its severe complications.
   a. Groups targeted for influenza vaccination include
      (1) Persons 50 years of age and older.
      (2) Persons with chronic cardiopulmonary disease (including asthma).
      (3) Persons requiring medical care for chronic metabolic diseases (eg, diabetes), renal dysfunction, or immunosuppression.

(4) Residents of nursing homes and other long-term care facilities.
(5) Persons who can transmit influenza to high-risk individuals (eg, health care workers, employees of nursing homes and chronic care facilities, household members of persons at risk).

b. A live, attenuated influenza A vaccine, given intranasally, is available for healthy adults and children.

INFLUENZA

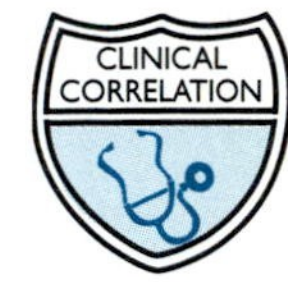

- *Influenza ranks among the top 10 causes of death in the United States because of its remarkable capacity for antigenic variation, ensuring continual circulation in the population and requiring annual vaccination.*

V. Filoviridae Family

A. Filoviruses

1. Filoviruses are **viral zoonoses** that cause severe hemorrhagic fever in humans.
2. Filoviruses have a highly pleomorphic, filamentous (threadlike) morphology.
3. Ebola virus and Marburg virus are the important human pathogens.

B. Ebola and Marburg Viruses

1. **Clinical manifestations:** Ebola and Marburg viruses cause severe hemorrhagic fever characterized by sudden onset of fever, headache, joint and muscle pain, followed by vomiting, diarrhea, and abdominal pain.
   - **a.** Symptoms become increasingly severe with bleeding into the skin, mucous membranes, and visceral organs.
   - **b.** Death is due to multiorgan failure and shock.
2. **Transmission/epidemiology:** Human-to-human transmission occurs by direct contact with contaminated body fluids (ie, blood or secretions from an infected individual).
   - **a.** Ebola and Marburg viruses have a greater than 90% mortality rate.
   - **b.** The natural reservoir for Ebola and Marburg viruses is unknown.
3. **Pathogenesis:** The viruses initially infect macrophages and then spread systemically via lymphatics and blood to infect and cause necrosis of the liver, spleen, and lymph nodes. Tissue destruction and large quantities of cytokines cause vascular permeability, hemorrhage, and shock.
4. **Virulence factors:** In Ebola virus infection, the viral glycoprotein acts as a determinant of vascular cell cytotoxicity and injury. In Marburg virus infection, no virulence factors are known.
5. **Laboratory diagnosis:** Ebola or Marburg virus antigen can be detected in tissues by immunohistochemistry or antigen capture EIA.
   - **a.** Polymerase chain reaction is used to detect viral RNA in clinical specimens.
   - **b.** Serologic detection of virus-specific IgM or IgG can be used for diagnosis.
6. **Treatment:** There is no specific treatment for Ebola or Marburg hemorrhagic fever.
7. **Prevention:** There are no vaccines for Ebola or Marburg hemorrhagic fever.
   - **a.** Patients with suspected or confirmed infections should be isolated.
   - **b.** Barrier techniques should be used to prevent direct physical contact with the patient and patient blood or body fluids.

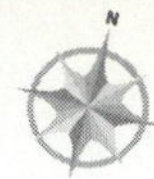

EBOLA HEMORRHAGIC FEVER

CLINICAL CORRELATION

- *Outbreaks of hemorrhagic fever caused by Ebola virus are associated with high mortality rates.*
- *Containment of these lethal outbreaks is an urgent public health problem.*
- *Efforts to develop a vaccine against Ebola offer a possible intervention to limit the spread of the disease.*

VI. Bunyaviridae Family

A. Bunyaviruses

1. The Bunyaviridae family has more than 300 serologically distinct viruses.
2. The viral genome consists of 3 segments of circular ss (–) RNA.
3. The Bunyaviridae family contains 2 medically important genera in the United States.
   a. The *Bunyavirus* genus is represented by California encephalitis virus and LaCrosse virus.
   b. The *Hantavirus* genus is represented by hantavirus.

B. California Encephalitis (CE) and LaCrosse Virus

1. **Clinical manifestations:** Most infections with CE or LaCrosse virus are subclinical or result in a mild, febrile illness.
   a. Encephalitis caused by CE or LaCrosse virus is characterized by a sudden onset of fever, headache, malaise, nausea, and vomiting.
   b. Seizures occur in about 50% of patients with encephalitis.
   c. Disease usually resolves in 5–7 days.
   d. Death is uncommon, but seizure disorders may be a sequela in some patients.
2. **Transmission/epidemiology:** CE or LaCrosse virus is an **arbovirus** (arthropod-borne) and transmitted by the bite of infected mosquitoes. CE (LaCrosse disease) is endemic in the Midwest.
3. **Pathogenesis:** The bite of an infected mosquito initiates a viremia. Establishment of a secondary viremia allows dissemination of the virus to CNS target tissue.
4. **Virulence factors:** No virulence factors are known.
5. **Laboratory diagnosis:** Diagnosis is generally established by serologic testing for IgM and IgG antibodies to CE or LaCrosse virus.
6. **Treatment:** There is no specific treatment for CE or LaCrosse viral infections.
7. **Prevention:** No vaccine is available. Insecticides are important in mosquito vector control.

C. Hantavirus

1. **Clinical manifestations:** Hantavirus causes **hantavirus pulmonary syndrome (HPS),** which is characterized by a brief influenzalike prodromal illness consisting of fever, myalgia, headache, cough, and gastrointestinal symptoms.
   a. The disease rapidly progresses to shortness of breath, pulmonary edema, thrombocytopenia, and hypotension.
   b. The majority of patients require mechanical ventilation.
   c. HPS has a high mortality rate (>50%) in previously healthy adults.
2. **Transmission/epidemiology:** Hantavirus is transmitted by aerosol inhalation of infected rodent excreta.
   a. The **deer mouse** is the rodent reservoir for HPS.
   b. Person-to-person transmission of hantavirus has not been observed in the United States.

c. HPS is a **viral zoonosis.**
d. Sin Nombre virus is the most important hantavirus in the United States and Canada.

3. **Pathogenesis:** Hantavirus multiplies in pulmonary capillary endothelial cells, where viral antigens and viral inclusions can be detected (by immunocytochemistry or electron microscopy).
   a. At autopsy, patients with HPS had bilateral pleural effusions with interstitial infiltrates of mononuclear cells.
   b. Immune injury of virus-infected endothelial cells may be a component of HPS pathogenesis.
   c. Humoral and cell-mediated immunity is believed to be responsible for recovery and protection from repeat infection.
4. **Virulence factors:** No virulence factors have been identified.
5. **Laboratory diagnosis:** Diagnosis is established by serologic testing to hantavirus IgM and IgG in serum. Hantavirus antigen by immunohistochemistry or viral RNA by reverse transcriptase-polymerase chain reaction can be detected in lung tissue.
6. **Treatment:** No specific treatment is available. Immediate intensive care is essential once symptoms of HPS develop.
7. **Prevention:** No vaccine is available. Control is by avoiding close contact with infected deer mice or their excreta.

HANTAVIRUS IS DEADLY

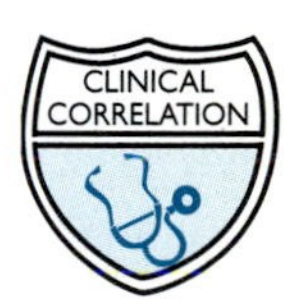

- *Because of its rapid downhill course and high fatality rate, HPS should be considered in patients who present with fever, moderate to severe myalgia, and recent exposure to mice.*
- *Rapid hantavirus-specific IgM serologic assays can aid in the clinical diagnosis.*

VII. Arenaviridae Family

A. Arenaviruses

1. Arenaviruses cause chronic infections in rodents and **zoonotic** infections in humans.
2. The viral genome consists of 2 segments of circular ss (–) RNA.
3. Prototype arenaviruses are Lassa fever virus and lymphocytic choriomeningitis virus (LCMV).

B. Lassa Fever Virus

1. **Clinical manifestations:** Lassa fever virus causes severe hemorrhagic fever characterized by fever, myalgia, and severe prostration.
   a. Hemorrhagic and CNS symptoms develop later.
   b. Hearing loss and spontaneous abortion are common complications.
2. **Transmission/epidemiology:** Virus is transmitted by aerosol inhalation or direct contact with excreta of infected rodents.
   a. Lassa fever may also spread through person-to-person contact with blood, tissue, secretions, or excretions of an infected individual.
   b. The field rat is the rodent reservoir of infection.
   c. Lassa fever is endemic to West Africa.
   d. The mortality rate is 15–20% in hospitalized patients.

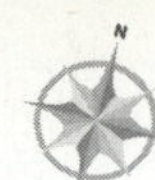

3. **Pathogenesis:** Virus gains entry via inhalation or skin abrasion and replicates in regional lymph nodes before producing a viremia.
   a. Virus infects macrophages and spreads systemically.
   b. Cytokine release from infected macrophages contributes to pathology and is correlated with mortality.
4. **Virulence factors:** No virulence factors are known.
5. **Laboratory diagnosis:** Serologic testing for virus-specific IgM or IgG by EIA is the standard laboratory method for diagnosis.
6. **Treatment:** Ribavirin is useful in the treatment of patients with severe Lassa fever. Convalescent serum, from patients who have recovered from the disease, has been found to be useful in some cases.
7. **Prevention:** No vaccine is available. Rodent control and strict infection control practices are important in prevention.

C. Lymphocytic Choriomeningitis Virus

1. **Clinical manifestations:** Asymptomatic infections with LCMV are common.
   a. Symptomatic infections may present with an influenzalike syndrome with fever, headache, myalgia, and malaise.
   b. LCMV causes aseptic meningitis characterized by fever, headache, and stiff neck in a minority of individuals.
   c. Most patients recover completely.
   d. CNS complications such as weakness, depression, and difficulty concentrating may persist for weeks.
   e. Pregnancy-related infection has been associated with spontaneous abortion, chorioretinitis, congenital hydrocephalus, and mental retardation.
2. **Transmission/epidemiology:** Virus is transmitted by aerosol inhalation, ingestion of contaminated food, or direct contact with excreta of infected rodents.
   a. Person-to-person transmission has not been reported.
   b. The common house mouse is the rodent reservoir of infection.
   c. LCMV has a wide geographic distribution.
   d. The mortality rate associated with LCMV is less than 1%.
3. **Pathogenesis:** The virus gains entry via aerosol inhalation, ingestion, or skin abrasions and replicates in lymph nodes before producing a viremia.
   a. The virus replicates in macrophages and spreads systemically.
   b. Tissue damage in meningitis is linked to release of cytokines and cytotoxic T-cell–induced immunopathology.
4. **Virulence factors:** No virulence factors are known.
5. **Laboratory diagnosis:** Serologic testing for virus-specific IgM or IgG by EIA is the routine method of diagnosis. An immunofluorescent antibody test is an alternative diagnostic tool.
6. **Treatment:** No specific treatment is available.
7. **Prevention:** No vaccine is available. Rodent control is essential for prevention.

LCMV AND CONGENITAL INFECTIONS

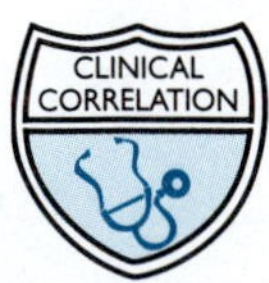

- *LCMV is an underdiagnosed congenital infection.*
- *This diagnosis, along with laboratory confirmation, should be considered for infants with unexplained chorioretinitis and hydrocephalus.*

CLINICAL PROBLEMS

A 70-year-old woman with a history of congestive heart failure has an abrupt onset of fever and cough that requires hospitalization. Two days later, she experiences increasing cough and shortness of breath. Chest x-ray reveals lung infiltrates consistent with viral pneumonia. Rapid antigen test results of nasopharyngeal washings are positive for influenza A virus.

1. Which of the following options would have been the best method to prevent influenza in this patient?

A. Prophylaxis with amantadine

B. Prophylaxis with zanamir

C. Influenza vaccine

D. Hyperimmune influenza immune globulin

A 6-week-old infant is brought to the pediatric clinic in respiratory distress. Physical examination is significant for diffuse expiratory wheezing and mild cyanosis. The chest x-ray is suggestive of bilateral pneumonia. The infant is admitted to the intensive care unit. A nasopharyngeal swab and nasopharyngeal washings are sent for culture and direct examination. The laboratory reports finding multinucleated giant cells in a smear from the swab, and the EIA result is positive for viral antigen.

2. The infection is *most likely* caused by:

A. Adenovirus

B. RSV

C. Influenza virus

D. Herpes simplex virus

E. Rhinovirus

3. The antiviral agent best suited for treating this infant is:

A. Acyclovir

B. Amantadine

C. Ribavirin

D. Ganciclovir

E. Zanamivir

A 20-year-old man seeks care at the hospital emergency department after being bitten by a bat while trying to chase it out of his apartment.

4. Proper treatment of this patient should include:

A. Immunocytochemical staining of a biopsy specimen from the wound site with rabies antibody

B. Histologic examination of tissue biopsied from the wound site for Negri bodies

C. Thorough washing of the wound site with soap and water and reporting the incident to the health department animal control division

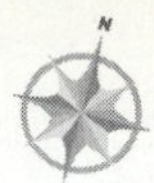

D. Passive administration of rabies immune globulin into the wound and active immunization with rabies vaccine

E. Culture of the wound site for rabies virus isolation and identification

A 3-year-old girl is seen in the emergency department with a high fever, cough, and conjunctivitis. Physical examination reveals small vesicular lesions on an inflamed buccal mucosa and a maculopapular rash on her face that is spreading to her trunk. There is no vaccination record.

5. The virus most likely responsible for this disease is:

A. Paramyxovirus

B. Filovirus

C. Orthomyxovirus

D. Bunyavirus

E. Arenavirus

6. Which of the following is a significant complication of this disease, especially in developing countries?

A. Hepatitis

B. Cellulitis

C. Encephalitis

D. Orchitis

E. Epiglottitis

ANSWERS

1. The answer is C. Influenza vaccination is the most effective method to prevent influenza and its complications.

2. The answer is B. Clinical and laboratory findings in this 6-week-old infant with respiratory distress confirm RSV infection.

3. The answer is C. Ribavirin is used in the treatment of infants hospitalized with severe RSV infection.

4. The answer is D. Postexposure prophylaxis to prevent rabies virus infection is based on the timely administration of a combination of rabies virus hyperimmune globulin directly around the wound site and active immunization with rabies virus vaccine. Choices A, B, and E are laboratory diagnostic procedures inappropriate for patient treatment. Thorough washing of the wound site is insufficient by itself for rabies postexposure prophylaxis.

5. The answer is A. The physical signs and symptoms are characteristic of childhood infection by measles virus, a paramyxovirus.

6. The answer is C. Encephalitis is a severe complication of measles virus infection with significant mortality and morbidity.

CHAPTER 14
DOUBLE-STRANDED RNA VIRUSES

I. Key Concepts

A. **Reoviridae** is the one family of double-stranded (ds) RNA viruses that infects humans and causes human disease.

B. **Reoviruses** are icosahedral, nonenveloped, **segmented ds RNA** viruses that replicate in the cytoplasm.

C. Reoviruses contain an **RNA-dependent RNA polymerase** as part of the virion structure.

D. **Genetic reassortment** of RNA segments promoting antigenic variation is a feature of reoviruses.

E. Medically important reovirus family members are **rotavirus** (11 RNA segments) and **Colorado tick fever (CTF) virus (CTFV)** (12 RNA segments).

II. Reoviridae Family

A. Rotavirus

1. **Clinical manifestations:** Rotavirus causes **acute viral gastroenteritis,** primarily in infants and young children.
   - a. Rotavirus infection is characterized by the sudden onset of nausea, low-grade fever, vomiting, and nonbloody, watery diarrhea lasting 4–5 days.
   - b. Dehydration and electrolyte loss are major complications of severe diarrhea.
   - c. Patients with malnutrition and associated immunodeficiencies are at an increased risk of developing severe rotavirus infections.
2. **Transmission/epidemiology:** Rotavirus is transmitted by the **fecal-oral** route.
   - a. Rotavirus infection occurs worldwide with an estimated 1 million infant deaths due to severe diarrhea, particularly in developing countries.
   - b. Rotavirus gastroenteritis occurs in all age groups, with the peak incidence of severe illness in children 6–24 months of age.
   - c. Rotavirus diarrhea exhibits a marked seasonality in temperate climates. In the United States, the rotavirus season lasts 1–4 months each winter.
   - d. Rotaviruses are divided into 7 groups (A–G), of which group A is the most common cause of diarrheal disease in infants and young children.
3. **Pathogenesis:** After ingestion, rotaviruses infect and lyse epithelial cells (enterocytes) of the small intestine.
   - a. Damaged enterocytes subsequently slough, resulting in stunted villi.
   - b. Damage to the enterocytes is associated with a flux of extraintestinal fluid across the intestinal membrane, resulting in net sodium and protein loss in some patients.

c. Mucosal injury results in a decreased absorptive surface area of the small intestine and decreased production of digestive enzymes (eg, disaccharidases).
d. These deficiencies result in a malabsorptive state leading to a hyperosmotic effect that causes diarrhea.
e. Viral clearance and subsequent immunity are correlated with serum antibody.
f. Intestinal secretory IgA response is correlated with immunity to reinfection.

4. **Virulence factors:** Rotavirus nonstructural protein, NSP4, functions as a viral enterotoxin capable of inducing diarrhea. The segmented genome facilitates genetic reassortment and antigenic shift in rotavirus infections.
5. **Laboratory diagnosis:** Detection of rotavirus antigen in stool by enzyme immunoassay is the method routinely used for diagnosis of infection.
6. **Treatment:** There is no specific therapy for rotavirus infection. Oral rehydration is required in severe cases to replace fluids and electrolytes.
7. **Prevention:** No vaccine for rotavirus infection is currently available.
   a. A live, attenuated virus vaccine was approved but later withdrawn because of an increased incidence of intussusception (ie, bowel obstruction) in vaccinated infants.
   b. Improved sanitation measures and practice of good hygiene, including proper hand washing, are important methods of control.

ACUTE VIRAL GASTROENTERITIS

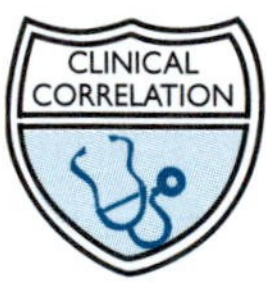

- *Rotavirus infections cause approximately 1 million deaths annually, especially in malnourished children.*
- *In the United States, rotavirus causes approximately 300,000 hospitalizations each year among children younger than 5 years of age.*
- *The development of a rotavirus vaccine is an important strategy for controlling rotavirus disease.*

B. Colorado Tick Fever Virus

1. **Clinical manifestations:** CTF is an acute febrile illness characterized by fever, myalgia, chills, headache, malaise, abdominal pain, and vomiting.
   a. A "saddle-back" fever pattern, consisting of a 2- to 3-day febrile period followed by an afebrile period and subsequent return of the fever, is seen in approximately half of affected patients.
   b. Encephalitis or hemorrhagic fever is a complication of CTFV infection, especially in children.
   c. Fatalities are rare.
2. **Transmission/epidemiology:** CTFV is an **arbovirus** transmitted by the bite of an infected wood tick, *Dermacentor andersoni.*
   a. CTFV is endemic throughout the western United States.
   b. The natural reservoir for CTFV is small mammals (eg, squirrels, chipmunks).
   c. CTF is a **viral zoonosis.**
3. **Pathogenesis:** CTFV enters the skin via a tick bite and infects and replicates in hematopoietic cells, including erythrocyte precursors.
   a. Direct cytopathic effects of the virus on stem cells are likely to account for the frequently observed leukopenia and thrombocytopenia.
   b. The virus persists in mature erythrocytes masked from immune clearance.
   c. Recovery is associated with elevated levels of neutralizing antibody and immunity to reinfection.
4. **Virulence factors:** Residence of CTFV in erythrocytes affords protection from the immune response.

5. **Laboratory diagnosis:** CTFV antigens can be detected on the surface of erythrocytes by direct immunofluorescent staining of blood smears. Serologic testing for virus-specific IgM or IgG by enzyme immunoassay can be used for diagnosis of CTFV infection.
6. **Treatment:** There is no specific therapy for CTFV.
7. **Prevention:** No vaccine is available. Protection from ticks, especially in endemic areas, is the best control method.

CLINICAL PROBLEMS

A 10-month-old infant is admitted to the pediatric unit with a 2-day history of fever; vomiting; and watery, nonbloody diarrhea. Physical examination reveals a mildly dehydrated infant with a temperature of 38 C but who is otherwise normal. A 3-year-old sister attends a daycare center and had a mild episode of diarrhea a week ago.

1. The virus most likely responsible for this diarrheal illness has a:
   A. Segmented, negative-strand RNA genome
   B. Segmented, double-stranded RNA genome
   C. Segmented, circular, negative-strand RNA genome
   D. Nonsegmented, negative-strand RNA genome
   E. Nonsegmented, positive-strand RNA genome
2. The virus most likely responsible for this illness is transmitted by:
   A. The fecal-oral route
   B. Respiratory droplets
   C. Aerosol inhalation of rodent excreta
   D. The bite of an infected arthropod
   E. Blood

A 40-year-old businessman is seen in the emergency department with fever, chills, headache, muscle aches, abdominal pain, and vomiting. He returned the previous week from a hiking trip in Utah and reported being bitten by a tick. He is admitted to the hospital, where his temperature cycles from febrile to afebrile over the next several days. Laboratory findings of significance are a moderate leukopenia and thrombocytopenia.

3. What is the most likely diagnosis?
   A. Rocky Mountain spotted fever
   B. Enterovirus infection
   C. CTF
   D. Lyme disease
   E. Typhoid fever

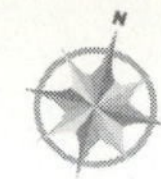

4. The agent responsible for this infection evades immune defense by:
   A. Antigenic shift
   B. The high mutation rate of error-prone RNA polymerase
   C. Downregulation of MHC class I antigens
   D. Cell-to-cell spread mediated by the viral fusion protein
   E. Persistence in mature erythrocytes

An 18-month-old infant is admitted to the hospital with symptoms of diarrhea, vomiting, fever, and dehydration. Blood and leukocytes were absent on the fecal smear.

5. The epidemiologic, clinical, and laboratory findings are characteristic of a gastrointestinal infection most likely caused by:
   A. Enteroinvasive *Escherichia coli*
   B. *Salmonella*
   C. *Shigella*
   D. Rotavirus
   E. Norovirus

ANSWERS

1. The answer is B. The clinical and epidemiologic features of this case are consistent with those of rotavirus infection.
2. The answer is A. Rotaviruses are spread by the fecal-oral route.
3. The answer is C. The clinical ("saddle-back fever") and epidemiologic features coupled with a tick bite exposure are consistent with those of CTF.
4. The answer is E. CTFV replicates in hematopoietic cells and escapes immune clearance by residing in mature erythrocytes. The other mechanisms of immune evasion are characteristic of viruses but not CTFV.
5. The answer is D. Rotavirus infections are more common in infants, whereas norovirus infection is more common in older children and adults. The presence of fecal leukocytes and blood in stool specimens is a diagnostic feature of bacterial gastrointestinal infections by enteroinvasive *E coli, Salmonella,* and *Shigella.* These findings are absent in acute viral gastroenteritis.

CHAPTER 15
RETROVIRUSES

I. Key Concepts

A. The retroviruses are a large group of icosahedral, enveloped viruses with two copies of single-stranded, positive-sense RNA (diploid genome).

B. The hallmark of retroviruses is virion-associated **reverse transcriptase (RT)** (RNA-dependent DNA polymerase) that converts the RNA genome into double-stranded DNA that becomes integrated into cellular DNA.

C. Retroviruses establish persistent lifelong infections.

D. Medically important members of the **Retroviridae** family are the **lentiviruses,** which include **HIV-1 and HIV-2,** and the **deltaretroviruses,** which include **human T-cell lymphotropic virus 1 and 2 (HTLV-1 and 2).** One other human family member (Spumavirus) is not associated with human disease.

E. HIV-1 and 2 lentiviruses are **cytopathic** and destroy target cells.

F. HTLV-1 and 2 deltaretroviruses are not cytolytic but are **transforming** and capable of cell immortalization leading to malignancy.

G. HIV-1 and 2 and HTLV-1 and 2 are characterized as complex retroviruses because they encode axillary proteins that have regulatory functions essential for viral replication or accessory functions essential for virus production in vivo. Properties of HIV and HTLV are compared in Table 15–1.

H. This chapter focuses on HIV-1 and HTLV-1. HIV-2 is of lower virulence than HIV-1, and infection is largely confined to West Africa. HTLV-2 disease association remains uncertain.

II. Retroviridae Family

A. HIV-1

1. Clinical manifestations: HIV-1 causes **AIDS.**

- **a.** HIV disease is characterized by an acute phase in 50–70% of infected persons days or weeks after infection with a "flulike" or infectious mononucleosislike syndrome. Infected persons may exhibit fever, pharyngitis, malaise, myalgia, headache, or generalized lymphadenopathy.
- **b.** The acute phase is followed by an asymptomatic phase of clinical latency with a median time of 10 years to development of AIDS.
- **c.** During the asymptomatic phase, patients may sporadically present with fatigue, weight loss, night sweats, or lymphadenopathy.

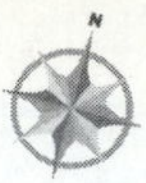

TABLE 15–1. Comparison of HIV and HTLV.

Property	HIV-1 & 2	HTLV-1 & 2
Structure by EM	Cone-shaped core	Spherical core
Cytopathic	Yes	No
Oncogenic	No	Yes
Basic genome structure gag-pol-env	Yes	Yes
Encoded regulatory proteins	Tat, Rev	Tax, Rex
Encoded accessory proteins	Nef, Vif, Vpr, Vpu	—
Cellular targets	CD4+ T lymphocytes & macrophages	CD4+ T lymphocytes

EM, electron microscopy.

   d. The symptomatic phase and AIDS is the end stage of HIV disease.
   e. AIDS is characterized by a CD4+ T lymphocyte count below 200/mL (normal = 800–1200/mL); opportunistic protozoal, fungal, bacterial, and viral infections; and malignancies (Table 15–2).

2. **Transmission/epidemiology:** HIV-1 is transmitted by sexual contact, blood, intravenous drug use, and from infected mother to child either across the placenta or perinatally at the time of delivery.
   a. HIV-1 and infected cells are present in semen and vaginal secretions of infected individuals and are transmitted by either homosexual or heterosexual intercourse.
   b. Homosexual contact is the major mode of HIV-1 transmission in the United States. Heterosexual transmission is most common in the rest of the world.
   c. Unprotected receptive anal intercourse carries the highest risk of sexual transmission.
   d. The risk of perinatal transmission of HIV-1 is 15–40%.
   e. Body fluids that contain a high concentration of mononuclear cells are most likely to transmit HIV-1.
3. **Pathogenesis:** HIV-1 gains entry by attachment of the virion surface glycoprotein gp120 to the **CD4 molecule** on the surface of helper T lymphocytes and monocytes-macrophages.
   a. The glycoprotein gp120 also interacts with a second cellular coreceptor, a **chemokine receptor** (CXCR4 on T cells or CCR5 on macrophages), that facilitates efficient fusion of the viral envelope with the cell plasma membrane and entry.
   b. Chemokine coreceptors dictate the cell tropism of different HIV-1 strains (eg, T-cell–tropic or monocyte-macrophage [M]–tropic strain).

Table 15–2. Opportunistic infections and associated diseases in patients with HIV or AIDS.

Infection	Disease
Protozoal	
Toxoplasma gondii	Disseminated toxoplasmosis
Cryptosporidium species	Cryptosporidiosis diarrhea
Isospora belli	Diarrhea
Fungal	
Pneumocystis jiroveci[a]	*P jiroveci* pneumonia
Candida albicans	Oral (thrush) & vaginal candidiasis
Cryptococcus neoformans	Cryptococcosis meningitis
Histoplasma capsulatum	Disseminated histoplasmosis
Bacterial	
Mycobacterium tuberculosis	Tuberculosis
Mycobacterium avium-intracellulare	Disseminated tuberculosis
Viral	
Herpes simplex virus	Recurrent oral & genital herpes
Cytomegalovirus	Retinitis, disseminated cytomegalovirus disease
Epstein-Barr virus	B cell lymphoma
Kaposi's sarcoma herpesvirus (HHV-8)	Kaposi's sarcoma
JC polyomavirus	Progressive multifocal leukoencephalopathy
Human papillomavirus	Anogenital cancer

[a]Formerly known as *Pneumocystis carinii.*

 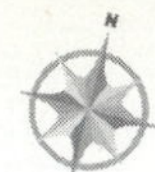

c. Individuals with homozygous mutations in the CCR5 gene are resistant to HIV-1 infection, demonstrating the physiologic importance of the chemokine receptor.
d. Mucosal dendritic cells can also be infected by HIV-1. Dendritic cells bind HIV-1 via a specific lectin receptor and transport virus to T cells or macrophages in draining lymph nodes.
e. HIV-1 may infect both activated and nonactivated CD4+ T cells in the draining lymph node.
f. Virus remains latent in nonactivated (ie, resting) T cells but replicates in T cells activated by infection or cytokines or both.
g. Free virus and virus-infected cells leave the lymph node and spread to other lymphoid organs, blood, and other tissues.
h. The loss of CD4+ T lymphocytes is the primary defect in AIDS pathogenesis. This is due to direct killing of CD4+ T cells by virus and a cytotoxic T-cell response to HIV-infected cells.
i. Latently infected T cells serve as a reservoir for HIV-1 and escape immune detection.
j. Latently infected T cells can switch to viral gene expression and release of infectious virus after antigen activation.
k. Ultimately, the decline in CD4+ T cells leads to a generalized failure of cell-mediated immunity, leaving the patient vulnerable to opportunistic infections and certain types of cancer.

4. **Virulence factors:** Integration of HIV-1 DNA into infected cells results in persistent infection and a reservoir of infected cells that are not detected by the immune system.
   a. HIV-1 RT has no proofreading capacity and, thus, a high error rate that generates many viral mutants with different biologic properties.
   b. The envelope glycoprotein gp120 gene has a high mutation rate, resulting in the generation of viral clones that escape immune recognition by neutralizing antibodies or virus-specific cytotoxic T cells.
   c. The Nef accessory protein reduces CD4 levels to enhance viral infectivity and downregulates MHC class I protein expression to escape cytotoxic T-cell recognition.
   d. The Vpr accessory protein facilitates transport of HIV-1 DNA into the nucleus of nondividing cells for subsequent integration into cellular DNA.
   e. The Vpu accessory protein facilitates degradation of CD4 molecules and promotes release of viral particles from infected cells.
   f. The Vif accessory protein increases infectivity of HIV-1.
5. **Laboratory diagnosis:** HIV and AIDS are diagnosed by the detection of antibodies to HIV-1 antigens by enzyme immunoassay (EIA) (screening test) and confirmed by the Western blot assay, which detects antibodies to specific HIV-1 proteins.
   a. RT-PCR is used to quantitate the amount of HIV-1 in plasma (viral load) and to monitor disease progression and response to antiretroviral therapy.
   b. RT-PCR is used to diagnose pediatric HIV-1 infection in babies born to HIV-1–positive mothers because passively transferred maternal antibodies could result in a false-positive EIA and Western blot.

6. **Treatment:** Currently available antiretroviral drugs target HIV-1 RT and viral protease and inhibit fusion of the viral envelope with the cell membrane.
   a. RT inhibitors include the nucleoside analogue RT inhibitors (NRTIs) and nonnucleoside RT inhibitors (NNRTIs). Both classes of inhibitors block RT activity and inhibit viral DNA synthesis.
   b. Selected examples of NRTIs are zidovudine (azidothymidine or AZT), didanosine (ddI), zalcitabine (ddC), lamivudine (3TC), and stavudine (d4T).
   c. Selected examples of NNRTIs are nevirapine, delavirdine, and efavirenz.
   d. Protease inhibitors (eg, ritonavir, indinavir, saquinavir, nelfinavir) block the HIV-1–encoded protease and, by interfering with viral polyprotein processing, result in the production of noninfectious viruses.
   e. The fusion inhibitor, enfuvirtide (T-20), specifically blocks fusion of HIV-1 envelope glycoprotein with CD4+ cells.
   f. Combinations of 3 classes of antiretroviral drugs administered together, termed **highly active antiretroviral therapy (HAART),** aim to attack HIV-1 replication at different targets to avoid emergence of viral mutants resistant to drug therapy.
   g. Perinatal administration of zidovudine (AZT) to HIV-1–infected pregnant women and their newborn infants can reduce the transmission of HIV-1 from 25 to 8%.
   h. The antiretroviral drugs and their mechanisms of action are summarized in Chapter 10.
7. **Prevention:** No vaccine against HIV-1 is available.
   a. Screening of blood for HIV-1 antibody has prevented HIV transmission by blood transfusion.
   b. Maternal-infant transmission of HIV-1 can be reduced significantly by AZT therapy for the pregnant mother and newborn infant.
   c. Educating society about methods to prevent transmission (eg, having only monogamous sex with uninfected partner, using barrier contraceptives, not sharing needles by intravenous drug users) is a critical public health objective.
   d. Universal precautions prevent HIV-1 transmission in health care workers.

B. HTLV-1

1. **Clinical manifestations:** HTLV-1 is the causative agent of **adult T-cell leukemia (ATL)** and a neurologic disorder called **HTLV-1–associated myelopathy-tropical spastic paraparesis (HAM-TSP).**
   a. ATL is characterized by a long asymptomatic incubation period of 20–50 years, increased numbers of leukemia cells with characteristic morphology, skin lesions, systemic lymphadenopathy, hepatosplenomegaly, and hypercalcemia.
   b. The lifetime risk for development of ATL in an infected individual is 3–5%.
   c. HAM-TSP is characterized by a shorter incubation period than ATL (2–4 years), demyelination of the long motor neurons of the spinal cord, muscle weakness in the legs, progressive spasticity, back pain, urinary incontinence, hyperreflexia, sensory disturbances, and impotence in men.
   d. The lifetime risk of having HAM develop is about 1%.
   e. ATL and HAM-TSP are endemic in southern Japan, the Caribbean Islands, South America, and parts of Africa.

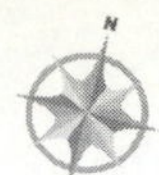

2. **Transmission/epidemiology:** HTLV-1 is highly cell-associated and transmitted primarily by HTLV-1–infected cells, not virus particles.
   a. HTLV-1 is transmitted from mother to infant by infected lymphocytes in breast milk and is the most common means of childhood infection.
   b. HTLV-1 is transmitted sexually by infected lymphocytes in semen. Male to female is the most efficient means of transmission.
   c. HTLV-1 is transmitted by blood transfusion and intravenous drug use.
3. **Pathogenesis:** HTLV-1 infects primarily CD4+ T lymphocytes but also can infect other cell types. The cellular receptor for HTLV-1 has not been identified.
   a. After infection, a DNA copy of the RNA genome is synthesized by RT and integrated randomly into the target cell chromosomal DNA.
   b. The HTLV-1–encoded regulatory protein **Tax** stimulates the growth and mitogenesis of CD4+ T cells by inducing cellular transcription factors that activate cellular growth factors and growth factor receptors (eg, interleukin-2 [IL-2] and IL-2 receptor).
   c. Tax can functionally inactivate the P53 tumor suppressor protein.
   d. Activation of T-cell growth factors and receptors and inactivation of P53 tumor suppressor protein stimulate T-cell proliferation and increase genetic instability, thereby providing a pool of target cells with the probability of accumulating additional cellular mutations required for malignant transformation.
   e. HAM-TSP pathogenesis is characterized by a CNS infiltration of HTLV-1–infected lymphocytes and a marked cytotoxic lymphocyte response with collateral damage to neurologic tissues.
4. **Virulence factors:** Integration of HTLV-1 DNA into cellular DNA is an evasion strategy to establish persistent infection.
   a. The virus utilizes the Tax protein to transactivate the expression of cellular growth promoting genes that contribute to its pathogenesis.
   b. The Tax protein activates or suppresses a variety of host cell genes that control cell division.
5. **Laboratory diagnosis:** HTLV-1 infection is detected by EIA for virus-specific antibody.
6. **Treatment:** There is no specific antiviral therapy for HTLV-1.
7. **Prevention:** No vaccine is available for HTLV-1.
   a. Screening of blood can prevent transmission by transfusion.
   b. Prevention measures established for HIV infection are applicable for HTLV-1: having safe sex and not sharing needles by intravenous drug users.
   c. Elimination of breastfeeding by HTLV-1–infected mothers would prevent maternal-infant transmission of HTLV-1.

AIDS

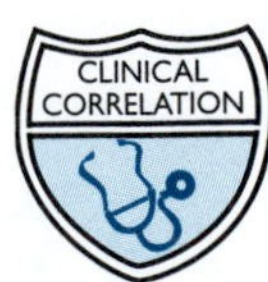

- *In 2003, an estimated 38 million people were living with HIV or AIDS, making the HIV-AIDS pandemic a crisis of global proportions.*
- *Urgent and intensified action is needed to provide medical care, expand prevention programs and increase understanding of HIV, and evaluate interventions to prevent further spread of HIV.*

CLINICAL PROBLEMS

A 7-month-old male infant is brought to the pediatric clinic because of severe, chronic diarrhea and failure to thrive. On examination, the child is febrile and malnourished and has oral thrush, hepatosplenomegaly, and generalized lymphadenopathy. His CD4+ cell count is decreased. His mother had died of AIDS 2 months after giving birth.

1. The laboratory test that would confirm HIV-1 infection is:

A. EIA for HIV-1 antibody

B. Western blot for HIV-1 antibody

C. HIV-1 isolation by cell culture

D. HIV-1 neutralization assay

E. RT-PCR for HIV-1 viral RNA

2. Transmission of HIV-1 from infected mother to infant might have been prevented by treatment of the pregnant mother and infant with:

A. High-titer HIV-1 antibody

B. HIV-1 vaccine

C. HIV-1 protease inhibitors

D. Zidovudine (AZT)

E. Interferon

A group of female commercial sex workers have normal CD4+ T-cell counts and no evidence of HIV or AIDS despite multiple exposures to HIV-1.

3. The most likely explanation for their resistance to HIV infection is:

A. The presence of serum-neutralizing antibodies to HIV-1

B. A mutation in the CCR5 chemokine receptor gene

C. A generalized loss of dendritic cells that transport HIV-1 to lymph nodes

D. Production of specific antibodies to RT that block viral integration

E. Elevated levels of mucosal immunity to HIV-1

4. A retrovirus that infects and kills CD4+ T lymphocytes and is transmitted sexually best describes:

A. HIV-1

B. HTLV-1

C. Hepatitis B virus

D. Cytomegalovirus

E. Human endogenous retrovirus

A 60-year-old man from the Caribbean Islands is diagnosed with ATL. Serologic testing confirms a viral etiology.

 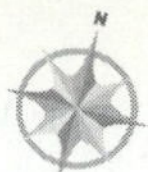

5. The viral protein that drives proliferation and transformation of target T lymphocytes leading to ATL is:
   A. Tat
   B. Nef
   C. Rex
   D. Tax
   E. gp120

ANSWERS

1. The answer is E. RT-PCR is used in the context of pediatric HIV-1 infections in which maternally transferred HIV-1 antibodies in infant's serum disappear slowly and remain detectable by EIA and Western blot for up to 15 months. Virus isolation is technically difficult, time-consuming, and not suitable for routine diagnosis. There are no serum neutralization assays for HIV-1.
2. The answer is D. Zidovudine administered to HIV-1–infected, pregnant women and newborn infants can reduce the perinatal transmission of HIV-1 significantly. Passive immunization with HIV-1 antibody is not a valid choice, and there is no HIV-1 vaccine. There is no evidence to support the use of protease inhibitors or interferon to block perinatal HIV-1 infection.
3. The answer is B. Individuals with mutations in the CCR5 chemokine receptor, a co-receptor required for HIV-1 entry, have a decreased susceptibility to HIV-1 infection.
4. The answer is A. HIV-1 is CD4+, T-cell tropic, and cytolytic. Sexual contact is one means of transmission. HTLV-1 is not cytolytic. Hepatitis B virus and cytomegalovirus are not retroviruses. Human endogenous retrovirus is not associated with any disease.
5. The answer is D. HTLV-1 Tax transactivates cellular growth promoting genes, and inactivates tumor suppressor proteins.

CHAPTER 16

SLOW INFECTIONS AND PRIONS

I. Key Concepts

A. Slow infections include a group of diseases that have a prolonged incubation period (months to years) and a slowly progressive clinical course ending in death.

B. The protracted course of slow infections requires that the causative agent be able to evade host defenses and establish a persistent infection.

C. Central nervous system involvement is a hallmark of slow infections. The central nervous system acts as a sanctuary for virus sequestration.

D. Slow infections are classified as

1. Diseases associated with conventional viruses.
2. Diseases associated with unconventional agents known as **prion** (pronounced "pree-on") diseases (Table 16–1).

E. Medically important slow virus diseases caused by conventional viruses are **progressive multifocal leukoencephalopathy (PML)** and **subacute sclerosing panencephalitis (SSPE).**

F. Medically important slow diseases caused by prions are the **transmissible spongiform encephalopathies.**

G. Figure 16–1 is a concept map of the slow infections discussed in this chapter.

II. Slow Infections Caused by Conventional Viruses

A. Progressive Multifocal Leukoencephalopathy

1. **Clinical manifestations:** PML is a demyelinating disease of the brain caused by human **polyomavirus, JC virus (JCV).**
   - **a.** PML occurs in adults with immunosuppressive diseases, particularly individuals with HIV infection, in whom PML is an AIDS-defining illness.
   - **b.** Disease onset is insidious. Early signs include speech and vision abnormalities and alteration in mental function.
   - **c.** The clinical course of PML is progressive, culminating in coma and death, usually within 6 months of onset.
2. **Transmission/epidemiology:** JCV is transmitted by **respiratory tract droplets.**
   - **a.** JCV is widespread. Infections occur during childhood, and 70–80% of adults have antibodies to JCV.

Table 16–1. Slow infections caused by conventional viruses and prions.

Disease	Host	Virus/Agent	Brain Lesion
Conventional viruses			
Subacute sclerosing panencephalitis	Human	Defective measles virus	Demyelination, inflammation
Progressive multifocal leukoencephalopathy	Human	JC polyomavirus	Demyelination, inflammation
Prions			
Creutzfeldt-Jakob disease	Human	Prion	TSE
Kuru	Human	Prion	TSE
Gerstmann-Sträussler-Scheinker disease	Human	Prion	TSE
Fatal familial insomnia	Human	Prion	TSE
Scrapie	Sheep & goats	Prion	TSE
Bovine spongiform encephalopathy	Cattle	Prion	TSE

TSE, transmissible spongiform encephalopathy.

b. Latent infections are reactivated in immunocompromised individuals, such as in
   (1) The elderly with immunodeficiency states.
   (2) Patients undergoing immunosuppressive therapy for organ transplantation or chemotherapy for cancer.
   (3) Patients with AIDS.

c. JCV is a human polyomavirus member of the Polyomaviridae family.

d. JCV is an icosahedral, nonenveloped, circular, double-stranded DNA virus that replicates in the nucleus.

3. Pathogenesis: JCV is likely acquired via the respiratory route and spread by viremia to establish latent infection in the kidney, lungs, and reticuloendothelial system.

a. In immunocompromised individuals, JCV is activated, spreads to the brain, and causes PML.

b. Polyomavirus particles can be detected by electron microscopy in brain tissue of patients with PML, and JCV can be isolated from biopsy and autopsy specimens.

c. JCV causes lytic infection of the **oligodendrocyte,** with intranuclear inclusions of viral capsids and myelin loss seen by pathology. The oligodendrocyte is the major myelin-producing cell in the central nervous system.

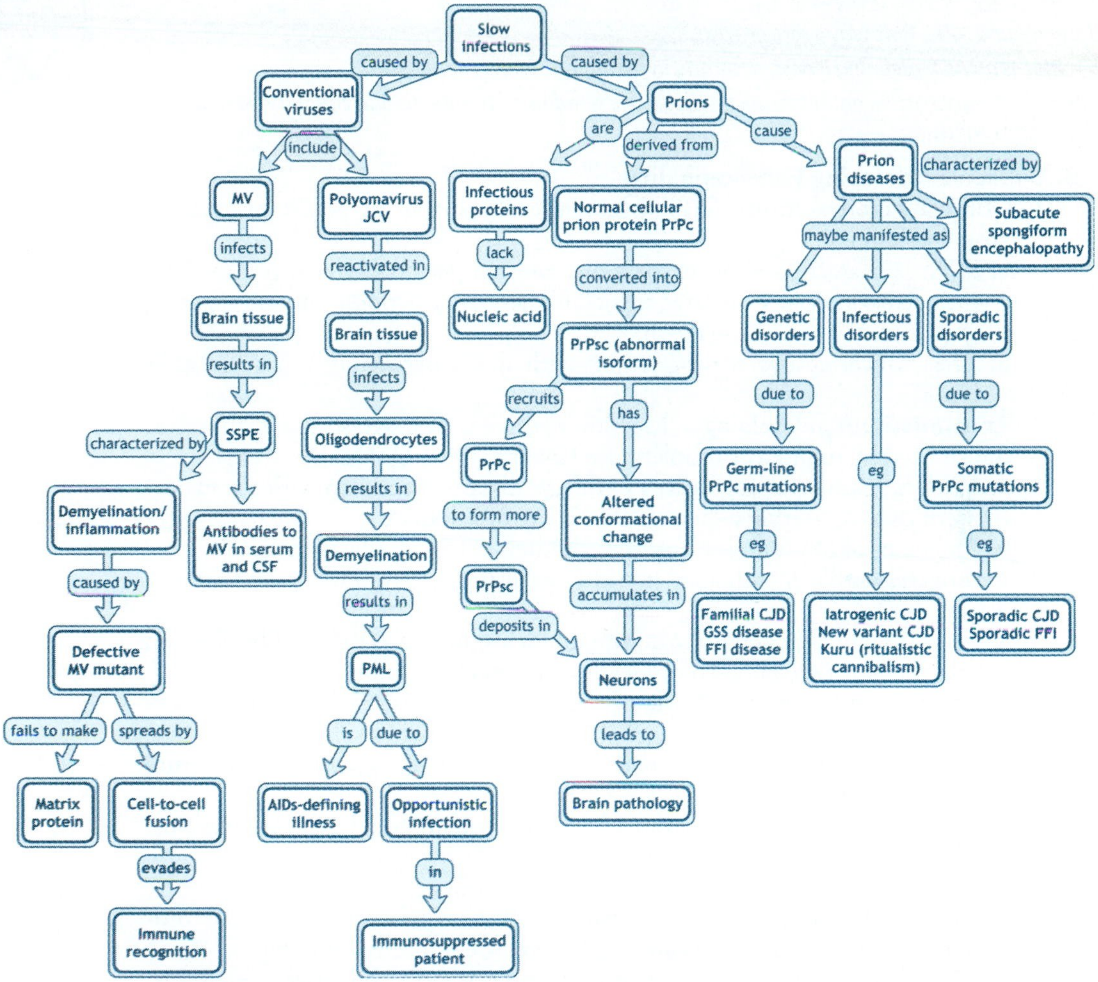

Figure 16–1. Concept map of slow infections.

d. The mechanism of immune evasion is **opportunism** in the immunosuppressed patient.

4. **Virulence factors:** JCV has the capacity to establish latent infections and to reactivate in the immunocompromised host.
5. **Laboratory diagnosis:** JCV infection can be detected by polymerase chain reaction in the cerebrospinal fluid (CSF) of patients with PML. JCV DNA can also be detected by polymerase chain reaction or in situ DNA hybridization in brain biopsy specimens.
6. **Treatment:** There is no specific treatment for PML.
7. **Prevention:** No vaccine for JCV is available.

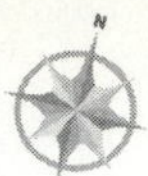

PROGRESSIVE MULTIFOCAL LEUKOENCEPHALOPATHY

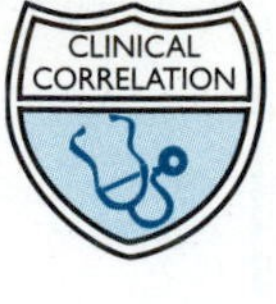

- *Before HIV and AIDS, PML was a rare disease.*
- *Now, PML is an AIDS-defining illness, occurring in about 5% of patients with AIDS.*
- *In the age of highly active antiretroviral therapy, PML remains a life-threatening condition with a relatively poor prognosis.*

B. Subacute Sclerosing Panencephalitis

1. **Clinical manifestations:** SSPE is a rare complication of persistent **measles virus** infection.
   - **a.** SSPE is characterized by an insidious onset of personality changes, intellectual deterioration, with later myoclonic jerks (ie, periodic muscle spasms), spasticity, blindness, and death.
   - **b.** The clinical course is progressive, with death occurring 1–3 years after onset.
2. **Transmission/epidemiology:** Measles virus is a negative-strand RNA virus transmitted by respiratory droplets (see Chapter 13, II.D. Measles Virus).
   - **a.** SSPE is a rare, late progressive neurologic disease of children with the majority of cases appearing 6–8 years after acute measles.
   - **b.** Incidence of SSPE in unvaccinated children is 1 in 1 million cases.
3. **Pathogenesis:** Brain pathology in SSPE consists of demyelination and inflammation.
   - **a.** Neurons and oligodendrocytes contain inclusion bodies detected by electron microscopy and composed of measles virus nucleocapsids.
   - **b.** Measles virus defective in virion production can be isolated from brain cells of patients with SSPE.
   - **c.** Patients with SSPE have elevated levels of measles virus antibodies in serum and CSF.
   - **d.** Patients with SSPE have elevated levels of antibody to all measles virus proteins, except the matrix (M) protein.
   - **e.** The M protein is not detected in brain tissue of patients with SSPE.
   - **f.** The measles virus variants that cause SSPE have mutations in the M protein. The M protein is responsible for viral assembly and budding.
   - **g.** The absence of a functional M protein results in nonproductive infection by SSPE measles virus.
   - **h.** MV escapes immune surveillance by **cell-to-cell fusion.**
4. **Virulence factors:** MV evades host antibody by direct cell-to-cell spread mediated by the fusion (F) protein.
5. **Laboratory diagnosis:** Patients with SSPE are diagnosed by the detection of high measles virus antibody levels in serum and CSF.
6. **Treatment:** There is no specific treatment for measles virus infection.
7. **Prevention:** Live, attenuated measles virus vaccine is highly effective in preventing measles and has reduced markedly the incidence of SSPE.

SLOW VIRUS INFECTION

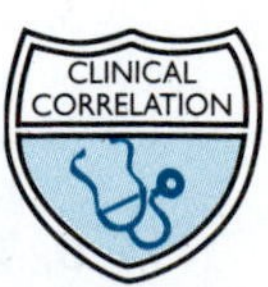

- *In otherwise uncomplicated cases of measles, the virus can invade neurons and oligodendrocytes in the central nervous system and cause SSPE.*
- *The chronic infection and the associated brain pathology that evolves over the course of years are invariably fatal.*

III. Slow Infections Caused by Transmissible Spongiform Encephalopathies: Prion Diseases

A. Characteristics of Prion Diseases

1. Prion diseases have a long preclinical phase (incubation period) leading to progressive, ultimately fatal, neurodegenerative diseases of humans and other animals (Table 16–1).
2. Human prion diseases are termed transmissible spongiform encephalopathies because they have been transmitted to primates and other animals through cell-free injections of infected brain tissue and exhibit similar brain pathology.
3. Brain pathology consists of subacute spongiform encephalopathy with progressive vacuolization of neurons and spongiform degeneration.
4. Prion diseases are caused by unconventional agents termed **prions: novel *pro*teinaceous *in*fectious particles that lack nucleic acids.**
5. The hallmark of all prion diseases is the accumulation of conformationally altered (misfolded) prion proteins in the brain and subsequent pathology.
6. Prion diseases of **humans** can be divided into infectious, sporadic, and familial and include Creutzfeldt-Jakob disease (CJD), kuru, Gerstmann-Sträussler-Scheinker disease, and fatal familial insomnia (Table 16–2).
7. Prion diseases of animals include scrapie in sheep and bovine spongiform encephalopathy or mad cow disease in cattle (Table 16–2). Similar diseases in mink, deer, and elk are caused by prions.

B. Creutzfeldt-Jakob Disease

1. **Clinical manifestations:** CJD is a progressive, neurodegenerative disease with onset usually between ages 50–70 years.
   a. CJD is characterized clinically by dementia, myoclonus (involuntary movements), and ataxia.
   b. The disease progresses to severe dementia and death within 6 months to 1 year.
2. **Transmission/epidemiology:** About 10–15% of CJD cases are familial. In contrast, Gerstmann-Sträussler-Scheinker and fatal familial insomnia are known hereditary prion diseases.
   a. The familial form of prion disease is due to mutations in the PrP gene on chromosome 20.
   b. Sporadic CJD accounts for most cases (85%).
   c. Transmission of CJD from person to person by ingestion or inoculation of infected brain tissue has been documented and includes
      (1) Transplantation of contaminated corneal grafts, dura mater grafts, or injection of human pituitary–derived growth hormone.
      (2) Use of contaminated medical devices (brain electrodes) incompletely sterilized between patients.
      (3) Ingestion of infected tissue (new variant CJD), which is thought to be acquired by ingestion of bovine spongiform encephalopathy–contaminated beef.
   d. CJD is a rare disease with an annual incidence of one case per 1 million people.
3. **Pathogenesis:** Prions have unique physical and biologic properties that distinguish them from conventional viruses (Table 16–3).
   a. Prion diseases are believed to occur from the accumulation in neurons of a protease-resistant isoform of a normal cellular protein (prion protein, PrP^{c})

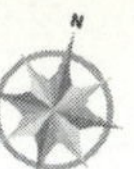

Table 16–2. Prion diseases.

Disease	Natural Host	Cause of Disease
Kuru	Humans	Acquired infection
CJD		
sCJD (sporadic)	Humans	Somatic mutation in PrP gene
iCJD (iatrogenic)	Humans	Acquired infection from prion-contaminated medical equipment, corneal grafts, human growth hormone
nvCJD (new variant)	Humans	Ingestion of bovine prions
fCJD (familial)	Humans	Germline mutations in PrP gene
Gerstmann-Sträussler-Scheinker disease	Human	Germline mutations in PrP gene
Fatal familial insomnia	Human	Germline mutations in PrP gene
Scrapie	Sheep	Infection in genetically susceptible sheep
Bovine spongiform encephalopathy	Cattle	Infection with prion-contaminated meat and bone meal

CJD, Creutzfeldt-Jakob disease.
Adapted, with permission, from Prusiner SB. Shattuck lecture—neurodegenerative disease and prions. *N Engl J Med.* 2001;344:1516–1526.

that is conformationally altered and called PrP^{sc} (sc for scrapie, the prototype prion disease studied extensively in animals).

b. The abnormal PrP^{sc} binds normal PrP^{c} and acts as a template to induce a conformational change in PrP^{c}, converting it into the abnormal PrP^{sc} form.

c. This process continues in a cascadelike fashion until abnormal PrP^{sc} accumulates to levels associated with neuronal dysfunction and neuronal death.

d. Accumulation of PrP^{sc} in the brain is the pathognomonic feature with the formation of amyloidlike fibrils and plaques. Extensive vacuolation, neuronal loss, and gliosis are also seen by pathology.

e. Prions escape immune surveillance because they are **nonantigenic** host proteins.

4. **Virulence factors:** No virulence factors are known.
5. **Laboratory diagnosis:** Prion diseases are generally diagnosed by the constellation of clinical findings. Histopathologic examination of brain sections at autopsy shows characteristic spongiform changes characterized by a "spongy" appearance (ie, holes in the tissue).

Table 16–3. Comparison of viruses and prions.

Property	Virus	Prion
Filterable infectious agent	Yes	Yes
Contains nucleic acid	Yes	No
Virion structure by EM	Yes	No
Inactiviated by: UV or ionizing radiation	Yes	No
100° C for 60 min	Yes	No
Autoclaving at 121° C for 90 min	Yes	No
3.7% formaldehyde	Yes	No
2N NaOH for 60 min	Yes	Yes
5% sodium hypochlorite	Yes	Yes
Induces:		
Cytopathic effect in cell culture	Most	No
Inflammatory response	Yes	No
Interferon	Yes	No
Immune response	Yes	No

EM, electron microscopy.

6. **Treatment:** There are no effective treatments for prion disease.
7. **Prevention:** No specific immunologic approaches are available to prevent prion diseases. Because of the unusually high resistance of prions to most disinfectants, strong surveillance and control programs are needed to prevent iatrogenic transmission and the risk of transmission via prion-contaminated food.

NEW VARIANT CRUETZFELDT-JAKOB DISEASE

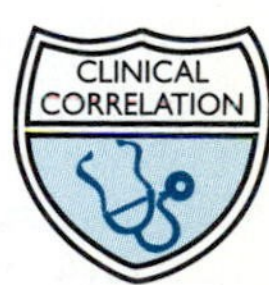

- *A new type of CJD, called new variant CJD (nvCJD or vCJD), was reported in the United Kingdom in 1996 and was caused by eating beef from cows with bovine spongiform encephalopathy.*
- *More than 153 cases of nvCJD have been reported as of December 2003. This is clear evidence that prions can jump the species barrier.*
- *Unlike classic CJD, nvCJD affects younger people and has atypical clinical features with prominent psychiatric symptoms.*

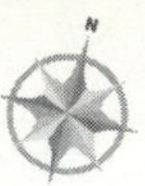

CLINICAL PROBLEMS

A 65-year-old man with chronic lymphatic leukemia experienced progressive deterioration of mental and neuromuscular function until death. At autopsy, the brain showed enlarged oligodendrocytes with intranuclear, naked, icosahedral virus particles.

1. The *most likely* diagnosis is:

A. Rabies

B. PML

C. Herpes encephalitis

D. CJD

E. AIDS dementia

A 12-year-old boy had been developing normally up to 10 years of age, when his teachers began noticing personality changes and a progressive deterioration in his schoolwork. He is brought to the emergency department after wandering into the street, apparently confused after falling off his bike. Screening results for alcohol and drugs are negative. Serologic results for CMV and HIV are negative. Antimeasles antibody titers are 640 in serum and 5120 in CSF.

2. The virus responsible for this disease:

A. Is missing the viral glycoprotein that mediates cell attachment

B. Lacks the virion-associated, RNA-dependent RNA polymerase

C. Is rapidly neutralized by anti–measles virus antibody

D. Is defective in nucleocapsid assembly and release from the infected cell

E. Is the vaccine strain of measles virus

A 67-year-old previously healthy woman experienced ataxia, slurred speech, and dementia. At autopsy, her brain shows spongiform changes, vacuolization of neurons, no inflammation, and no evidence of viral particles by electron microscopy or viral antigens.

3. The disease is *most likely* caused by:

A. An autoimmune response to a neuronal protein antigenically related to measles virus

B. Reactivation of an intranuclear DNA virus

C. An aberrant cellular protein with altered conformation

D. Cytolytic destruction of oligodendrocytes by Creutzfeldt-Jakob virus

E. HIV-1 replication in brain macrophages and microglia

4. Progressive multifocal encephalopathy is a demyelinating brain disease caused by:

A. Prions

B. Rubella virus

C. JC polyomavirus

D. Measles virus
E. Scrapie virus

5. SSPE is a demyelinating brain disease caused by:
   A. Mumps virus
   B. Rubella virus
   C. JC polyomavirus
   D. Measles virus
   E. LaCrosse virus

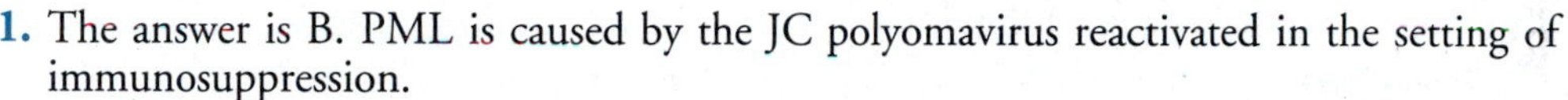

ANSWERS

1. The answer is B. PML is caused by the JC polyomavirus reactivated in the setting of immunosuppression.
2. The answer is D. This case of SSPE has the important diagnostic feature of high-titer measles virus antibody in serum and CSF. SSPE is caused by a defective measles virus that lacks the M protein essential for viral assembly and release.
3. The answer is C. Clinical history and laboratory findings are consistent with those of prion disease caused by a conformationally altered (misfolded) cellular protein.
4. The answer is C. JCV is the cause of PML.
5. The answer is D. Measles virus is the cause of SSPE.

CHAPTER 17
BASIC MYCOLOGY

I. Properties of Fungi: Key Concepts

A. Fungi are eukaryotic organisms and have a nucleus, unlike prokaryotic bacteria.

B. Fungi are not photosynthetic and have no chlorophyll pigment.

C. Fungi secrete enzymes that digest plant and animal tissue and utilize the soluble nutrients for growth.

D. Of the more than 100,000 species of fungi, fewer than 300 are routinely associated with human disease.

E. Nearly all fungal infections are derived from the environment. The exceptions are *Candida* and *Malassezia,* part of the normal flora.

II. Structure and Growth

A. Fungal cells have several components.

1. A **plasmalemma** (or **cell membrane**) encloses the cytoplasm and is composed of glycoproteins, lipids, and **ergosterol** in contrast to cholesterol found in mammalian cell membranes.
2. The **cell wall** exterior to the plasmalemma is composed of **chitin,** a polymer of *N*-acetyl glucosamine, in contrast to peptidoglycan found in bacterial cell walls.
3. **Mannans** and **glucans** are polysaccharides that complex with surface proteins and surround the cell wall to provide cell wall rigidity and make up the **capsule** in some species.

B. Fungi can be grouped morphologically as either **yeasts** or **molds.**

1. Yeasts grow as single cells and reproduce by budding.
2. Molds are multicelled, filamentous forms of fungi composed of threadlike, branching filaments termed **hyphae** that form an intertwined mass called a **mycelium** or mold.

C. Hyphae may be divided by partitions, termed **septate,** or be **nonseptate,** structural features that aid in laboratory diagnosis.

D. Some fungi are thermally dimorphic and can exist as either hyphal forms at ambient temperature (25°C) or yeast forms in infected tissue (37°C), such as *Blastomyces, Coccidioides,* and *Histoplasma.*

E. Fungi reproduce asexually and sexually by the formation of **spores,** specialized structures for dissemination and survival under adverse conditions.

F. Most fungal spores are asexual and of two general types: **conidia** and **sporangiospores.**
   1. Conidia are formed externally by mitosis on a specialized hyphal structure called the **conidiophore. Macroconidia** and **microconidia** denote the size and complexity of conidia.
   2. Sporangiospores are produced internally within specialized structures termed sporangia.

III. Fungal Pathogenesis and Host Response

A. Mechanisms of fungal pathogenesis are poorly understood.

B. Fungal surface mannoproteins mediate adherence to target cells in some species of fungi.

C. Most human fungal infections are mild and self-limited because of a high level of innate immunity to fungi.

D. Progressive and life-threatening fungal diseases are a common theme in immunocompromised patients.

E. Host resistance is due to the fatty acid content, pH, epithelial cell turnover, and normal bacterial flora of the skin, as well as the pH of mucosal surfaces and cilia of the respiratory tract.

F. Host responses to systemic fungal infection result in the formation of a **granuloma,** characterized by an inflammatory cell infiltrate and macrophages that phagocytize fungi, resulting in a localized nodule that acts to contain the infection.

G. Neutrophils function to phagocytize and kill fungi. Capsular polysaccharides of some fungi are antiphagocytic.

H. T-cell–mediated immunity is a key determinant in protection from disease.

I. Fungal mannoproteins elicit strong T- and B-cell responses.

IV. Laboratory Diagnosis

A. Detection and identification of fungi can be made by culture and nonculture methods.

B. Fungi grow slowly in culture with a long doubling time (hours) compared with bacteria (minutes).

C. Sabouraud's medium, commonly used to culture fungi, is selective for fungal growth because of acid pH and high sugar content.

D. Nonculture methods include direct microscopic examination, antigen detection by enzyme immunoassay or latex agglutination, and nucleic acid detection by polymerase chain reaction.

E. Fungi are Gram-positive but difficult to stain with the Gram stain.

F. Gomori methamine silver and the periodic acid–Schiff stain are special stains used to detect yeast cells and hyphae in tissues.

G. Clinical specimens, treated with 10% potassium hydroxide (KOH) that digests tissue material but leaves fungal cell walls intact, are examined microscopically as wet mounts to detect fungi.

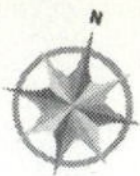

Table 17–1. Properties of selected antifungal agents.

Agent	Mode of Action	Treatment	Clinical Use
Grisans			
Griseofulvin	Disrupts microtubules; mitotic poison	Systemic	Dermatophytes
Polyenes			
Amphotericin B (AmB)	Binds to ergosterol & disrupts membrane integrity	Systemic	Most fungi
Liposomal AmB	Same as AmB	Systemic	Most fungi; less toxic than AmB
Azoles			
Fluconazole	Targets lanosterol demethylase part of the ergosterol biosynthesis pathway	Systemic	*Candida* species *Cryptococcus*
Itraconazole	Same as fluconazole	Systemic	*Candida* species *Aspergillus* *Sporothrix* *Histoplasma* *Blastomyces*
Voriconazole	Same as fluconazole	Systemic	All *Candida* species *Aspergillus* *Fusarium* *Scedosporium*
Nucleoside analogues			
5-Fluorocytosine (Flucytosine)	Inhibits RNA & DNA synthesis	Systemic	*Candida* species *Cryptococcus*
Allylamines			
Terbinafine	Inhibits ergosterol biosynthesis via inhibition of squalene epoxidase	Systemic Topical	Dermatophytes; especially onychomycosis
Echinocandins			
Caspofungin	Inhibits glucan synthesis	Systemic	*Candida* species *Aspergillus*
Potassium iodide	Unknown	Systemic	*Sporothrix schenckii*
Tolnaftate	Inhibits ergosterol biosynthesis similar to allylamines	Topical	Dermatophytes

V. Antifungal Therapy

A. Selected antifungal agents and their mechanism of action, route of treatment, and clinical use are summarized in Table 17–1.

B. Increased use of antifungal drugs has led to increased drug resistance.

C. Novel antifungal drugs in development and combination drug therapy are important antifungal drug strategies.

CHEMOTHERAPY OF FUNGAL INFECTIONS

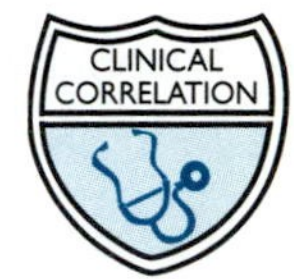

- *The frequency of fungal infections has increased dramatically since 1980, largely because of an expanding population of immunocompromised patients.*
- *Patients undergoing bone marrow transplantation, solid-organ transplantation, or cancer chemotherapy or those with HIV or AIDS are highly susceptible to fungal infections with increased morbidity and mortality.*
- *The documented increase in systemic and localized mycoses has fueled the development of antifungal drugs with a broader spectrum of activity, reduced toxicity, and fewer drug interactions.*

CLINICAL PROBLEMS

1. Fungal infections most likely result in systemic disease in patients with:

A. T-cell immunodeficiency
B. B-cell immunodeficiency
C. Autoimmune disease
D. Allergic disease
E. Complement deficiency

2. A component of the fungal cell wall is:

A. Teichoic acid
B. Chitin
C. Peptidoglycan
D. Ergosterol
E. Keratin

3. The antifungal agent that inhibits glucan synthesis and blocks cell wall synthesis is:

A. Amphotericin B
B. Griseofulvin
C. Itraconazole
D. Flucytosine
E. Caspofungin

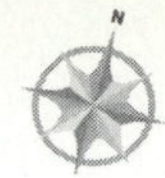

4. The fungal cell structures that mediate transmission of fungi by aerosolization are called:

A. Hyphae

B. Mycelial

C. Conidia

D. Capsules

E. Mannans

5. A laboratory method commonly used to detect and diagnose fungal infections rapidly is:

A. Culture on Sabouraud's medium

B. Gram stain

C. Acid-fast stain

D. Direct microscopic examination in KOH preparation

E. Serologic rise in fungus-specific antibody titer

ANSWERS

1. The answer is A. Patients with decreased T-cell immunity are at risk for life-threatening mycoses. The other choices are not significant risk factors for systemic fungal infections.

2. The answer is B. Chitin is a component of the fungal cell wall. Teichoic acid and peptidoglycan are components of the bacterial cell wall. Ergosterol is a component of the fungal cell membrane. Keratin is a cytoskeletal protein of epithelial cells.

3. The answer is E. Caspofungin causes cessation of cell wall synthesis by blocking the synthesis of glucan, a component of the cell wall. Amphotericin B binds to ergosterol and disrupts membrane integrity. Griseofulvin is a mitotic poison. Itraconazole inhibits ergosterol synthesis. Flucytosine is an inhibitor of DNA and RNA synthesis.

4. The answer is C. Conidia are the fungal structures that mediate aerosol dissemination and transmission of fungi. Hyphae are filamentous forms of fungi, and a mass of hyphae is termed a mycelium. The capsule and its component polysaccharides, mannans, complex with and surround the cell wall and are antiphagocytic in some fungal species.

5. The answer is D. Direct microscopic examination of clinical specimens in a 10% KOH preparation is commonly used to detect hyphal and yeast forms. KOH digests host tissue material, but fungal structures are resistant. Culture of fungi is important in identification but not rapid because fungi grow slowly. Fungi stain poorly with the Gram stain and are not acid-fast. A rise in antibody titer is not a rapid method and can be used to diagnose fungal infections retrospectively.

CHAPTER 18
SUPERFICIAL, CUTANEOUS, AND SUBCUTANEOUS MYCOSES

I. Fungal Diseases: Key Concepts

A. Diseases caused by fungi (mycoses) are categorized into groups (superficial mycoses, cutaneous mycoses, subcutaneous mycoses, and systemic mycoses) based on the type of tissue they colonize and the disease produced.

B. Superficial mycoses are limited to the outermost layers of the skin or hair with little tissue damage and generally no inflammatory response.

C. Medically important superficial mycoses are pityriasis versicolor, tinea nigra, black piedra, and white piedra.

D. Cutaneous mycoses are limited to keratinized tissues of the skin, hair, or nails without penetration of deeper tissues and elicit a host inflammatory response.

E. Medically important cutaneous mycoses are the dermatophyte infections, classically called tinea or ringworm.

F. Subcutaneous mycoses are limited to the deeper skin structures often associated with traumatic inoculation of subcutaneous tissue.

G. Medically important subcutaneous mycoses are mycetoma, chromoblastomycosis, sporotrichosis, rhinosporidiosis, and lobomycosis.

II. Superficial Mycoses

A. Pityriasis Versicolor

1. **Clinical manifestations:** Pityriasis versicolor is caused by *Malassezia furfur,* a lipophilic yeast.
   - **a.** Pityriasis versicolor is characterized by dry, scaly, hyperpigmented, or hypopigmented lesions on the torso, arms, and abdomen.
   - **b.** *M furfur* can cause rare systemic disease in patients receiving intravenous intralipid therapy and seborrheic dermatitis in patients with AIDS.
2. **Transmission/epidemiology:** *M furfur* is part of the normal flora and transmitted by direct contact. Pityriasis versicolor is a common infection with worldwide distribution and a higher prevalence in the tropics, in patients who have undergone renal transplant, and in patients with AIDS.
3. **Pathogenesis/virulence factors:** Pityriasis versicolor is not associated with a host immune response, and no virulence factors are known.

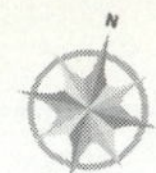

4. **Laboratory diagnosis:** Direct microscopic examination of scaly lesions in a potassium hydroxide (KOH) preparation reveals a characteristic "spaghetti and meatballs" appearance of yeast and hyphae.
5. **Treatment/prevention:** Pityriasis versicolor is treated topically with selenium sulfide or miconazole. Good hygiene is important in prevention.

B. Tinea Nigra

1. **Clinical manifestations:** Tinea nigra is caused by *Exophiala werneckii,* a melanin-producing, dimorphic fungus. Tinea nigra is characterized by flat brown to black, nonscaly macular lesions of the palms and soles and other areas less often.
2. **Transmission/epidemiology:** *E werneckii* is found in the soil and often transmitted by injury. Tinea nigra is endemic in the tropics.
3. **Pathogenesis/virulence factors:** Tinea nigra does not elicit a host immune response, and no virulence factors are known.
4. **Laboratory diagnosis:** Direct microscopic examination of skin scrapings in a KOH preparation reveals brown pigmented yeast cells and hyphae. Culture confirmation reveals black colonies.
5. **Treatment/prevention:** Tinea nigra is treated topically with salicylic acid. Good hygiene is an important preventive measure.

C. Black Piedra and White Piedra

1. **Clinical manifestations:** Black piedra is an infection of the scalp hair caused by *Piedraia hortae* and characterized by hard, brown to black nodules attached to the hair shaft.
   a. White piedra is an infection of the scalp, moustache, beard, or pubic hair caused by *Trichosporon asahii* (formerly *T beigelii*) and characterized by cream-colored, soft nodules on the hair shaft.
   b. *T asahii* can cause disseminated trichosporonosis, mainly in neutropenic and immunocompromised patients.
2. **Transmission/epidemiology:** Black and white piedra are transmitted by infected hairs on shared combs or hairbrushes. Both black and white piedra are more common in young adults in tropical areas.
3. **Pathogenesis/virulence factors:** Black and white piedra do not elicit a host immune response, and no virulence factors are known.
4. **Laboratory diagnosis:** Direct microscopic examination of hairs in a KOH preparation reveals dark pigmented nodules containing dark septate hyphae on the hair shaft (black piedra) or white to light brown nodules with septate hyphae on the hair shaft (white piedra).
5. **Treatment/prevention:** Piedra is treated by shaving the hairs combined with good personal hygiene.

III. Cutaneous Mycoses

A. Dermatophyte Infections

1. Dermatophyte infections are usually restricted to the skin, hair, and nails.
2. Dermatophyte infections are the second most common skin disease of adults and the third most common in children.
3. Dermatophytes belong to 3 genera: *Microsporum, Trichophyton,* and *Epidermophyton.*

4. Dermatophytes are grouped by their natural habitat or reservoir as either **anthropophilic** (human skin pathogens), **zoophilic** (animal skin pathogens), or **geophilic** (soil).
5. Dermatophyte infections are clinically called ringworm or tinea along with the involved anatomic site (eg, tinea capitis [scalp], tinea pedis [feet], tinea barbae [beard, hair], tinea cruris [groin], tinea unguium [nails], and tinea manuum [hands]).

B. Tinea or Ringworm

1. **Clinical manifestations:** Tinea is an infection of the skin, hair, or nails caused by a group of dermatophytes (*Microsporum, Trichophyton, Epidermophyton*).
   a. **Tinea capitis or scalp ringworm** is caused predominately by *Trichophyton tonsurans* and the zoophilic *Microsporum canis.* It is characterized by dry, ringlike, scaly, itchy, erythematous lesions on the scalp and may present as areas of alopecia.
   b. **Tinea cruris ("jock itch")** is usually caused by *Trichophyton rubrum* or *Epidermophyton floccosum* and characterized by scalloped, scaly, erythematous lesions in the groin area.
   c. **Tinea pedis ("athlete's foot")** is usually caused by *T rubrum, T mentagrophytes,* or *E floccosum* and characterized by itchy, peeling, erythematous, painful lesions between the toes.
   d. **Tinea barbae** is usually caused by the zoophilic *T verrucosum* and characterized by inflammatory vesicopustular eruptions and areas of alopecia in the beard and moustache area.
   e. **Tinea unguium (onychomycosis)** is usually caused by *T rubrum* and characterized by thickened, friable, and discolored nails with distal subungual debris accumulation. Proximal subungual onychomycosis is uncommon in the general population but frequent in patients with AIDS.
2. **Transmission/epidemiology:** Tinea infections are transmitted directly by close contact with infected humans or animals (zoophilic species) or indirectly by contact with detached skin or hair in items such as clothing, towels, combs, and brushes.
   a. Tinea capitis is predominately a disease of children and can spread rapidly in a family or school.
   b. Onychomycosis affects 20% of the adult US population with significant social morbidity.
   c. In onychomycosis, infected nails are the reservoir for seeding other areas of the body.
3. **Pathogenesis/virulence factors:** Dermatophytes are **keratinophilic** with infection localized to the skin, hair, and nails.
   a. Dermatophytes secrete **keratinase** that digests keratin.
   b. Dermatophyte infections evoke an inflammatory response that limits infection.
   c. Deeper tissue invasion is rare because of nonspecific host defense mechanisms in skin and T-cell immunity.
   d. Patients with defects in cell-mediated immunity are at risk for chronic or disseminated dermatophyte infections.
4. **Laboratory diagnosis:** Direct microscopic examination of skin, hair, or nails in a KOH preparation demonstrates hyphae and conidia characteristic of the dermatophyte. A Wood's ultraviolet lamp can be used to detect certain fungi that fluoresce (*Microsporum*).

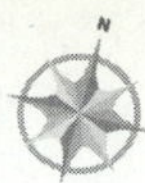

5. **Treatment/prevention:** Dermatophyte infections are treated topically with tolnaftate and terbinafine.
   a. Onychomycosis is treated systemically with itraconazole or terbinafine.
   b. Good personal hygiene is important in prevention.

ONYCHOMYCOSIS

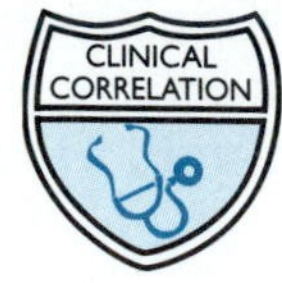

- *Onychomycosis affects approximately 20% of the US population, increases with age, and is more frequent in men than women.*
- *Onychomycosis is very difficult to treat because nails, especially toenails, grow slowly, and the location of the infection is poorly accessible.*
- *New antifungal agents (terbinafine and itraconazole) have markedly changed treatment of onychomycosis with cure rates around 80%, owing to the ability of these agents to be absorbed into the nail matrix, where they remain active for months.*

IV. Subcutaneous Mycoses

A. Characteristics of the Subcutaneous Mycoses

1. Fungi that cause subcutaneous mycoses gain entry to subcutaneous tissue via trauma to the skin.
2. The source of the causative agent is the soil or vegetation.
3. Human-to-human transmission does not occur with the subcutaneous mycoses.
4. Subcutaneous mycoses are characterized by a chronic and indolent growth pattern.

B. Sporotrichosis

1. **Clinical manifestations:** Sporotrichosis is caused by the dimorphic fungus *Sporothrix schenckii* and characterized by nodules and ulcers at the site of inoculation and along the draining lymphatic chain.
2. **Transmission/epidemiology:** Sporotrichosis is transmitted from the soil or decaying vegetation by occupational or recreational exposure to the organism via a puncture wound (eg, thorn prick).
   a. Sporotrichosis is frequently seen in gardeners.
   b. Rose thorns, sphagnum moss, and baled hay are sources of infection.
3. **Pathogenesis/virulence factors:** Sporotrichosis is a localized infection that induces an inflammatory response.
   a. Production of melanin by *S schenckii* may inhibit killing by neutrophils.
   b. Cell-mediated immunity is the major host defense mechanism.
4. **Laboratory diagnosis:** Diagnosis is made by culture demonstration of dimorphism (ie, a mold at 25 °C and yeast at 37 °C).
5. **Treatment/prevention:** Sporotrichosis is treated orally with potassium iodide (less common) or systemically with itraconazole or amphotericin B. Preventive measures include wearing gloves and protective clothing when handling rose bushes, sphagnum moss, hay bales, and wood splinters.

C. Chromoblastomycosis

1. **Clinical manifestations:** Chromoblastomycosis is caused by multiple soil fungi (*Fonsecaea, Cladosporium, Phialophora*) and characterized by the slow development of wartlike lesions that progress to a cauliflowerlike appearance at the inoculation site.
2. **Transmission/epidemiology:** The organisms responsible for chromoblastomycosis are found in the soil, endemic in the tropics, and rarely seen in the United States. Most infections occur on the feet and legs of barefoot workers.

3. **Pathogenesis/virulence factors:** Chromoblastomycosis lesions exhibit an inflammatory response with keratinolytic microabscesses and epithelial cell hyperplasia.
4. **Laboratory diagnosis:** Skin scrapings in a KOH preparation reveal copper-colored cells called sclerotic (muriform) bodies that are pathognomonic for chromoblastomycosis.
5. **Treatment/prevention:** Chromoblastomycosis is treated by surgical excision or with flucytosine or itraconazole. Wearing shoes is a preventive measure.

D. Mycetoma

1. **Clinical manifestations:** Mycetoma (also called Madura foot) is a chronic infection of subcutaneous tissue caused by a variety of saprophytic fungi in the soil.
   a. Mycetoma is characterized by localized abscess formation, edema, induration, and draining sinuses most often of the foot after a traumatic injury.
   b. The granulomas can extend to muscle and bone and result in deformities.
2. **Transmission/epidemiology:** The agents of mycetoma are ubiquitous and transmitted by inoculation due to injury most commonly in individuals who go barefoot. Mycetoma is common in the tropics but rare in the United States.
3. **Pathogenesis/virulence factors:** The granulomatous lesions of mycetoma contain sclerotia (granules, grains) that consist of a compact mass of hyphae.
4. **Laboratory diagnosis:** Diagnosis is made by macroscopic identification of granules from sclerotia. The size, shape, and color of the granules help to identify the etiologic agent.
5. **Treatment/prevention:** Treatment is by surgical debridement often combined with antifungal drugs depending on the etiologic agent. Wearing shoes is a preventive measure.

E. Rhinosporidiosis

1. **Clinical manifestations:** Rhinosporidiosis is caused by *Rhinosporidium seeberi* and characterized by the development of painless, pedunculated nasal polyps.
2. **Transmission/epidemiology:** Rhinosporidiosis is associated with divers and traumatic inoculation.
   a. Fish are the natural reservoir for rhinosporidiosis.
   b. Most cases are reported from India and Sri Lanka.
3. **Pathogenesis/virulence factors:** Lesions of rhinosporidiosis are characterized by an inflammatory cell infiltrate with abscess formation and tissue necrosis.
4. **Laboratory diagnosis:** Direct microscopic examination of excised tissue or nasal discharge in a KOH preparation reveals large spherules and endospores.
5. **Treatment/prevention:** Treatment of rhinosporidiosis is surgical removal or local injections of amphotericin B.

F. Lobomycosis

1. **Clinical manifestations:** Lobomycosis is caused by *Loboa loboi* and characterized by hard, painless nodules (keloids) on the upper extremities, face, and ear.
2. **Transmission/epidemiology:** Lobomycosis is associated with traumatic inoculation of the etiologic agent. *L loboi* is a natural infection of dolphins.
3. **Pathogenesis/virulence factors:** Lobomycosis lesions are similar to the lesions of chromoblastomycosis and mycetoma.
4. **Laboratory diagnosis:** Direct microscopic examination of excised tissue in a KOH preparation reveals yeast cells in long chains.
5. **Treatment/prevention:** Surgical excision is curative for lobomycosis.

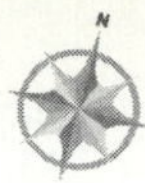

MULTISTATE OUTBREAK OF SPOROTRICHOSIS

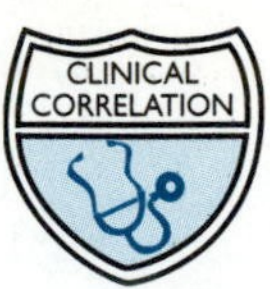

- *Sporotrichosis usually occurs sporadically as isolated cases.*
- *A multistate outbreak of sporotrichosis in the United States in 1988 affected 84 people who handled sphagnum moss.*
- *S schenckii was cultured from multiple samples of sphagnum moss.*
- *Contact with sphagnum moss should be recognized as a risk factor for infection with S schenckii.*

CLINICAL PROBLEMS

A 30-year-old man has multiple hypopigmented lesions on his chest and back. On examination, the lesions have a dry, scaly appearance. A KOH preparation reveals yeast cells and hyphae that look like spaghetti and meatballs.

1. What fungus is most likely responsible for the infection?

A. *Malassezia furfur*

B. *Exophiala werneckii*

C. *Piedraia hortae*

D. *Trichosporon asahii*

E. *Trichophyton rubrum*

A 50-year-old man living in a homeless shelter has cream-colored, soft nodules on the hair shafts of his moustache. Microscopic examination of hairs in a KOH preparation reveals white nodules on the hair shaft containing septate hyphae.

2. What fungus is most likely responsible for the infection?

A. *Malassezia furfur*

B. *Exophiala werneckii*

C. *Piedraia hortae*

D. *Trichosporon asahii*

E. *Trichophyton rubrum*

An 11-year-old boy has patchy alopecia of the scalp. He has a dog that sleeps with him nightly. Scrapings of the scalp lesions revealed hair that fluoresced under ultraviolet light and hyphae by microscopic examination.

3. What organism is most likely responsible for the infection?

A. *Trichophyton tonsurans*

B. *Microsporum canis*

C. *Epidermophyton floccosum*

D. *Trichophyton rubrum*

E. *Trichophyton verrucosum*

A 40-year-old man has thickened, friable, discolored fingernails on both hands.

4. This clinical presentation is characteristic of:

A. Pityriasis versicolor

B. Black piedra

C. Onychomycosis

D. Tinea manuum

E. Tinea nigra

A 60-year-old master gardener has an ulcerative lesion on her thumb and several nodular lesions on her arm along the lymphatic chain. She reports being pricked with a rose thorn 2 weeks earlier.

5. What organism is responsible for the infection?

A. *Phialophora* species

B. *Sporothrix schenckii*

C. *Rhinosporidium seeberi*

D. *Loboa loboi*

E. *Trichosporon asahii*

ANSWERS

1. The answer is A. *M furfur* is the cause of this case of pityriasis versicolor, and fungal structures that look like spaghetti and meatballs are seen microscopically. *E werneckii* is the cause of tinea nigra. *P hortae* is the cause of black piedra. *T asahii* is the cause of white piedra. *T rubrum* is the common cause of athlete's foot and onychomycosis.

2. The answer is D. *T asahii* is the cause of this case of white piedra characterized by the white nodules containing hyphae on the hair shafts. *M furfur* is the cause of pityriasis. *E werneckii* is the cause of tinea nigra. *P hortae* is the cause of black piedra. *T rubrum* is the common cause of athlete's foot and onychomycosis.

3. The answer is B. The zoophilic *M canis* is the cause of this case of tinea capitis or scalp ringworm. It is likely that the ringworm was transmitted from the pet dog to the boy. *Microsporum* fluoresces under ultraviolet light (Wood's lamp). *T tonsurans* is an anthropophilic dermatophyte that causes tinea capitis but does not fluoresce with ultraviolet light. *E floccosum* is a cause of tinea cruris ("jock itch"). *T rubrum* is the common cause of athlete's foot and onychomycosis. *T verrucosum* is the cause of tinea barbae.

4. The answer is C. The case presentation is typical of a dermatophyte infection of the nails. Pityriasis versicolor is a superficial fungal infection localized to the torso and arms. Black piedra is an infection of the scalp hair. Tinea manuum is an infection of the hands. Tinea nigra is an infection most often of the palms and soles.

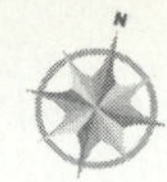

5. The answer is B. This is a classic case presentation of sporotrichosis caused by *S schenckii* introduced into subcutaneous tissue by a rose thorn contaminated with the organism. *Phialophora* species is one of the fungi responsible for chromoblastomycosis. *R seeberi* is the cause of nasal polyps seen in rhinosporidiosis. *L loboi* is the lobomycosis that presents with nodules on the face and ears. *T asahii* is the cause of white piedra, which is an infection of the hair shaft.

CHAPTER 19

SYSTEMIC (GEOGRAPHIC) MYCOSES AND OPPORTUNISTIC MYCOSES

I. Fungal Diseases: Key Concepts

A. Fungi that cause systemic infections are inherently virulent and capable of causing disease in otherwise healthy persons.

B. Medically important systemic mycoses are **histoplasmosis, blastomycosis, coccidioidomycosis,** and **paracoccidioidomycosis.**

C. Systemic fungal pathogens cause endemic disease in defined geographic areas.

D. Systemic fungal pathogens are **thermally dimorphic,** growing as the mycelial form in the soil and the yeast form at body temperature.

E. Systemic fungal pathogens are transmitted by the inhalation of spores that germinate in the lungs. There is no human-to-human transmission.

F. Opportunistic fungi primarily cause disease in immunocompromised or debilitated individuals.

G. Opportunistic fungi cause a diverse spectrum of diseases determined by the immunologic and physiologic state of the individual.

H. Medically important opportunistic mycoses are **candidiasis, cryptococcosis, aspergillosis, zygomycosis, hyalohyphomycosis,** and **pneumocystosis.**

II. Systemic Mycoses

A. Histoplasmosis

1. **Clinical manifestations:** Histoplasmosis is caused by *Histoplasma capsulatum.*
   a. Most infections (>90%) are asymptomatic, are self-limiting, and involve immunocompetent individuals.
   b. Chronic pulmonary and progressive histoplasmosis occurs in 1% of cases, usually in the immunocompromised person or because of exposure to a large inoculum of the organism.
   c. Disseminated histoplasmosis is rare but may develop in immunocompromised patients with T-cell defects (eg, in patients with AIDS) and solid-organ transplant recipients.
   d. Disseminated histoplasmosis has a mortality rate of about 10% in patients with HIV or AIDS.

 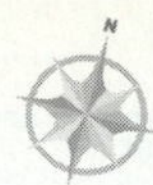

2. **Transmission/epidemiology:** Histoplasmosis is transmitted by **inhalation** of aerosolized **spores (microconidia)** after disturbance of contaminated soil.
   a. Histoplasmosis occurs worldwide but is **endemic** in the **Ohio and Mississippi River valleys** of the United States.
   b. *H capsulatum* grows in the soil, particularly in soil containing bird (especially starlings) and bat droppings.
3. **Pathogenesis/virulence factors:** Inhaled microconidia of *H capsulatum* are phagocytized by and grow in alveolar **macrophages,** where they undergo conversion to the yeast form.
   a. Yeast cells multiply intracellularly in macrophages and continue to grow until an immune response is elicited, resulting in a localized granuloma.
   b. Disseminated histoplasmosis involves invasion of cells of the reticuloendothelial system (liver, spleen, lymph nodes, bone marrow).
   c. *H capsulatum* survives phagolysosomal killing by inducing a rise in lysosomal pH, thereby inactivating degradative enzymes of the phagolysosome.
4. **Laboratory diagnosis:** Direct microscopic examination of clinical specimens (sputum, tissue) stained with Giemsa or Wright stain reveals yeast within macrophages.
   a. Culture of the organism at 25 °C shows hyphae with characteristic tuberculate macroconidia and conversion to the yeast form when incubated at 37 °C.
   b. A *H capsulatum*-specific polysaccharide antigen can be detected by enzyme immunoassay in blood and urine of patients with disseminated disease.
5. **Treatment/prevention:** No treatment is required for primary infections that are usually self-limited.
   a. Itraconazole and amphotericin B are used to treat histoplasmosis.
   b. There is no vaccine for the prevention of histoplasmosis.
   c. Avoidance of exposure in high endemic areas is a preventive measure.

B. Blastomycosis

1. **Clinical manifestations:** Blastomycosis is caused by *Blastomyces dermatitidis.*
   a. Symptomatic infection is common (50% of cases) with pulmonary symptoms of chest pain, sputum production, and fever.
   b. Clinical features are similar to histoplasmosis and may mimic tuberculosis or lung cancer.
   c. Progressive disseminated blastomycosis may involve secondary sites, most commonly the skin (70%), bone (33%), genitourinary tract (25%), and central nervous system (CNS) (10%).
2. **Transmission/epidemiology:** Blastomycosis is transmitted by the **inhalation** of aerosolized **spores (conidia)** after disturbance of contaminated soil.
   a. Blastomycosis is **endemic** in the **Ohio and Mississippi River valley** regions as well as in the **Missouri and Arkansas River basins** of the United States.
   b. Soil enriched with organic matter is the reservoir of infection.
   c. The typical patient is a middle-aged male with extensive outdoor occupational or recreational exposure.
   d. Blastomycosis is an important veterinary disease with natural disease in dogs and horses.
3. **Pathogenesis/virulence factors:** After inhalation of *Blastomyces* conidia, a mixed inflammatory response occurs with infiltration of macrophages and neutrophils and granuloma formation. Cell-mediated immunity is an important determinant in recovery from infection.

4. **Laboratory diagnosis:** Direct microscopic examination of sputum, exudates, or tissues in a potassium hydroxide (KOH) preparation reveals the characteristic **broad-base budding yeast** cells of *Blastomyces dermatitidis.* Culture identification of thermal dimorphism (mold at 25 °C, yeast at 37 °C) is prolonged.
5. **Treatment/prevention:** Itraconazole is used to treat non–life-threatening disease, and amphotericin B is used for life-threatening, disseminated blastomycosis.
   a. There is no vaccine for the prevention of blastomycosis.
   b. Avoidance of exposure in high endemic areas is a means of prevention.

C. Coccidioidomycosis

1. **Clinical manifestations:** Coccidioidomycosis is caused by *Coccidioides immitis.*
   a. Infection is largely asymptomatic, but about 40% develop pulmonary disease that is self-limited in most.
   b. Disseminated extrapulmonary coccidioidomycosis occurs in about 5% of cases and involves the skin, bone, and CNS with meningitis.
   c. Untreated disseminated disease has a mortality of 50%.
2. **Transmission/epidemiology:** Coccidioidomycosis is transmitted by **inhalation** of aerosolized **arthroconidia** after contaminated soil is disturbed by humans (excavation) or nature (dust storms, earthquakes).
   a. Coccidioidomycosis is **endemic** in arid regions of the **southwestern United States, parts of Mexico, and South America.**
   b. In the United States, endemic areas are Arizona, Nevada, New Mexico, western Texas, and parts of central and southern California.
   c. Travelers to areas of endemic disease may become infected and develop symptoms after returning home.
   d. Maximum transmission in endemic areas is in the dry summer and autumn and increases after heavy seasonal rains.
   e. Groups at high risk for infection are blacks and Asians, pregnant women during the third trimester, and immunocompromised individuals.
3. **Pathogenesis/virulence factors:** Inhaled arthroconidia germinate in the lung to form spherules filled with endospores.
   a. Organisms are phagocytized by macrophages and neutrophils.
   b. Proteases and components of the spherule outer wall contribute to virulence.
   c. Cell-mediated immunity is a key determinant to disease resolution.
4. **Laboratory diagnosis:** Direct examination of clinical specimens (sputum, tissue) in a KOH preparation reveals characteristic **spherules.**
   a. *C immitis*–specific serum IgM response is indicative of acute infection.
   b. Skin test reactivity to fungal extracts (coccidioidin and spherulin) is used to diagnose exposure to infection but may become negative in disseminated disease.
   c. Eosinophilia has been noted as a useful laboratory marker of coccidioidomycosis.
5. **Treatment/prevention:** Amphotericin B, fluconazole, and itraconazole are used to treat coccidioidomycosis.
   a. Fluconazole is effective for disease-associated meningitis because of its improved CNS penetration.
   b. There is no vaccine to prevent coccidioidomycosis.
   c. Avoidance of travel to endemic areas and activities that generate dust exposure in endemic areas are preventive measures.

 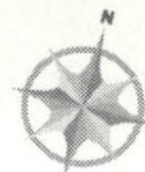

D. Paracoccidioidomycosis

1. **Clinical manifestations:** Paracoccidioidomycosis is caused by *Paracoccidioides brasiliensis.*
   a. Asymptomatic infections are common.
   b. Symptomatic infections present as primary and chronic pneumonia characterized by fever, cough, sputum production, and chest pain, symptoms similar to those of histoplasmosis and blastomycosis.
   c. Disseminated extrapulmonary disease is rare but usually presents as oral, nasal, and facial nodular ulcerative lesions and submandibular lymphadenopathy.
2. **Transmission/epidemiology:** Paracoccidioidomycosis is transmitted by the **inhalation** of aerosolized **conidia** after contaminated soil is disturbed.
   a. Paracoccidioidomycosis is restricted to **Central and South America.**
   b. Symptomatic and progressive paracoccidioidomycosis is 9 times more common in males than females because of the estrogen-mediated inhibition of mycelial-to-yeast conversion in vivo.
3. **Pathogenesis/virulence factors:** Inhaled conidia germinate in the lung to the pathogenic yeast form.
   a. A fungal, cytoplasmic, estrogen-binding protein inhibits the mold-to-yeast phase conversion in the presence of estrogen, accounting for the clinical disease predilection in males.
   b. Cell-mediated immunity is a primary determinant of recovery from infection.
4. **Laboratory diagnosis:** Direct microscopic examination of clinical specimens (sputum, bronchoalveolar lavage, tissue) in a KOH preparation reveals characteristic **yeast with multiple buds** in a "pilot wheel" configuration. Culture to demonstrate thermal dimorphism (mold at 25 °C, yeast at 37 °C) may be performed for confirmation.
5. **Treatment/prevention:** Itraconazole and amphotericin B are the drugs of choice for the treatment of paracoccidioidomycosis.
   a. There is no vaccine for the prevention of paracoccidioidomycosis.
   b. Avoidance of travel to endemic areas is a means of prevention.

COCCIDIOIDOMYCOSIS IN TRAVELERS TO ENDEMIC AREAS

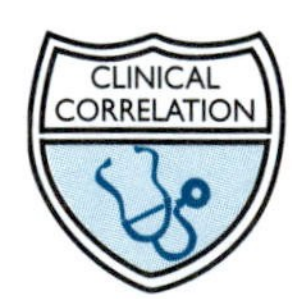

- *Outbreaks of coccidioidomycosis have been reported among travelers returning from Mexico, where the disease is endemic.*
- *Travel to Mexico for work or vacation has become more common and underscores the need for increased awareness about coccidioidomycosis, especially for those exposed to occupational or recreational activities in dusty environments.*
- *Health care workers should consider coccidioidomycosis in travelers returning from endemic areas experiencing an influenzalike illness with symptoms of fatigue, fever, and myalgia.*

III. Opportunistic Mycoses

A. Candidiasis

1. **Clinical manifestations:** Candidiasis, caused by *Candida albicans* and other *Candida* species, includes cutaneous, mucocutaneous, chronic mucocutaneous, and disseminated infections.
   a. **Cutaneous candidiasis** involves warm, moist skin folds and presents as localized erythema or rash (eg, diaper rash, skin folds of obese individuals) in healthy hosts.

b. **Mucocutaneous candidiasis** is seen as **oral thrush or oropharyngeal candidiasis,** usually in newborns, that presents as creamy, curdlike patches on the oral mucosa and tongue. **Vulvovaginal candidiasis** appears as thick, white, vaginal discharge accompanied by burning or itching.
c. Oral thrush and recurrent vulvovaginal candidiasis are common in patients with AIDS.
d. **Chronic mucocutaneous candidiasis** is a rare but severe infection of skin and mucous membranes but without invasive manifestations that is linked to a specific T-cell defect.
e. **Disseminated candidiasis** is limited to immunocompromised individuals and can involve nearly every organ (eg, esophagitis, renal and hepatosplenic infection, meningitis, endophthalmitis).

2. **Transmission/epidemiology:** *Candida* species are part of the **normal flora** of the mouth, vagina, and gastrointestinal tract and cause endogenous infections.
   a. *Candida* species are many and include *C albicans* (most common), *C tropicalis, C paralopsis, C krusei, C glabrata,* and *C lusitaniae,* among others.
   b. Nearly 75% of all women have at least one vaginal yeast infection in their lifetime.
   c. *Candida* species are an important cause of nosocomial bloodstream infections in the immunocompromised.
   d. Risk groups for disseminated disease are debilitated individuals in intensive care units, individuals with diabetes, patients with cancer with chemotherapy-induced neutropenia or mucositis, patients with depressed cell-mediated immunity (HIV-AIDS), and individuals receiving broad-spectrum antibiotics that alter the normal microbial flora.
3. **Pathogenesis/virulence factors:** Candidiasis occurs when host immune defenses are impaired because of disease or iatrogenic intervention (eg, antibiotics, chemotherapy, steroids), allowing *Candida* overgrowth.
   a. The switch from the yeast to hyphal form is associated with virulence of *C albicans.*
   b. Hyphal cell wall protein promotes attachment of *C albicans* to epithelial cells.
   c. Other *C albicans* virulence factors include surface integrinlike molecules that mediate binding to the extracellular matrix, proteases that facilitate invasion, and a receptor that binds complement.
   d. Neutrophils, humoral immunity, and cell-mediated immunity are important defense mechanisms against *Candida* infections.
4. **Laboratory diagnosis:** Direct microscopic examination of clinical specimens in a KOH preparation demonstrates **budding yeast** and **pseudohyphae** (ie, elongated yeast cells that resemble hyphae). *C albicans* is identified by the formation of **germ tubes** (ie, hyphal outgrowths from yeast cells) when incubated in serum at 37 °C.
5. **Treatment/prevention:** Fluconazole and itraconazole are used to treat thrush and vulvovaginal candidiasis.
   a. *C krusei* and *C glabrata* are resistant to fluconazole.
   b. Cutaneous infections are treated with topical antifungals (eg, miconazole).
   c. Amphotericin B is used to treat systemic disease.
   d. There is no vaccine for the prevention of *Candida* infections.

 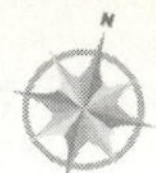

B. Cryptococcosis

1. **Clinical manifestations:** Cryptococcosis, caused by *Cryptococcus neoformans,* presents with a slow onset of CNS symptoms that progress to chronic **meningitis** in patients with AIDS.
   a. *C neoformans* can cause a mild or asymptomatic pneumonia that is usually self-limited.
   b. Skin lesions and bone involvement are frequent in disseminated disease.
2. **Transmission/epidemiology:** Cryptococcosis is transmitted by the **inhalation** of yeast cells in soil and roosting sites contaminated with **pigeon droppings.**
   a. There is no human-to-human transmission of cryptococcosis.
   b. *C neoformans* is not dimorphic, existing only as the yeast form.
   c. *C neoformans* is the most common cause of meningitis in patients with AIDS.
   d. Groups at risk for infection are the immunocompromised, especially patients with HIV and AIDS, and those who have undergone an organ transplant.
3. **Pathogenesis/virulence factors:** The organism gains access to the lungs by inhalation followed by hematogenous spread to the brain and meninges.
   a. The polysaccharide **capsule** of *C neoformans* inhibits phagocytosis by neutrophils and macrophages in the lung, promoting dissemination.
   b. T-cell–mediated immunity is the primary determinant of resistance.
4. **Laboratory diagnosis:** Detection of **cryptococcal polysaccharide antigen** in cerebrospinal fluid or serum by latex agglutination is highly sensitive and specific for the diagnosis of cryptococcosis. **India ink stain** of cerebrospinal fluid demonstrates **encapsulated yeast,** visualized as cells surrounded by a clear halo, in about 50% of cases.
5. **Treatment/prevention:** Amphotericin B plus flucytosine is used to treat disseminated cryptococcosis.
   a. Fluconazole is used to prevent disease relapse in patients with AIDS.
   b. There is no vaccine to prevent cryptococcosis.
   c. Avoidance by immunocompromised patients of areas with pigeon excreta is a preventive measure.

C. Aspergillosis

1. **Clinical manifestations:** Aspergillosis is caused by *Aspergillus* species, including *A fumigatus* (most common), *A flavus,* and *A niger.*
   a. In immunocompromised persons, *Aspergillus* is a common cause of fungal **sinusitis** and **allergic bronchopulmonary aspergillosis** characterized by asthma, eosinophilia, and elevated IgE antibodies.
   b. *Aspergillus* causes **fungus balls (aspergillomas),** a noninvasive mass of hypae that colonizes an old cavity (eg, a tuberculous cavity) in the lungs of debilitated individuals. Hemoptysis (ie, coughing up blood) is the most common symptom.
   c. *Aspergillus* species cause invasive **pulmonary aspergillosis** that may disseminate to any organ in patients with hematologic malignancies, bone marrow or solid-organ transplant recipients, and in patients receiving high doses of immunosuppressive drugs.
2. **Transmission/epidemiology:** Aspergillosis is transmitted by the **inhalation** of aerosolized **conidia** in the soil or dust exposure during building construction.
   a. *Aspergillus* species are not dimorphic, existing only as the mold form.
   b. Invasive aspergillosis is the second most common fungal infection, requiring hospitalization in the United States.

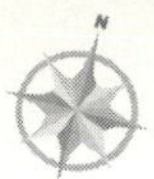

c. Severe, protracted neutropenia is the major risk factor for the development of aspergillosis.
d. Aspergillosis is one of the most common causes of infection and related death in patients with hematologic malignancies.
e. Aspergillosis is uncommon in patients with HIV and AIDS.

3. **Pathogenesis/virulence factors:** Inhaled conidia germinate in the lung alveoli into angioinvasive filamentous hyphae that produce hemorrhage, infarction, and necrosis and disseminate to distal sites.
   a. In immunocompetent individuals, alveolar macrophages and neutrophils are the first line of defense against invasive aspergillosis, acting to ingest and kill conidia and hyphae.
   b. These innate cellular defense mechanisms are impaired in underlying disease or corticosteroid and cytotoxic therapy, rendering patients neutropenic and susceptible to invasive aspergillosis.
   c. Activation of T-cell immunity is critical in the control of infection.
   d. *Aspergillus* secretes proteases and phospholipases that may contribute to tissue injury and invasion.
4. **Laboratory diagnosis:** Detection of *Aspergillus* **antigen** (galactomannan) in serum by enzyme immunoassay is a sensitive assay for the diagnosis of invasive aspergillosis.
   a. Direct microscopic detection of **septate hyphae** in tissue biopsy specimens provides a presumptive diagnosis of invasive fungal disease, but culture confirmation is required for identification.
   b. Polymerase chain reaction detection of *Aspergillus* nucleic acid in bronchoalveolar lavage and blood specimens is a promising method for early detection of invasive aspergillosis.
5. **Treatment/prevention:** Therapy for invasive aspergillosis is difficult and highly individualized and includes amphotericin B, itraconazole, voriconazole, and caspofungin. Surgical removal of the fungus ball is a therapeutic option.

D. Zygomycosis (Mucormycosis)

1. **Clinical manifestations:** Zygomycosis is a fungal infection caused most commonly by *Rhizopus, Absidia,* and *Mucor* species and characterized by rhinocerebral, pulmonary, or cutaneous disease.
   a. **Rhinocerebral zygomycosis,** most common in patients with **diabetes,** originates in the paranasal sinus and spreads to the orbit, hard palate, and brain with a high mortality rate.
   b. **Pulmonary** and **cutaneous zygomycoses** are seen in immunocompromised and debilitated individuals and characterized by pulmonary lesions or necrotic skin ulcers often associated with leukemia, organ transplantation, or burns.
2. **Transmission/epidemiology:** Zygomycosis is transmitted by the **inhalation** of aerosolized **spores** that exist in the soil or on food. Groups at risk for zygomycosis are patients with diabetes with ketoacidosis and individuals with leukopenia or who are undergoing treatment with immunosuppressive drugs.
3. **Pathogenesis/virulence factors:** Inhaled spores germinate in the lung into angioinvasive, filamentous hyphae that result in tissue infarction, necrosis, and hemorrhage. Cell-mediated immunity is the major determinant of resistance to zygomycosis.
4. **Laboratory diagnosis:** Zygomycosis is diagnosed by the detection of nonseptate, "ribbonlike" hyphae in biopsy specimens and confirmed by culture identification.

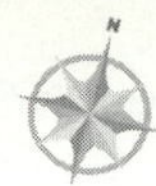

5. **Treatment/prevention:** Surgical debridement and amphotericin B are the treatment options for zygomycosis.

E. Hyalohyphomycosis

1. **Clinical manifestations:** Hyalohyphomycosis denotes a group of opportunistic fungi distinguished by the presence of filamentous hyphae without cell wall pigmentation, notably *Fusarium, Scedosporium,* and *Penicillium.*
   a. **Fusariosis,** caused by *Fusarium,* exhibits a wide range of clinical symptoms, including cutaneous lesions (most common), rhinocerebral syndrome, endophthalmitis, pneumonia, and disseminated infection, particularly in neutropenic, burn, and transplant patients.
   b. ***Scedosporium*** is characterized by sinusitis, endophthalmitis, and pneumonia with dissemination to the CNS in debilitated and immunocompromised patients similar to that of *Aspergillus.*
   c. **Penicilliosis,** caused by *Penicillium marneffei,* is characterized by multiple skin lesions and disseminated infection of the lung and liver in **patients with AIDS in Thailand** and Southeast Asia.
   d. Cases of penicilliosis in the United States are linked to patients who have visited endemic areas.
2. **Transmission/epidemiology:** Fusariosis, *Scedosporium,* and penicillinosis are transmitted by the **inhalation** of aerosolized **spores** that exist in the soil. *P marneffei* is the third most common cause of disseminated infection in patients with AIDS in Thailand.
3. **Pathogenesis/virulence factors:** Histopathology and pathogenesis of fusariosis and *Scedosporium* are similar to those of aspergillosis.
   a. *P marneffei* germinates in tissue to form yeast.
   b. Cell-mediated immunity is the major determinant of resistance to hyalohyphomycosis.
4. **Laboratory diagnosis:** Direct examination of tissue biopsy specimens from patients with fusariosis and *Scedosporium* reveals hyphae that resemble *Aspergillus.* Definitive diagnosis requires culture identification. Detection of intracellular yeast in biopsy specimen of bone marrow or skin lesions provides a presumptive diagnosis of *P marneffei* infection.
5. **Treatment/prevention:** Fusariosis has variable responses to amphotericin B or azoles.
   a. *Scedosporium* is resistant to amphotericin B but susceptible to azoles.
   b. *P marneffei* is treated with amphotericin B or itraconazole with lifelong maintenance therapy to prevent disease relapse.

F. Pneumocystosis

1. **Clinical manifestations:** Pneumocystosis is a lethal pneumonia of patients with AIDS caused by *Pneumocystis jiroveci* (formerly known as *Pneumocystis carinii*) and characterized by a fever, nonproductive cough, and progressive dyspnea.
   a. Extrapulmonary disease occurs in a minority (<3%) of cases involving the lymph nodes, spleen, bone marrow, and liver.
   b. *P jiroveci* pneumonia (PCP) is also seen in premature, malnourished infants.
2. **Transmission/epidemiology:** PCP is transmitted by the **airborne route,** but the reservoir of transmission is unknown.
   a. *P jiroveci* is classified as a fungus based on nucleic acid and biochemical analysis.

   b. The organism is ubiquitous, with more than 80% of individuals seropositive for *P jiroveci* antibodies by the age of 4 years.
   c. PCP is the most common opportunistic infection and the leading cause of death in patients with AIDS.
3. **Pathogenesis/virulence factors:** *P jiroveci* attaches to alveolar pneumocytes, accumulates in the lumen, and induces an inflammatory cell infiltrate, effectively blocking gas exchange in the lung. Cell-mediated immunity is the primary determinant of disease resolution.
4. **Laboratory diagnosis:** Gomori methenamine-silver stain of induced sputum or bronchoalveolar lavage material is used to detect morphologic forms of *P jiroveci.*
5. **Treatment/prevention:** PCP is treated with a combination of trimethoprim and sulfamethoxazole (TMP-SMX), also used prophylactically to prevent PCP in patients with AIDS.

OPPORTUNISTIC MYCOSES

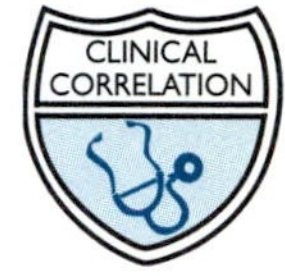

- *Medical advances in cancer chemotherapy, allogeneic bone marrow, and solid organ transplantation coupled with the AIDS epidemic have expanded the proportion of immunocompromised patients at risk for life-threatening opportunistic fungal infections.*
- *Rapid diagnostic tests, immune reconstitution strategies, and improved antifungal drugs are pressing needs for the development of more effective treatment strategies for opportunistic mycoses.*

CLINICAL PROBLEMS

A 45-year-old man is seen in the emergency department reporting fatigue, fever, myalgia, chest pain, and shortness of breath that have lasted a week. He recently returned from a mission trip to Acapulco, Mexico, where he helped to construct a church. On physical examination, he had a fever of 101 °F, a deep cough, and tender joints. Laboratory workup revealed eosinophilia. Microscopic examination of a sputum specimen detected spherules.

1. The most likely diagnosis is:

   A. Histoplasmosis
   B. Blastomycosis
   C. Coccidioidomycosis
   D. Paracoccidioidomycosis
   E. Cryptococcosis

A 50-year-old man from rural Arkansas experiences symptoms of chest pain and fever. He is a former smoker and works as a guide for a local hunt club. Chest x-ray revealed a right lower lobe, masslike lesion suggestive of lung cancer. Cytologic examination of the lung tissue showed broad-based budding yeast.

 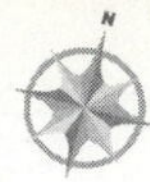

2. The most likely diagnosis is:

A. Histoplasmosis

B. Blastomycosis

C. Coccidioidomycosis

D. Paracoccidioidomycosis

E. Pneumocystosis

A 55-year-old man with acute myelogenous leukemia had prolonged neutropenia and fever develop after chemotherapy despite broad-spectrum antimicrobial therapy. Lung lesions were apparent on computed tomography scan, and 1 week later, he had an episode of hemoptysis. Biopsy of one of the lesions showed septate hyphae, and laboratory test results for galactomannan antigen were positive.

3. The fungus most likely responsible for this infection is:

A. *Candida albicans*

B. *Cryptococcus neoformans*

C. *Rhizopus*

D. *Aspergillus*

E. *Pneumocystis jiroveci*

A 55-year-old woman with diabetes is seen in the emergency department with severe ketoacidosis. One week after hospital admission, she had a persistent headache and eye pain develop. Physical examination revealed an ulcerative lesion on the hard palate and biopsy results showed "ribbonlike" hyphae on microscopic examination.

4. The fungus most likely responsible for this clinical presentation is:

A. *Aspergillus fumigatus*

B. *Rhizopus*

C. *Fusarium*

D. *Scedosporium*

E. *Penicillium marneffei*

An HIV-infected woman is seen in the clinic reporting a severe headache and increasing disorientation. Two weeks before this visit, she helped clean out an abandoned house that was inhabited by pigeons. She was admitted to the hospital, where an India ink stain of a lumbar puncture revealed budding yeast surrounded by a capsule.

5. The fungus most likely responsible for the infection is:

A. *Candida albicans*

B. *Histoplasma capsulatum*

C. *Cryptococcus neoformans*

D. *Penicillium marneffei*

E. *Pneumocystis jiroveci*

ANSWERS

1. The answer is C. Coccidioidomycosis is a systemic fungal infection endemic in parts of Mexico and linked with the inhalation of spores in dust created by construction. Eosinophilia is a marker of coccidioidomycosis, and morphologically characteristic spherules are diagnostic of *C immitis.*

2. The answer is B. Blastomycosis is a geographic fungal infection found in the midwestern United States and frequently associated with outdoor occupational and recreational activity. Detection of broad-based budding yeast in clinical specimens is characteristic of blastomycosis.

3. The answer is D. *Aspergillus* species cause opportunistic infections in patients with neutropenia with hematologic malignancies. This patient had a fungus ball develop and exhibited the common symptom of hemoptysis. A positive antigen test result for *Aspergillus*-specific galactomannan is diagnostic for *Aspergillus* infection.

4. The answer is B. Diabetic ketoacidosis is a strong risk factor for zygomycosis caused by *Rhizopus.* Laboratory detection of "ribbonlike" hyphae in the tissue biopsy specimen reinforces the clinical presentation of *Rhizopus* infection.

5. The answer is C. *C neoformans* is the most common cause of meningitis in patients with AIDS. The history of exposure to pigeon excreta likely aerosolized during cleaning coupled with encapsulated yeast detection on cerebrospinal fluid India ink examination strongly implicates infection by *C neoformans.*

CHAPTER 20
BASIC PARASITOLOGY

I. Classification

A. The medically important parasites are classified into 2 major groups: protozoa and worms.

B. There are 4 different classes within the phylum Protozoa.

1. The **Sarcodina,** better known as **amebae,** include *Entamoeba histolytica* and *Naegleria fowleri.*
2. The **Mastigophora,** commonly referred to as **flagellates,** include *Giardia lamblia, Trichomonas vaginalis, Leishmania* (*L donovani, L tropica, L mexicana,* and *L braziliensis*), and *Trypanosoma* (*T brucei* [rhodesiense and gambiense], *T cruzi*).
3. The **Ciliata,** better known as the **ciliates,** have one primary human pathogen, *Balantidium coli.*
4. The **Sporozoa** are characterized with alternating cycles of sexual and asexual reproduction and include *Plasmodium species* (*P vivax, P ovale, P malariae,* and *P falciparum*), *Toxoplasma gondii,* and *Cryptosporidium parvum.*

C. The worms are divided into 2 phyla, **Aschelminthes** and **Platyhelminthes.**

1. Within the Aschelminthes, the class **Nematoda** (ie, roundworms) includes *Enterobius vermicularis, Ascaris lumbricoides, Trichuris trichiura, Ancylostoma duodenale, Necator americanus, Strongyloides stercoralis, Trichinella spiralis, Wuchereria bancrofti, Onchocerca volvulus, Toxocara canis,* and *Toxocara cati.*
2. The Platyhelminthes have 2 classes, **Cestoda** and **Trematoda.**
   - **a.** Cestodes, better known as the **tapeworms,** are **segmented flatworms** and include *Taenia solium, Taenia saginata, Diphyllobothrium latum, Echinococcus granulosus,* and *Hymenolepis nana.*
   - **b.** Trematodes, also known as the **flukes,** are **nonsegmented flatworms** and include the *Schistosoma* (species *S mansoni, S japonicum,* and *S haematobium*).

II. Hosts, Transmission, and Life Cycles

A. A **parasite** is, by definition, an organism that lives upon or within another organism (the host) at the expense of that host organism.

1. A **definitive host** harbors the sexually mature or adult form of the parasite.
2. In an **intermediate host,** a parasite develops to a certain stage but can progress no further without transmission to the definitive host to complete its life cycle.
3. A **reservoir host** parallels a human host in the life cycle of a parasite.
4. A human becomes a **dead-end host** when infected with a parasitic form that cannot be transmitted back to the definitive host.

5. A **vector,** often also a host, is important in the transmission of parasites from one host to another.

B. There are 4 primary modes of **transmission** of parasitic infections.
   1. **Ingestion** of parasites, cysts, or eggs is extremely common for both protozoa (eg, *E histolytica* and *G lamblia*) and worm organisms (eg, *A lumbricoides* and *T trichiura*) and usually involves fecal-oral transmission.
   2. **Direct skin penetration** occurs with several different parasites (eg, *Schistosoma* species, hookworms, and *S stercoralis*).
   3. **Direct person-to-person** transmission occurs by sexual contact (eg, *T vaginalis*) or oral-anal contact (eg, *E histolytica, G lamblia,* and *C parvum*).
   4. **Arthropods** are important not only as hosts, but also as vectors of transmission (eg, *Plasmodium* species, *Leishmania* species, *Trypanosoma* species, *W bancrofti,* and *O volvulus*).

C. The life cycle of a parasite can involve a single host or multiple hosts.
   1. When only a single host is involved, parasites are passed from person to person, usually either by direct contact or by coming in contact with human fecal waste.
   2. When multiple hosts are required to complete the life cycle, transmission is sometimes limited to geographic areas that harbor all hosts.
   3. Humans can be a definitive host, an intermediate host, or a dead-end host depending on the parasitic infection.

III. Pathogenesis

A. The pathogenesis caused by parasitic infections is often directly related to the **parasite burden** (ie, number of parasites) and can be classified into 7 different general mechanisms.

B. The presence of parasites within the intestine, various ducts, and lymphatics can result in physical **obstruction** (eg, *Ascaris* obstruction of bile ducts and *Wuchereria* obstruction of lymphatics leading to elephantiasis).

C. Invasion into host cells and tissues results in **cell and tissue destruction** (eg, *Plasmodium* destruction of erythrocytes).

D. Some parasites **compete with the host for nutrients,** leading to nutrient deficiencies (eg, *D latum* and vitamin B_{12}).

E. The presence of parasites in large numbers in the intestine can cause host **malabsorption** (eg, *G lamblia*).

F. Attachment of parasites to the intestinal mucosa can lead to **blood loss and iron deficiencies** (eg, hookworm and whipworm infections).

G. Growth of parasites within a closed environment, such as the central nervous system, can cause **pressure-related pathogenesis** (eg, **hydatid** cysts of *E granulosus*).

H. The **host immunologic response** to infection often results in eosinophilia, nonspecific tissue destruction, hypersensitivity responses (anaphylaxis), immune complex deposition, and granuloma formation in vital organs.

PARASITE BURDEN AND PATHOGENESIS

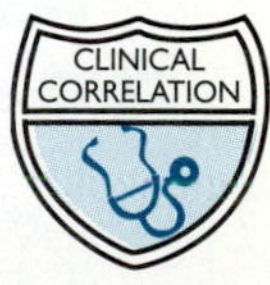

- *The parasite load or burden is directly related to the severity of pathogenesis.*
- *Unlike most protozoa, many worm infections do not result in a replication-induced increase in parasitic burden within the host.*

 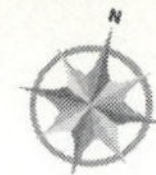

- *Because many worms are extremely long lived (some for decades), reinfection results in a gradual increase in parasite load within an individual.*
- *Some treatment strategies are aimed at reducing parasite burden rather than curing infection.*

IV. Treatment

A. Because parasites are eukaryotes, treatment must rely on differential toxicity using strategies to target preferential uptake, differential susceptibility, or drug modification by the parasite.

B. Quinolines (**chloroquine, primaquine, mefloquine, quinine,** and **quinidine**) are preferentially accumulated in parasitized host cells, where they interfere with DNA replication.

C. Arsenic and antimonial drugs, such as **melarsoprol** and **sodium stibogluconate,** bind to sulfhydryl groups on proteins and enzymes and are particularly effective in parasitic cells with high metabolic activity.

D. Many protozoa need to synthesize folic acid for purine biosynthesis and are therefore sensitive to inhibitors of folic acid synthesis, such as **pyrimethamine, trimethoprim,** and **sulfonamides.**

E. Nitroimidazoles, such as **metronidazole,** are converted to toxic intermediates by parasites and are thought to work at the level of inhibition of DNA synthesis, possibly through DNA alkylation.

F. Benzimidazoles, such as **mebendazole, thiabendazole,** and **albendazole,** are broad-spectrum antihelmintic agents that inhibit tubulin polymerization and the formation of microtubules.

G. Paralytic agents—including tetrahydropyrimidines (eg, **pyrantel pamoate**), piperazines (eg, **piperazine** and **diethylcarbamazine**), and avermectins (eg, **ivermectin**)—stimulate neuromuscular paralysis, facilitating the expulsion of worms from the host intestinal tract.

H. Pyrazinoisoquinolines, such as **praziquantel,** alter the balance of intracellular calcium, causing tetanic muscle contraction and alterations in the parasite tegument leading to increased susceptibility to host immune killing.

V. Prevention and Control

A. Most parasitic infections are associated either with arthropod vectors or with poor sanitation and poverty, leading to conditions in which humans come in contact regularly with human and animal fecal material.

B. Education concerning parasite transmission and measures to improve sanitation can go a long way toward breaking the continuous cycle of infection, transmission, and reinfection.

C. Control of vector-borne parasite transmission includes measures designed to reduce arthropod vectors and use of physical barriers to prevent human exposure.

D. Chemoprophylactic measures are effective for certain parasitic infections, including malaria.

CLINICAL PROBLEMS

A 6-year-old boy is infected with *Plasmodium* and is exhibiting symptoms of malaria.

1. In the parasitic life cycle of *Plasmodium* species, the boy represents the:
   A. Definitive host
   B. Intermediate host
   C. Vector host
   D. Dead-end host

A 30-year-old man with a bowel obstruction as a consequence of infection with *A lumbricoides* is treated with pyrantel pamoate.

2. The general mechanism by which this drug works is:
   A. Worm paralysis facilitating expulsion
   B. Inhibition of tubulin polymerization
   C. Alteration of intracellular calcium
   D. Inhibition of folic acid synthesis

Antiprotozoal agents often target high metabolic activity and DNA replication.

3. Which of the following antiparasitic agents would most likely be effective in a protozoa infection?
   A. Ivermectin, melarsoprol, and sodium stibogluconate
   B. Melarsoprol, metronidazole, and diethylcarbamazine
   C. Sodium stibogluconate, metronidazole, and melarsoprol
   D. Ivermectin, diethylcarbamazine, and metronidazole

4. The class Sporozoa differs from the class Sarcodina in that the Sporozoa:
   A. Have both sexual and asexual cycles of reproduction
   B. Are single-host parasites
   C. Have only sexual cycles of reproduction
   D. Require arthropod hosts to complete their reproductive cycle

A 23-year-old man is infected with a beef tapeworm, *T saginata.*

5. Which of the following properties correctly describe this parasite?
   A. It is a nonsegmented flatworm, and cattle are the definitive host.
   B. It is a segmented flatworm, and humans are the definitive host.
   C. It is a nonsegmented flatworm, and humans are the definitive host.
   D. It is a segmented flatworm, and cattle are the definitive host.

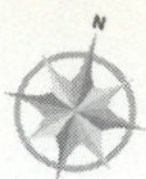

ANSWERS

1. The answer is B. *Plasmodium* completes its sexual development in the *Anopheles* mosquito, which is the definitive host and vector of transmission. Humans are the intermediate host.

2. The answer is A. Pyrantel pamoate is a paralytic agent.

3. The answer is C. Sodium stibogluconate and melarsoprol are heavy metal drugs that target parasites with high metabolic activity. Metronidazole is a DNA synthesis inhibitor. Ivermectin and diethylcarbamazine are paralytic agents that are more widely effective in treating worm infections.

4. The answer is A. Sporozoa are protozoa that have both sexual and asexual reproductive cycles. The Sarcodina, which include amebae, reproduce asexually. Some members of the Sporozoa class, such as *Plasmodium* species, require mosquito hosts for transmission and to complete the sexual life cycle. Others, such as *T gondii,* use a feline definitive host and do not require an arthropod vector.

5. The answer is B. *T saginata* is a member of the Cestoda class, which are segmented flatworms. Humans become infected by ingesting contaminated beef. Adult forms develop in the human intestine and produce eggs, making humans the definitive host.

CHAPTER 21
PROTOZOA

I. Key Concepts

A. The protozoan parasites important to human disease are broadly classified as **amebae, flagellates, ciliates,** and **sporozoa.**

B. The clinical manifestations of infection caused by these parasites vary but fall into 2 general groups based on their major sites of pathogenesis.
   1. **Intestinal and urogenital** manifestations result from infections with amebae (*Entamoeba histolytica*), flagellates (*Giardia lamblia* and *Trichomonas vaginalis*), ciliates (*Balantidium coli*), and sporozoa (*Cryptosporidium parvum.*)
   2. **Blood and tissue** manifestations result from infections with amebae (*Naegleria fowleri*), flagellates (*Leishmania* species and *Trypanosoma* species), and sporozoa (*Plasmodium* species and *Toxoplasma gondii*).

C. Amebae exist in 2 forms: **trophozoite** and **cyst.**
   1. The trophozoite is the active form and the cyst is the quiescent form and often more resistant to the environment.
   2. Cysts often contain multiple nuclei, giving rise to multiple trophozoites.

D. Flagellates multiply by binary fission and are motile by means of flagella.

E. Ciliates are distinguished by their cilia covering, which aids in locomotion.

F. Sporozoa are intracellular parasites with alternating cycles of sexual (sporogony) and asexual (schizogony) reproduction.

II. Amebae: *Entamoeba* and *Naegleria*

A. Two amebae important to human disease are *E histolytica* and *N fowleri.*

B. ***E histolytica*** is an obligate parasite of the human alimentary tract.
   1. **Clinical manifestations:** Three manifestations occur after *E histolytica* infection.
      a. **Asymptomatic** infection is common, giving rise to a carrier state.
      b. **Amebic dysentery** is characterized by cramps, flatulence, tenesmus, and stools containing **blood** and **mucus.**
      c. **Systemic disease** results in abscesses, particularly in **liver.**
   2. **Transmission/epidemiology:** Cysts shed in stool by asymptomatic carriers are a major source of **fecal-oral** transmission.
      a. Cysts contaminate food and water and are resistant to chlorination.
      b. **Oral-anal** transmission is common in homosexuals.

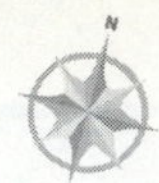

3. **Pathogenesis/virulence factors:** Mature cysts contain 4 nuclei.
   a. Following ingestion of a cyst, excystation occurs, resulting in a trophozoite with 4 nuclei that divides, giving rise to 8 individual trophozoites.
   b. Trophozoites infect the **large intestine,** resulting in characteristic **flask-shaped ulceration** and tissue destruction.
   c. Further invasion results in systemic spread and abscess formation.
4. **Laboratory diagnosis:** Trophozoites, often containing ingested erythrocytes, can be found in diarrheal stool and lesions.
   a. Formed stool contains cysts with 4 nuclei.
   b. It is important to distinguish *E histolytica* from nonpathogenic species such as *Entamoeba coli.*
      (1) Trophozoite nucleus has a characteristic morphology.
      (2) The cyst nucleus of *E coli* has 8 nuclei in contrast to the 4 nuclei of *E histolytica.*
5. **Treatment:** Current guidelines should be consulted, but, depending on the severity of symptoms, treatment generally includes metronidazole and luminal amebicides, such as iodoquinol and diloxanide furoate.
6. **Prevention:** Good hygiene and sanitation coupled with education about transmission are strategies for prevention.

C. ***N fowleri*** is an opportunist causing a highly fatal meningoencephalitis.
   1. **Clinical manifestations: Primary amebic meningoencephalitis** is characterized by rapid-onset headache, stiff neck, fever, vomiting, disorientation, and often altered odor and taste sensations.
      a. Progression to coma and death can occur within 4–6 days.
      b. Primary amebic meningoencephalitis is a highly fatal disease with few documented survivors.
   2. **Transmission/epidemiology:** Trophozoites usually infect humans while they are **swimming** in warm, contaminated fresh water. Cysts are resistant to chlorination.
   3. **Pathogenesis/virulence factors:** Trophozoites enter through nasal mucosal and invade the central nervous system (CNS) through the cribriform plate.
   4. **Laboratory diagnosis:** Examination of cerebrospinal fluid shows neutrophils, erythrocytes, and trophozoites. Amebae can be cultured on a lawn of gram-negative rods (food for the amebae).
   5. **Treatment:** Current guidelines should be consulted, but treatment with amphotericin B in combination with rifampin and miconazole has met with some success.

III. Flagellates: *Giardia, Trichomonas, Leishmania,* and *Trypanosoma*

A. The most important flagellates causing human disease include 2 intestinal or urogenital parasites (*Giardia* and *Trichomonas*) and 2 invasive blood and tissue parasites (*Leishmania* and *Trypanosoma*).

B. ***G lamblia*** causes a noninvasive disease of the gastrointestinal tract.
   1. **Clinical manifestations:** Giardiasis symptoms begin 1–3 weeks after exposure.
      a. Many individuals are asymptomatic but may become carriers, shedding cysts in the stool.
      b. Mild disease is characterized by watery diarrhea.
      c. More severe disease presents as **malabsorption syndrome.**
         (1) Symptoms include abdominal cramps, foul-smelling stools, flatulence, and **steatorrhea** (ie, fat in stool).
         (2) Symptoms can last as long as 4 weeks.

2. **Transmission/epidemiology:** *G lamblia* infection is transmitted by ingestion of cysts.
   a. Fecal contamination of water, especially mountain streams, by infected **beavers,** muskrats, humans, and other mammals, is the source of infection in hikers and campers.
   b. **Fecal-oral** transmission accounts for outbreaks in daycare centers and institutions.
   c. **Oral-anal** transmission is common in homosexuals.
3. **Pathogenesis/virulence factors:** The **ventral sucking disk** of the trophozoite attaches to intestinal epithelial cells in the **duodenum** and **jejunum,** causing inflammation. *Giardia* organisms do not invade but block absorption, especially of fat.
4. **Laboratory diagnosis:** *G lamblia* contains both trophozoite and cyst forms.
   a. The pear-shaped trophozoite contains 4 flagella, 2 nuclei, and a ventral sucking disk.
   b. The cyst contains 4 nuclei, giving rise to 2 trophozoites.
   c. Microscopic examination of diarrheal stool may reveal trophozoites, whereas only cysts are seen in formed stool from asymptomatic carriers.
   d. The **string test** can be used to capture trophozoites from the duodenum for microscopic examination when stool results are negative.
   e. A variety of fecal antigen tests are also available.
5. **Treatment:** Current guidelines should be consulted, but metronidazole or quinacrine hydrochloride is generally used for treatment.
6. **Prevention:** Filtration, iodine treatment, or boiling water from mountain streams provides protection from this source of infection.

C. ***T vaginalis*** is a sexually transmitted urogenital parasite.
1. **Clinical manifestations:** Infection often is asymptomatic.
   a. **Vaginitis** is characterized by a watery, foul-smelling, greenish yellow discharge that may be accompanied by itching, burning, vaginal erythema, and cervical lesions.
   b. Most men are asymptomatic but may exhibit **prostatitis** or **urethritis.**
2. **Transmission/epidemiology:** *T vaginalis* is a sexually transmitted parasite, although infants can become infected at birth by passage through an infected birth canal.
3. **Pathogenesis/virulence factors:** *T vaginalis* **does not form cysts** and exists only in the trophozoite form. Contact with the trophozoite stimulates inflammation and epithelial cell destruction.
4. **Laboratory diagnosis:** Microscopic analysis of wet mounts reveal oval trophozoites, with 4 anterior flagella characterized by jerky movements. Antigen tests are also available.
5. **Treatment:** Current guidelines should be consulted, but in general, metronidazole is used for women with symptoms as well as their asymptomatic partners.
6. **Prevention:** Safe sex practices can reduce transmission.

D. Four different ***Leishmania*** species cause human disease: *L donovani, L tropica, L mexicana,* and *L braziliensis.*
1. **Clinical manifestations:** Disease manifestations vary depending on the species.
   a. **Visceral leishmaniasis,** also called **"kala azar,"** is caused by *L donovani.*
   b. **Cutaneous leishmaniasis,** also called **"oriental sore"** and **"chiclero ulcers,"** is caused by *L tropica* and *L mexicana,* respectively.

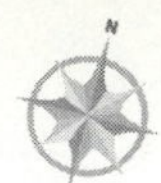

c. **Mucocutaneous leishmaniasis,** also called **espundia,** is caused by *L braziliensis.*

2. **Transmission/epidemiology:** Many mammals serve as reservoirs for infection, but the vector of transmission is the **sandfly.** The life cycle includes a flagellated form called the **promastigote** and a nonflagellated form called the **amastigote.**
3. **Pathogenesis/virulence factors:** *L donovani* invades macrophages, multiplies, and is carried to the spleen, liver, and bone marrow.
   a. The disease course has a gradual onset with fever, chills, liver and spleen enlargement, anemia, and leukopenia.
   b. The prolonged course of disease (months to years) can result in secondary infections, wasting, and death.
   c. *L tropica* and *L mexicana* induce a papule and ulceration at the site of infection.
   d. *L braziliensis* primarily affects soft tissue of the nose and palate, causing a disfiguring disease with common secondary infection complications.
4. **Laboratory diagnosis:** Diagnosis involves detection of amastigote forms in biopsy specimens of lymph nodes, spleen, or bone marrow (*L donovani*), or in specimens of skin lesions (*L tropica, L mexicana, L braziliensis*).
   a. Serologic tests are also available.
   b. Leishmanin skin test results are negative during active disease but positive after recovery.
5. **Treatment:** Current guidelines should be consulted, but pentavalent antimonials such as sodium stibogluconate are generally used for treatment.
6. **Prevention:** Infection is best prevented by measures to avoid sandfly bites, such as insect repellents and physical barriers.

E. ***Trypanosoma brucei*** (rhodesiense and gambiense) is transmitted by the **tsetse fly** and causes **African sleeping sickness.**

1. **Clinical manifestations:** West African sleeping sickness is caused by *T brucei* gambiense.
   a. Disease begins with an ulcer or chancre at the site of the tsetse fly bite.
   b. Acute disease progresses to a cyclic fever and characteristic **posterior cervical lymph node enlargement,** known as **Winterbottom's sign.**
   c. Chronic disease manifestations progress over several years and include CNS invasion (**demyelinating encephalitis**) that results in coma and death.
   d. East African sleeping sickness, caused by *T brucei* rhodesiense, is similar but more acute, rapidly progressive, and also highly fatal if untreated.
2. **Transmission/epidemiology:** The tsetse fly is the vector of transmission.
   a. *T brucei* gambiense is found in West and Central Africa, and there are no known animal reservoirs.
   b. *T brucei* rhodesiense is found in East Africa, and many domestic and wild animals serve as reservoirs.
   c. The only parasitic form in humans is the flagellated **trypomastigote.**
3. **Pathogenesis/virulence factors:** *T brucei* has a dramatic ability to alter the antigenic structure of its surface glycoproteins, resulting in effective evasion of the host humoral immune system.
   a. Antigenic variation accounts for the cyclic nature of the fever (similar to the mechanism of *B recurrentis*).
   b. Parasites can gain access to the CNS through the blood.

4. **Laboratory diagnosis:** Diagnosis involves examination of blood, cerebrospinal fluid, or lymph node aspirates for trypomastigotes. IgM levels are generally highly elevated.
5. **Treatment:** Current guidelines should be consulted, but generally suramin or pentamidine can be used for acute disease, and melarsoprol is used when the CNS is involved.
6. **Prevention:** Physical barriers can prevent bites by the tsetse fly and limit transmission.

F. ***Trypanosoma cruzi*** causes American trypanosomiasis, also called **Chagas disease.**

1. **Clinical manifestations:** Chagas disease begins with an erythematous **chagoma** at the site of the insect bite on the face and around the eyes or with **Romaña's sign** (swelling, conjunctivitis, and local lymphadenopathy) when the infection is in the eye.
   a. Acute disease symptoms include fever, chills, myalgia, hepatosplenomegaly, and lymphadenopathy.
   b. Chronic disease manifestations include myocarditis, megaesophagus, and megacolon.
   c. Meningoencephalitis may occur in young children and infants.
2. **Transmission/epidemiology:** *T cruzi* is transmitted by reduviid bugs (*Triatoma,* "kissing" bugs), mainly in Mexico and Central and South America.
   a. Mammals, including humans, can serve as reservoirs.
   b. Two forms of parasites are seen in humans.
      (1) The flagellated trypomastigote is extracellular and seen in blood.
      (2) The unflagellated amastigote is intracellular and found in tissues.
3. **Pathogenesis/virulence factors:** Trypomastigotes circulate in blood and infect many cells and tissues, particularly heart, muscle, and glial cells. Once inside cells, the amastigote form emerges, multiplies intracellularly, eventually killing the cell and releasing parasites that invade other cells and tissues.
4. **Laboratory diagnosis:** Diagnosis involves detection of flagellated trypomastigotes in thick or thin blood films.
   a. Amastigote forms can be seen in tissue biopsy specimens.
   b. **Xenodiagnosis,** in which a reduviid bug feeds on the patient and the bug becomes infected, can complement false negative blood tests.
5. **Treatment:** Current guidelines should be checked, but acute phase disease is usually treated with nifurtimox or benznidazole.
6. **Prevention:** Measures to control insect vectors will control transmission.

IV. Ciliates: *Balantidium*

A. There is only one **ciliate** that causes significant human disease, *B coli.*

B. ***B coli*** is an intestinal parasite that causes diarrhea.

1. **Clinical manifestations:** *B coli* causes a watery diarrhea with blood and mucus similar to that caused by *E histolytica.* Extraintestinal manifestations do not usually occur.
2. **Transmission/epidemiology:** Cysts are excreted in human and animal (especially **pig**) feces.
   a. Transmission is through ingestion of contaminated food or water.
   b. Fecal-oral spread human to human can also occur.

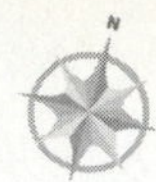

3. **Pathogenesis/virulence factors:** Trophozoites attach and invade the colon, resulting in ulceration.
4. **Laboratory diagnosis:** Diagnosis is by direct stool examination, which shows ciliated trophozoites or cysts.
5. **Treatment:** Current guidelines should be checked, but tetracycline is generally used for treatment.

V. Sporozoa: *Plasmodium, Toxoplasma,* and *Cryptosporidium*

A. The Sporozoa from the subclass **Coccidia** are intracellular parasites with alternating cycles of sexual and asexual reproduction.

B. **Malaria** is caused by 4 different *Plasmodium* species: ***P vivax, P ovale, P malariae,*** and ***P falciparum.***

1. **Clinical manifestations:** Acute disease is cyclic and involves 3 general stages.
   - **a.** The "cold stage" is characterized by shaking chills.
   - **b.** The "hot stage" follows, with fevers as high as 41 °C.
   - **c.** The "sweating stage," characterized by drenching sweats and exhaustion, follows.
   - **d.** Other common manifestations include splenomegaly, hepatomegaly, and anemia.
   - **e.** **Relapsing malaria** occurs with *P vivax* and *P ovale* months to years after the primary infection because of latent **hypnozoite** forms in the liver.
   - **f.** Severe complications are most common with *P falciparum* and result from massive capillary occlusion, which causes brain damage (cerebral malaria), kidney damage (blackwater fever), acute renal failure, and death.
2. **Transmission/epidemiology:** The life cycle of *Plasmodium* infections is diagrammed in Figure 21–1.
   - **a.** The definitive host is the female *Anopheles* mosquito.
   - **b.** The sexual cycle (sporogony) occurs in the mosquito host.
   - **c.** The asexual cycle (schizogony) occurs in the human intermediate host.
3. **Pathogenesis/virulence factors:** *Plasmodium*-induced pathogenesis results mainly from cyclic infection and destruction of erythrocytes (Table 21-1 and Figure 21–1).
   - **a.** Hepatocyte infection occurs rapidly after initial inoculation.
   - **b.** After 8–25 days, merozoites are released into the blood from hepatocyte schizonts.
     - *(1)* *P vivax* and *P ovale* also produce latent liver forms called hypnozoites.
     - *(2)* Hypnozoites cause relapsing malaria months to years after initial infection.
   - **c.** Merozoites in blood attach to and infect different populations of red blood cells (RBCs) (Table 21–1).
   - **d.** The trophozoite in the infected RBC matures, forming a schizont with 8–24 merozoites.
   - **e.** Rupture of the RBC releases merozoites into blood to infect new RBCs and is the cause of the malaria fever paroxysm.
   - **f.** Some trophozoites differentiate into male and female gametocytes that circulate in blood and are ingested by feeding *Anopheles* mosquitos.
4. **Laboratory diagnosis:** Microscopic examination of thick and thin blood smears is diagnostic.
   - **a.** Each species has characteristic microscopic characteristics (eg, *P falciparum* has banana-shaped gametocytes and may have more than one ring in a single RBC).
   - **b.** Speciation is necessary to guide treatment.

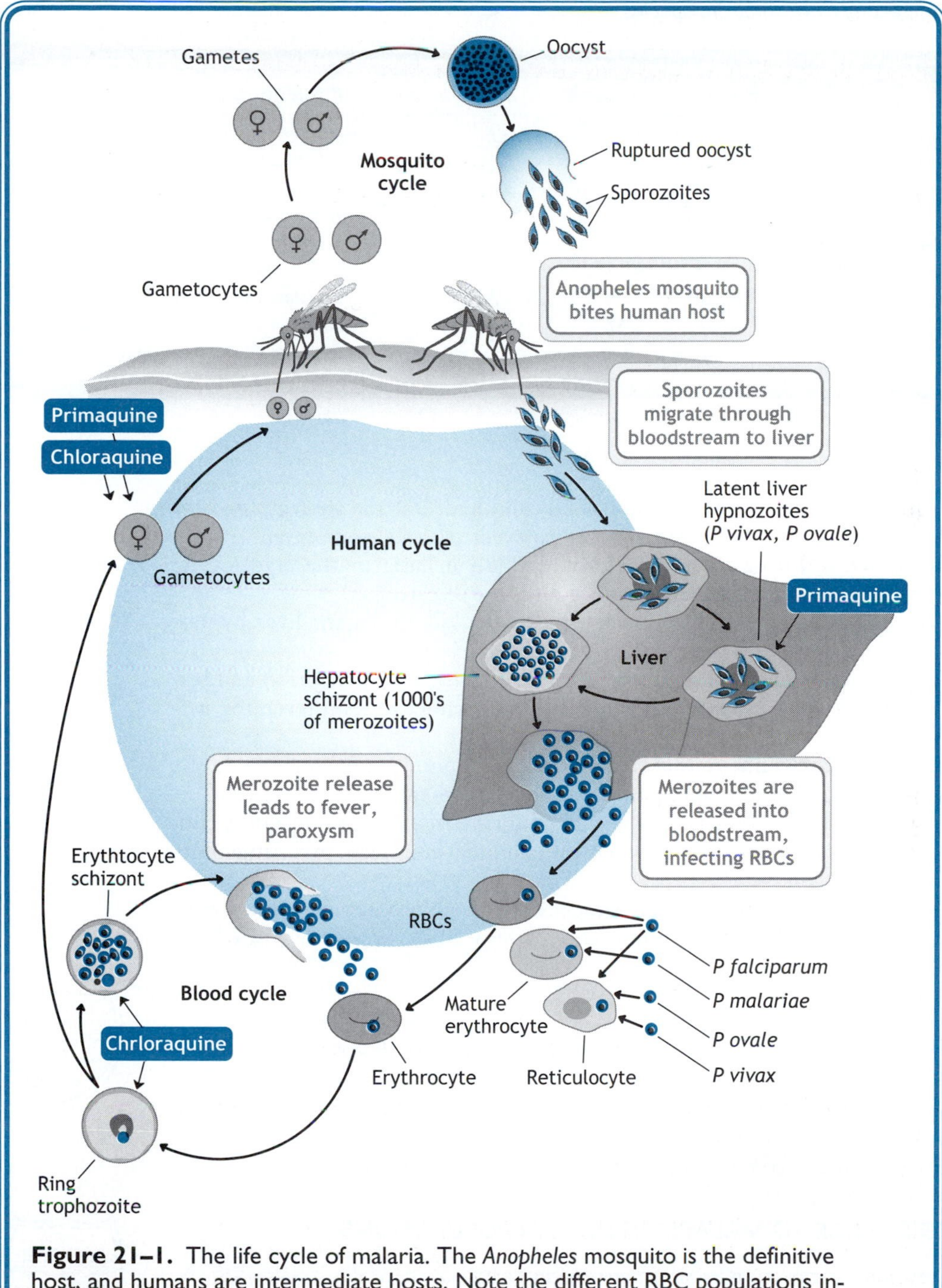

Figure 21–1. The life cycle of malaria. The *Anopheles* mosquito is the definitive host, and humans are intermediate hosts. Note the different RBC populations infected by various *Plasmodium* species (see also Table 21–1). The sites of action of chloroquine and primaquine are noted. Gametocytes of *P vivax, P ovale,* and *P malariae* are sensitive to chloroquine, whereas those of *P falciparum* require treatment with primaquine.

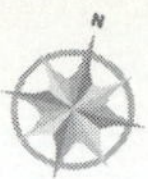

Table 21–1. Properties of *Plasmodium* species.

	P vivax	*P ovale*	*P malariae*	*P falciparum*
Latent liver hypnozoites	Yes	Yes	No	No
Reticulocytes	+	+	–	+
RBCs	–	–	–	+
Mature erythrocytes	–	–	+	+
Common disease course	Tertian (48 h), benign	Tertian (48 h), benign	Quartan (72 h)	Tertian (36–48 h), malignant (blackwater fever, cerebral malaria, acute renal failure)

5. **Treatment:** Current guidelines should be consulted, but the strategy used for treatment is to target the acute symptoms, prevent relapses, and prevent spread.
   a. Blood schizonticides such as chloroquine kill malaria in the erythrocytic stages and are the treatment of choice for acute disease.
   b. Primaquine, a tissue schizonticide, is used to kill the latent liver hypnozoites, preventing relapses.
   c. Gametocides such as chloroquine (*P vivax, P ovale,* and *P malariae*) and primaquine (*P falciparum*) are effective at killing gametocytes, preventing further spread.
   d. Because chloroquine-resistant malaria is common, treatment should be guided by known resistance patterns in the area where infection occurred.
   e. Agents that have been effective on chloroquine-resistant strains include mefloquine, Malarone (atovaquone/proguanil), quinine, quinidine, pyrimethamine-sulfadoxine, and others.
6. **Prevention:** Prophylaxis involves treatment with chloroquine or other antimalarials (depending on known resistance patterns in the area being visited).

MALARIA PROPHYLAXIS

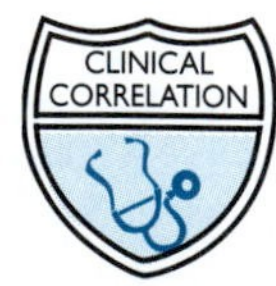

- *Chloroquine and other blood schizonticides are effective against only the erythrocytic forms of malarial disease.*
- *Prophylaxis with chloroquine is continued for 4 weeks after return from a malaria-endemic area to ensure that liver forms have progressed to the erythrocytic stage.*
- *Primaquine is given after return to destroy latent liver forms of* P vivax *and* P ovale.

NATURAL RESISTANCE TO MALARIA IN HUMAN POPULATIONS

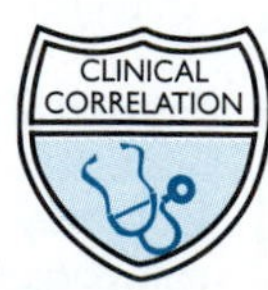

- *Human genetic resistance to malaria is found in many endemic areas.*
- *Individuals heterozygous for the sickle cell trait are protected because their erythrocytes do not support parasitic growth.*
- *Individuals lacking the Duffy blood group antigen, the receptor for* P vivax, *are naturally resistant to* P vivax *infection.*

C. *T gondii* is the causative agent of toxoplasmosis.

1. **Clinical manifestations:** Infection is extremely common, but most individuals are asymptomatic.
   a. Acute disease resembles mononucleosis (negative heterophil antibody) and is self-limiting.
   b. Congenital infections may be asymptomatic or severe, causing encephalitis, hydrocephalus, microcephalus, chorioretinitis, cerebral calcifications, stillbirths, and spontaneous abortions.
   c. Reactivation disease is seen in immunocompromised individuals, such as in patients with AIDS, and may be severe and include encephalitis and multifocal CNS lesions (with associated neurologic symptoms).
2. **Transmission/epidemiology:** Cats are the definitive host, and many animals, including humans, act as intermediate hosts.
   a. The 3 major recognized routes of transmission to humans are
      (1) Ingestion of undercooked, cyst-contaminated meat.
      (2) Exposure to oocysts in cat feces.
      (3) Transplacental spread to the fetus from a mother with an acute infection.
   b. Reactivation of endogenous cysts can occur in immunocompromised individuals.
3. **Pathogenesis/virulence factors:** After infection, excystation releases trophozoites that invade the intestinal wall and are ingested by macrophages, where they multiply.
   a. Trophozoites circulate and enter many tissues, especially brain, heart, liver, lungs, and eyes.
   b. Cysts form in tissue and remain viable for years.
   c. Transplacental spread occurs only during acute infection, when trophozoites are present.
   d. Antibodies protect against transplacental spread.
4. **Laboratory diagnosis:** Serology is used to detect IgM antibody.
   a. Cysts can be detected in tissue biopsies.
   b. Trophozoites may be seen during acute phase disease.
5. **Treatment:** Current guidelines should be checked, but, in general, pyrimethamine and sulfadiazine are used to treat both congenital and reactivation disease.
6. **Prevention:** Infection can be avoided by proper cooking of meat. Pregnant women should avoid cat litter boxes and undercooked foods.

D. ***C parvum*** causes cryptosporidiosis.

1. **Clinical manifestations:** A self-limiting watery diarrhea occurs in immunocompetent individuals. In immunocompromised patients (eg, those with AIDS), a chronic watery diarrhea with massive fluid loss (up to 15 L/d) results in electrolyte imbalance, malnutrition, and wasting.
2. **Transmission/epidemiology:** *C parvum* is transmitted by drinking water contaminated with oocysts from human or domestic animal reservoirs. Fecal-oral and oral-anal transmission can also occur.
3. **Pathogenesis/virulence factors:** The life cycle of *C parvum* contains both sexual and asexual stages.
   a. Oocysts are ingested and sporozoites are released.
   b. Sporozoites attach to epithelial cells in the jejunum and are transformed into asexual trophozoites.

 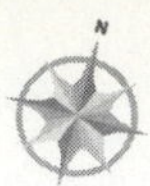

   c. Trophozoites divide asexually (schizogony) into merozoites, which eventually develop into sexual stages (gametocytes) to initiate sexual reproduction (sporogony).
   d. Fertilized zygotes develop into oocysts that are excreted in stool.
4. **Laboratory diagnosis:** Microscopy of fecal smears reveals acid-fast oocysts. Fecal antigen tests are also available.
5. **Treatment:** Diarrhea in immunocompetent individuals is usually self-limiting.
   a. Current guidelines should be consulted, but unfortunately there are no good treatments for immunocompromised individuals except for fluid replacement and supportive measures.
   b. Paromomycin may help reduce diarrhea.
6. **Prevention:** Infection is prevented through water purification and personal hygiene.

CLINICAL PROBLEMS

A 20-year-old woman complaining of vaginitis is seen by her primary care physician. A wet prep examination reveals parasitic organisms with "jerky" motility.

1. The organism most likely involved is:

   A. An ameba

   B. A flagellate

   C. A ciliate

   D. A sporozoa

A 30-year-old man is seen with complaints of abdominal pain, flatulence, and bloody diarrhea.

2. Organisms to consider in the differential diagnosis of this man's illness include:

   A. *Shigella sonnei, E histolytica, G lamblia*

   B. *C parvum,* enterotoxigenic *Escherichia coli,* Rotavirus

   C. *B coli, G lamblia,* Rotavirus

   D. *E histolytica, B coli, S sonnei*

Stool examination of this patient shows trophozoites with internalized erythrocytes.

3. The most likely organism is:

   A. *B coli*

   B. *G lamblia*

   C. *E histolytica*

   D. *C parvum*

One week after returning from a month-long trip to Africa, a 25-year-old man experiences cyclic episodes of chills, fever, and sweats about every 2 days. He is diagnosed with malaria, treated with chloroquine, and recovers. One year later, after he has been living continuously in Idaho, the symptoms reemerge.

4. What is the most likely explanation for this reemergence?

A. Anopheles mosquitoes are endemic in Idaho and were vectors of a new malarial infection.

B. His original infection most likely involved *P falciparum,* which often shows latent reactivation.

C. Antigenic variation of the outer envelope proteins resulted in reemergence of disease.

D. Hypnozoites latent in his liver are reactivated.

After returning from a 3-day camping trip, a 14-year-old boy exhibits abdominal cramps, flatulence, and steatorrhea. After 2 weeks of symptoms, the boy is taken to be examined. Stool examination reveals pear-shaped trophozoites with 2 nuclei.

5. What is the most likely parasitic agent causing this boy's illness?

A. *E histolytica*

B. *G lamblia*

C. *N fowleri*

D. *C parvum*

E. *B coli*

ANSWERS

1. The answer is B. The most likely organism is *T vaginalis,* which is a flagellate.

2. The answer is D. All 3 of these organisms cause diarrhea with blood, whereas the others do not.

3. The answer is C. Trophozoites with internalized RBCs are characteristic of *E histolytica.*

4. The answer is D. His malaria was most likely caused by *P vivax* or *P ovale* because of the reactivation. Both form hypnozoites that remain latent in the liver. Chloroquine only destroys the erythrocytic stages but not the liver stages. Reinfection in Idaho is unlikely since malaria is not endemic to most of the United States.

5. The answer is B. Giardiasis is characterized by fatty stools (steatorrhea) and a long course. He probably acquired the infection while camping and drinking contaminated water. Microscopic examination is consistent with *G lamblia. E histolytica* trophozoites have 1 nucleus and usually have ingested RBCs, *Naegleria* species are not usually intestinal parasites, cryptosporidia shed oocysts in stool, and *B coli* is ciliated.

CHAPTER 22
NEMATODES

I. Key Concepts

A. Nematodes are roundworms with complete digestive systems and both male and female forms.

B. Two general groups are categorized based on where they reside in the human host: **intestinal nematodes** and **tissue nematodes.**

1. Important intestinal nematodes include *Enterobius vermicularis, Ascaris lumbricoides, Trichuris trichiura, Ancylostoma duodenale, Necator americanus,* and *Strongyloides stercoralis.*
2. Tissue nematodes include *Trichinella spiralis, Wuchereria bancrofti, Onchocerca volvulus, Toxocara canis,* and *Toxocara cati.*

C. Pathogenesis relates to the worm load, destructive migration, and host inflammatory response.

D. Transmission is characteristic for each species and includes ingestion of eggs, ingestion of larvae, bites from mosquitoes or flies, and direct skin penetration (Figure 22–1).

E. **Eosinophilia** is a common manifestation in many nematode infections.

II. *Enterobius, Ascaris, Trichuris, Ancylostoma, Necator,* and *Strongyloides*

A. ***E vermicularis,*** the causative agent of **pinworms,** is the most common nematode infection in the United States.

1. **Clinical manifestations:** The main symptom of *E vermicularis* infection is perianal itching.
   - **a.** Intense scratching can lead to secondary bacterial infections.
   - **b.** Migration to the vagina can cause vaginitis.
2. **Transmission/epidemiology:** Pinworm infections start with the ingestion of eggs through fecal-oral transmission or by swallowing dust containing eggs.
   - **a.** Autoinfection occurs when fingers become contaminated with eggs after scratching and are then placed in the mouth.
   - **b.** Retroinfection can occur if larvae develop in the perianal area and then migrate back through the rectum.
   - **c.** Pinworm infections are easily spread through entire households.
3. **Pathogenesis/virulence factors:** The life cycle of *E vermicularis* lasts about 2 weeks (Figure 22-2).
   - **a.** Eggs are ingested and hatch in the small intestine.
   - **b.** Larvae migrate to the colon and differentiate into adults.

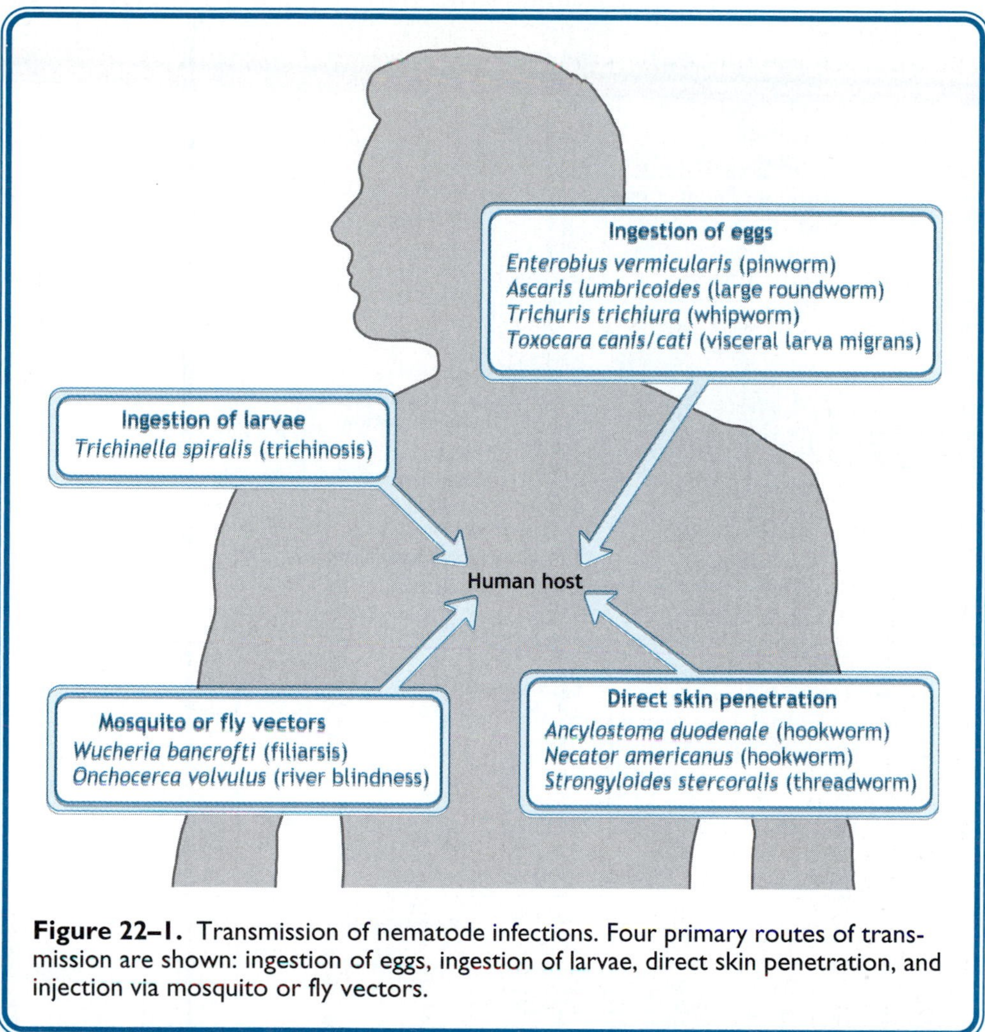

Figure 22–1. Transmission of nematode infections. Four primary routes of transmission are shown: ingestion of eggs, ingestion of larvae, direct skin penetration, and injection via mosquito or fly vectors.

   c. The female migrates from the colon out the anus at night to lay eggs in the perianal area.
   d. The eggs become embryonated in only a few hours and are again infectious.

4. **Laboratory diagnosis:** Eggs are generally not found in stool but can be found around the perianal area. Diagnostic eggs are recovered by perianal sampling using an applicator covered with adhesive tape (sticky side out).
5. **Treatment:** Current guidelines should be checked, but **pyrantel pamoate** or **mebendazole** generally is used to kill adult worms.
   a. A second course is given after 2 weeks to prevent reinfection.
   b. All family members should be treated simultaneously.
6. **Prevention:** Good personal hygiene and prompt treatment help limit infections.

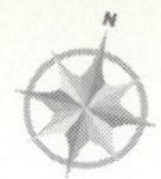

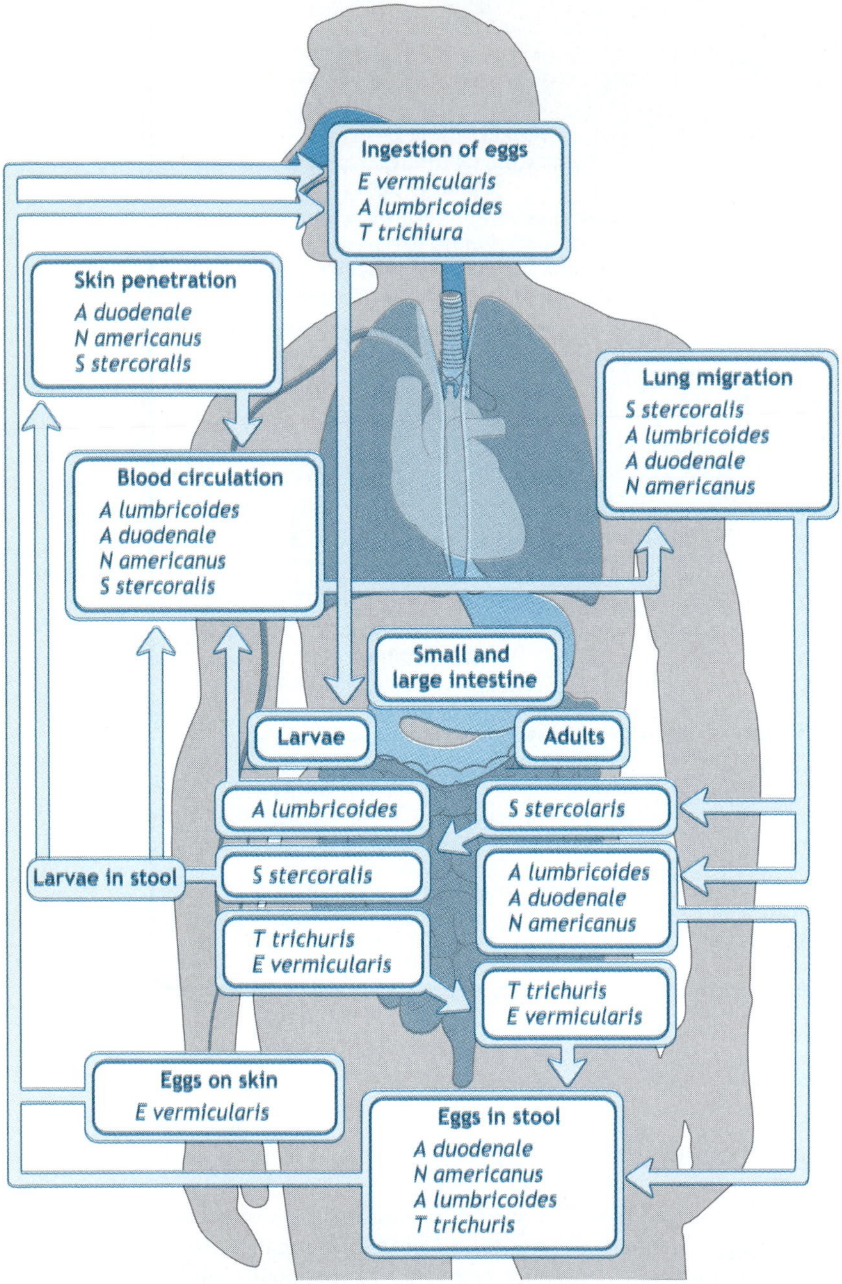

Figure 22–2. Life cycle of intestinal nematodes. Some nematodes require a lung migration before adult development, whereas others develop entirely within the intestinal tract. Note that *S stercoralis* can autoinfect from larvae that develop within the intestine.

B. ***A lumbricoides,*** the most common nematode infection worldwide, is a large roundworm that can reach lengths from 20 to 35 cm.

1. **Clinical manifestations:** *A lumbricoides* causes a variety of symptoms, the severity of which depends on the worm burden and the stage of infection.
   a. **Pneumonitis** is an early symptom in response to lung migration.
   b. **Bowel obstructions** and **malnutrition** result from large worm burdens.
   c. **Bowel perforations, blockages in bile ducts or gallbladder,** and **occlusion of the appendix** result from adult worm migrations.
2. **Transmission/epidemiology:** Infection begins with the ingestion of embryonated eggs that are found in soil contaminated with human feces (Figures 22–1 and 22–2).
   a. Larvae undergo a **lung migration.**
      (1) Larvae hatch, invade though the intestine, reach the bloodstream, and migrate through the liver, heart, and lung.
      (2) From the lung, the larvae penetrate alveoli and are coughed up and swallowed to return to the gastrointestinal tract.
   b. Adults live in the intestine, laying up to 200,000 eggs per day that are passed in stool.
   c. Eggs embryonate after incubation in soil for several weeks and become infectious.
3. **Pathogenesis/virulence factors:** The lung migration through the bloodstream results in **eosinophilia** and **pneumonitis.**
   a. Adult worms do not attach in the intestine but rather remain in place by constant movement.
   b. When the host has a fever or is treated with antibiotics, the **adult worms migrate,** sometimes lodging in ducts causing obstructions.
4. **Laboratory diagnosis:** During the lung migration, larvae and eosinophils can sometimes be seen in sputum.
   a. Diagnosis is most often made by finding characteristic eggs (ie, oval with a knobby surface) in stool.
   b. Worms are sometimes passed in stool.
5. **Treatment:** Current guidelines should be checked, but **mebendazole** or **pyrantel pamoate** typically is used for treatment.
6. **Prevention:** Proper sanitation, cleanliness, and proper human waste disposal are important measures for preventing infection.

C. ***T trichiura*** is also known as the whipworm.

1. **Clinical manifestations:** Symptoms vary depending on the worm load.
   a. Most individuals with small worm loads are asymptomatic.
   b. With larger worm burdens, symptoms include abdominal pain, **bloody diarrhea,** tenesmus leading to **rectal prolapse, anemia,** and **eosinophilia.**
   c. Severe cases may lead to significant blood loss.
2. **Transmission/epidemiology:** Infection begins with the ingestion of eggs from soil contaminated with human feces (Figures 22–1 and 22–2).
   a. Larvae hatch in the small intestine, migrate to the colon, and mature into adults, which can live 4–8 years.
   b. Adult females produce 3000 to 10,000 eggs per day that are passed in stool, contaminate soil, and become infectious after 2–3 weeks in soil.
   c. *T trichiura* is seen worldwide, including the southern United States, with many infections associated with use of human feces as fertilizer.

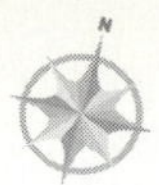

3. **Pathogenesis/virulence factors:** Adult worms attach to the colon, causing local ulceration.
4. **Laboratory diagnosis:** Stool examination reveals characteristic barrel-shaped eggs with a plug at each end.
5. **Treatment:** Current guidelines should be checked, but **mebendazole** generally is used for treatment.
6. **Prevention:** Ensuring proper human waste disposal, avoiding use of human waste as fertilizer, and following good personal hygiene will limit transmission.

D. ***A duodenale*** and ***N americanus*** both cause **hookworm** infections.

1. **Clinical manifestations:** Symptoms vary depending on worm burden.
   a. Most individuals have no symptoms.
   b. Some individuals have an **allergic rash** at the site of entry, often referred to as "ground itch."
   c. **Pneumonitis** may be seen during lung migration.
   d. Heavy worm burdens may induce **microcytic hypochromic anemia** resulting in fatigue, weight loss, and mental and physical retardation.
2. **Transmission/epidemiology:** Infection occurs by **direct skin penetration** (Figures 22–1 and 22–2).
   a. Eggs from human feces develop into filariform larvae.
   b. Filariform larvae in the soil penetrate skin, such as bare feet.
   c. Larvae then go through a **lung migration,** similar to that of *A lumbricoides,* and end up in the small intestine, where they attach.
   d. Adult hookworms may live 5 or more years and produce 10,000 or more eggs per day that are passed in stool, hatch in soil, and differentiate into infectious filariform larvae.
3. **Pathogenesis/virulence factors: Pneumonitis** and **eosinophilia** are associated with the larval lung migration.
   a. Adult worms feed on blood, resulting in blood loss.
   b. Blood loss can be as high as 0.2 mL per worm per day.
   c. Anemia and associated symptoms result from blood loss associated with high worm burdens.
4. **Laboratory diagnosis:** Characteristic eggs in stool are diagnostic.
5. **Treatment:** Current guidelines should be followed, but, in general, **pyrantel pamoate** or **mebendazole** is used to kill worms, and anemia is treated with iron supplementation or even blood transfusion.
6. **Prevention:** Proper sanitation and human waste disposal, education concerning transmission, and wearing shoes will help prevent infection.

E. ***S stercoralis,*** also called **threadworm,** is found in the southeastern United States and in tropical regions worldwide.

1. **Clinical manifestations:** Symptoms vary depending on the worm burden and the immunologic competence of the individual.
   a. Many individuals have no symptoms.
   b. With large worm burdens, symptoms include pneumonitis, watery diarrhea, abdominal pain, and blood in stool.
   c. **Hyperinfection syndrome,** in which larvae disseminate to many different organs, including lung, heart, and central nervous system (CNS), may occur, especially in immunocompromised individuals receiving corticosteroid therapy.
   d. Internal autoinfection can lead to **secondary bacterial sepsis.**

2. **Transmission/epidemiology:** Infection results from direct skin penetration of filariform larvae in soil contaminated with human feces (Figure 22–1 and 22–2).
   a. Larvae penetrate the feet and undergo a **lung migration,** similar to those of *Ascaris* and hookworm infections.
   b. Adults develop in the small intestine and produce eggs that hatch into larvae within the intestine.
   c. Larvae are passed in feces.
      (1) Larvae in soil can develop into adults, producing eggs and larvae outside of a host.
      (2) Some larvae develop to the filariform stage inside the intestine and can directly penetrate the intestine, resulting in **internal autoinfection** and a perpetuation of the infection.
   d. Filariform larvae that reach the perianal area can autoinfect externally.
3. **Pathogenesis/virulence factors:** Pathogenesis depends on the worm burden but in general results from larvae migration, host inflammation, larval dissemination, and secondary bacteria-induced sepsis from autoinfection.
4. **Laboratory diagnosis:** Larvae, not eggs, are found in stool.
5. **Treatment:** Current guidelines should be consulted, but **thiabendazole, mebendazole,** or **ivermectin** generally is used for treatment.
6. **Prevention:** Preventive measures are the same as for hookworm.

III. *Trichinella, Wuchereria, Onchocerca,* and *Toxocara*

A. ***T spiralis,*** the cause of **trichinosis,** has both intestinal and tissue stages.
1. **Clinical manifestations:** Two stages of disease symptoms occur with trichinosis.
   a. The intestinal stage includes common gastrointestinal symptoms such as nausea, vomiting, diarrhea, and abdominal pain.
   b. The tissue stage begins several weeks after the gastrointestinal stage and relates to the location and load of the migrating larvae.
      (1) Symptoms may include rash, fever, myalgia, conjunctival bleeding, periorbital edema, and splinter hemorrhages.
      (2) In heavy infections, respiratory arrest, cardiac symptoms (eg, congestive heart failure), and CNS disorders (eg, meningitis, encephalitis, psychosis) may occur.
2. **Transmission:** Infection begins with the ingestion of larvae, encysted in muscle, in undercooked meats, including pork, bear, deer, and seal (Figure 22–1).
   a. Larvae quickly become adults in the intestine.
   b. Intrauterine embryonation within the female occurs, giving rise to larvae that invade the intestinal wall and migrate through the bloodstream to many different organs.
   c. Larvae survive, develop, and encyst in striated muscle (eg, the diaphragm; tongue, deltoid, pectoral, extraocular muscle of the eye; and gastrocnemius muscles).
   d. Because eggs and infectious larvae do not pass in stool, humans are a dead-end host.
3. **Pathogenesis/virulence factors:** Pathogenesis results from the host inflammatory response (eosinophilic) and depends on the number and location of migrating larvae and muscle cysts.
4. **Laboratory diagnosis:** Serology, marked eosinophilia, and detection of larvae within striated muscle biopsy specimens or suspected meats, if still available, are used in diagnosis.

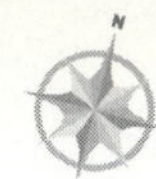

5. **Treatment:** Current guidelines should be consulted, but in general, **thiabendazole** or **mebendazole** is used to kill adult worms and halt the production of new larvae. There are **no effective treatments to kill tissue-encysted larvae,** but steroids can be used to reduce inflammation.
6. **Prevention:** The most effective means of prevention is to avoid eating undercooked meats, especially pork and bear.

B. ***W bancrofti*** causes **filariasis,** of which an extreme form is known as elephantiasis.

1. **Clinical manifestations:** Acute disease includes fever, chills, lymphadenitis, urticaria, and eosinophilia. A chronic inflammatory response to the organisms results in **lymph obstruction,** secondary bacterial infections, and, in extreme cases, **elephantiasis.**
2. **Transmission/epidemiology:** Infection is transmitted through the bite of a **mosquito** (eg, *Anopheles* and *Culex*) (Figure 22–1).
   a. Disease is endemic to Africa, South America, Asia, and parts of the southern Mediterranean.
   b. Larvae carried by mosquitoes penetrate skin and migrate through the lymphatics to regional lymph nodes.
      (1) After 6 months to 1 year, the larvae develop into adults and produce microfilariae larval forms that migrate into the blood at night.
      (2) The microfilariae are ingested by mosquitoes during a blood meal to perpetuate transmission.
      (3) Adult forms can persist for as long as 10 years.
3. **Pathogenesis/virulence factors:** Acute disease results from an inflammatory response to larvae.
   a. Chronic disease results from inflammation and granulomas in the lymphatics, which is worsened by heavy and repeated infections.
   b. Inflammation causes obstruction and edema, especially in genitals and legs.
   c. Bacterial superinfections, repeated infections, and chronic lymph obstruction can lead to elephantiasis.
4. **Laboratory diagnosis:** Because *Wuchereria* microfilariae migrate to the blood with a nocturnal periodicity, thick smear examination for microfilariae should be performed with blood samples taken between 10:00 PM and 4:00 AM.
5. **Treatment:** Current treatment guidelines should be consulted, but **diethylcarbamazine** typically is used to kill adults and microfilariae. Surgical therapy can help reduce enlarged extremities.
6. **Prevention:** Infection is prevented by mosquito control and methods to reduce personal exposure to mosquitoes in endemic areas, such as repellents and physical barriers.

C. ***O volvulus*** causes a disease known as **river blindness.**

1. **Clinical manifestations:** Acute and chronic inflammation results in skin rash, itching, large skin folds from loss of elasticity in subcutaneous tissue, and partial to total blindness.
2. **Transmission/epidemiology:** Infection is transmitted through bites of the *Simulium* **black fly** (Figure 22–1).
   a. Larvae enter the bite wound and migrate to subcutaneous tissue.
   b. Adult development occurs within fibrous nodules.
   c. Microfilariae are produced that migrate through the skin and subcutaneous tissue, where they are ingested by biting flies to continue the cycle.

   d. *Onchocerca* infections are found primarily in Africa and Central and South America.

3. **Pathogenesis/virulence factors:** Pathogenesis is caused by hypersensitivity to parasite antigens and to the acute and chronic inflammation associated with adults and migrating larvae. When adult dermal nodules are on the head or neck, migrating larvae often reach the eye, leading to ocular tissue destruction and, ultimately, blindness.
4. **Laboratory diagnosis:** In contrast to *Wucheria,* microfilariae do not circulate in blood. They may be seen on eye examination or from biopsy of affected skin.
5. **Treatment:** Current guidelines should be followed, but treatment generally involves surgical removal of nodules containing adult worms in combination with **ivermectin** to kill microfilariae and **suramin** to kill adults.
6. **Prevention:** Infection control involves methods to control black fly populations. In endemic areas, ivermectin may be given several times per year to reduce the microfilarial load.

D. ***T canis*** and ***T cati*** cause toxocariasis, also known as **visceral larva migrans.**

1. **Clinical manifestations:** Symptoms vary depending on larval load, location, and degree of inflammatory response by the host.
   a. Individuals may have no symptoms or may have abdominal pain, rash, fever, hepatomegaly, or eosinophilia.
   b. Retinal involvement, which may be mistaken for retinoblastoma, can lead to blindness.
   c. In severe cases, death can result from cardiac, respiratory, and CNS involvement.
2. **Transmission/epidemiology:** Dogs (*T canis*) and cats (*T cati*) are the definitive hosts and pass eggs in their stool (Figure 22–1).
   a. Humans are dead-end hosts and become infected by ingesting eggs.
   b. Larvae invade through the small intestine, reach the bloodstream, and are carried to a variety of organs, including liver, lungs, heart, kidney, muscle, eyes, and CNS, where the larvae die.
3. **Pathogenesis/virulence factors:** Toxocariasis is an inflammatory disease in which eosinophilic granulomas form in response to dead larvae. Pathogenesis relates to the number of larvae present, their location, and the severity of the inflammatory response.
4. **Laboratory diagnosis:** Clinical signs, serologic testing, and the presence of larvae in tissue can aid diagnosis. Pets can be checked for *Toxocara* eggs in their stool.
5. **Treatment:** Current guidelines should be checked, but, in general, **diethylcarbamazine** is used for treatment and corticosteroids are used to reduce inflammation.
6. **Prevention:** Pets should be dewormed and pet feces cleaned up.

WORM BURDENS AND PATHOGENESIS

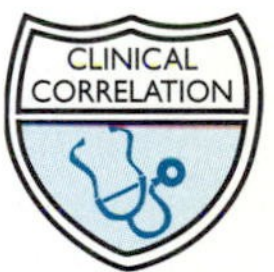

- *In contrast to protozoa, many nematodes do not normally replicate inside the human host.*
- *When humans are the definitive host, adult worms develop and lay eggs that are passed and become infectious outside of the host (exceptions are W bancrofti, O volvulus, and S stercoralis).*
- *Worm burdens are determined directly by the infectious dose (eg, eggs or larvae ingested, injected, or that penetrate) and the frequency of infection.*
- *The worm burden has a direct effect on determining the degree of pathogenesis and the severity of symptoms.*

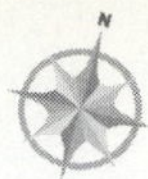

CLINICAL PROBLEMS

A 3-year-old boy has been having trouble sleeping because of intense perianal itching. His mother is instructed to collect a perianal specimen for examination with an applicator covered with adhesive tape (sticky side out).

1. The life cycle of the nematode most likely responsible for this child's symptoms:
   A. Involves a lung migration
   B. Begins with direct skin penetration
   C. Ends with cyst formation in striated muscle
   D. Involves migration of adult female worms from the colon out the anus to lay eggs

Many nematode infections involve lung migration as part of their life cycle.

2. Nematodes in this group include:
   A. *A lumbricoides, A duodenale,* and *S stercoralis*
   B. *T trichiura, A lumbricoides,* and *E vermicularis*
   C. *S stercoralis, T trichiura,* and *N americanus*
   D. *E vermicularis, S stercoralis,* and *N americanus*

A 30-year-old woman taking high-dose corticosteroids is suspected of having *S stercoralis*–induced hyperinfection syndrome.

3. What would a stool sample be expected to reveal?
   A. Barrel-shaped eggs with a plug on both ends
   B. Thin-walled oval eggs
   C. Adult worms
   D. Larvae

A 20-year-old woman with periorbital edema and marked eosinophilia reports eating rare pork regularly.

4. What nematode is most likely responsible for her symptoms?
   A. *A lumbricoides*
   B. *T spiralis*
   C. *T trichiura*
   D. *T cati*

A 2-year-old boy has received a new puppy for Christmas. After 3 weeks, the puppy is found to have *T canis* and is dewormed.

5. If transmission to the 2-year-old occurred, the worm larvae would:
   A. Develop into adults in the small intestine
   B. Undergo a lung migration before setting up residence in the colon

C. Invade the small intestine and disseminate through the bloodstream to different organs before dying

D. Differentiate into adults in the colon and migrate out the anus to lay eggs on the skin

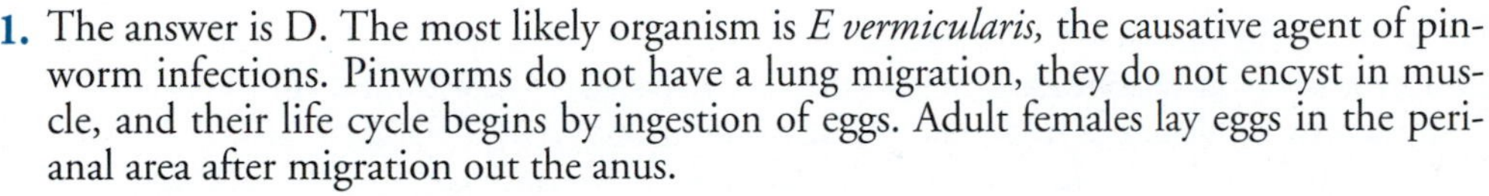

ANSWERS

1. The answer is D. The most likely organism is *E vermicularis,* the causative agent of pinworm infections. Pinworms do not have a lung migration, they do not encyst in muscle, and their life cycle begins by ingestion of eggs. Adult females lay eggs in the perianal area after migration out the anus.
2. The answer is A. Nematodes that have a lung migration include *A lumbricoides, A duodenale, N americanus,* and *S stercoralis.*
3. The answer is D. Strongyloides eggs hatch inside the host in the intestine, and larvae are passed in stool. This is important because larvae can autoinfect inside the host, increasing the worm burden and perpetuating infection.
4. The answer is B. Trichinosis results from ingestion of undercooked cyst containing pork and other meats. *T spiralis* is the causative agent of trichinosis. Infection by the other 3 organisms results from ingestion of eggs.
5. The answer is C. Humans are a dead-end host for *Toxocara.* Larvae do not differentiate to adults but rather die after dissemination.

CHAPTER 23
CESTODES AND TREMATODES

I. Key Concepts

A. Cestodes, also known as **tapeworms,** are segmented flatworms with 3 types of segments: the **scolex** or head, the neck, and the **strobila** or body.

1. The scolex is involved in attachment to intestinal cells.
2. The neck region is the point where new strobila proglottids form.
3. The strobila consists of one or more hermaphroditic **proglottids.**
4. Medically important **cestodes** include *Taenia solium, Taenia saginata, Diphyllobothrium latum, Echinococcus granulosus,* and *Hymenolepis nana.*

B. Trematodes, also known as **flukes,** are nonsegmented flatworms.

1. Snails serve as the intermediate host.
2. Depending on their location in the human body, trematodes are referred to as intestinal flukes, liver flukes, lung flukes, and blood flukes.
3. The **schistosomes,** also known as the blood flukes, are one of the most common causes of infectious disease mortality worldwide.

II. Cestodes: *Taenia, Diphyllobothrium, Echinococcus,* and *Hymenolepis*

A. *T solium* is also known as the **pork tapeworm.**

1. **Clinical manifestations:** Adult tapeworm infections are generally asymptomatic with mild gastrointestinal symptoms.
   a. **Cysticercosis** is a more serious manifestation that leads to formation of cysticerci in different tissues, including the eye, brain, muscle, and lungs.
   b. Symptoms vary depending on the location of the cysticerci (eg, meningoencephalitis, seizures, and other neurologic manifestations occur with cysticerci in the brain).
2. **Transmission/epidemiology:** The life cycle of *T solium* is outlined in Figure 23–1.
   a. Physical properties of *T solium* are summarized in Table 23–1.
   b. Transmission to humans results from ingestion of undercooked pork contaminated with cysticerci.
   c. Fecal-oral transmission of *T solium* eggs results in cysticercosis.
3. **Pathogenesis/virulence factors:** After ingestion of pork containing cysticerci, larvae attach to the intestine by way of the scolex and grow up to 5 m in length and, if untreated, survive for years to decades.
   a. Terminal proglottids containing eggs are passed in feces.
   b. Pigs ingest water or food contaminated with *T solium* eggs.
   c. Embryos hatch and larvae attach to intestinal cells, invade, and are spread through the bloodstream to skeletal muscle, where they develop into cysticerci.

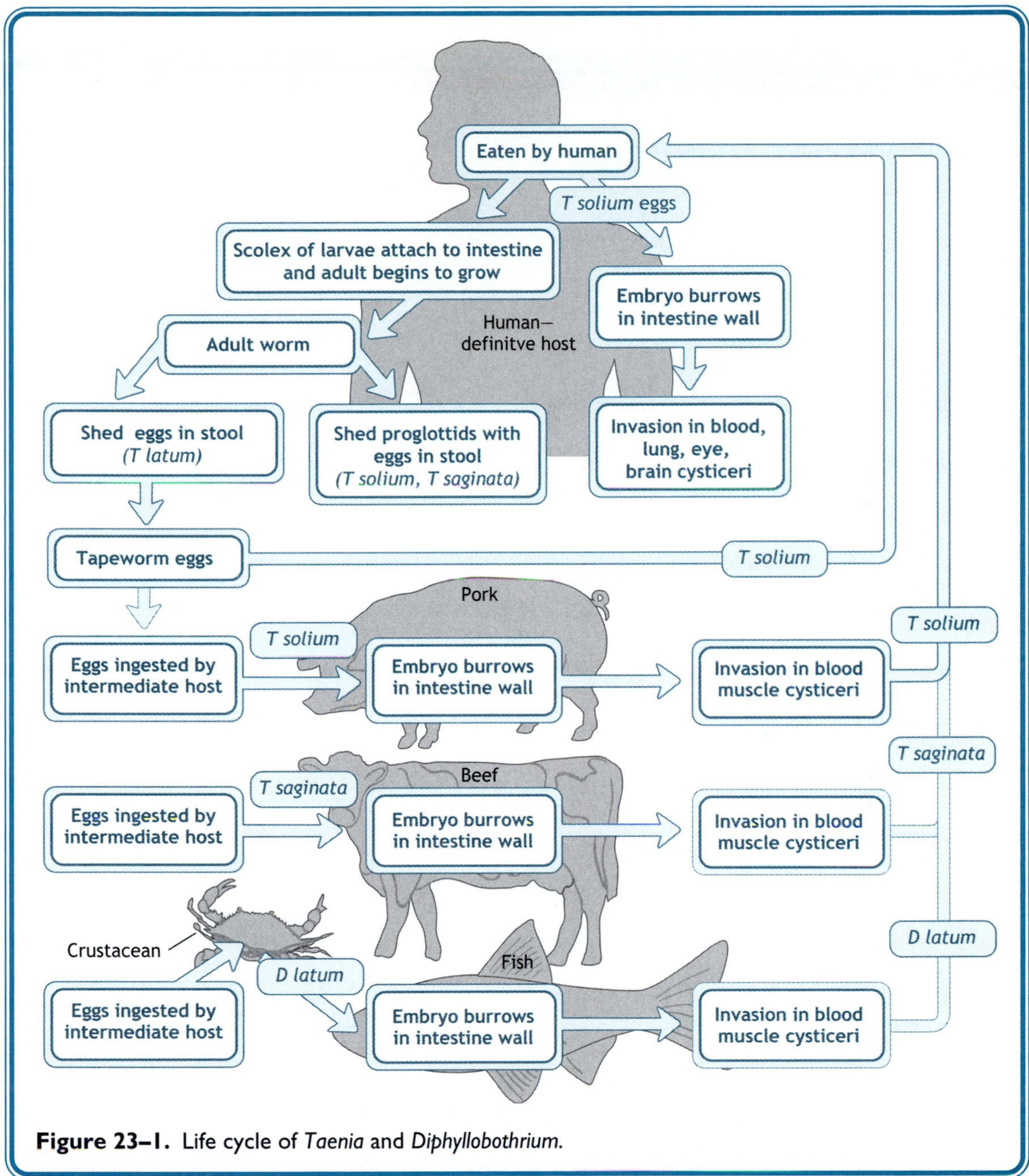

Figure 23–1. Life cycle of *Taenia* and *Diphyllobothrium*.

 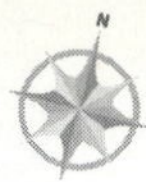

Table 23–1. Properties of cestodes.

	T solium	*T saginata*	*D latum*	*E granulosus*	*H nana*
Common name	Pork tapeworm	Beef tapeworm	Broad fish tapeworm		Dwarf tapeworm
Definitive host	Human	Human	Human	Canines	Human
Intermediate hosts	Pigs	Cattle	Crustaceans then fish	Sheep or human	None
Adult size	5 m	10 m	13 m	5 cm	2–4 cm
Scolex properties	4 suckers, hooks	4 suckers, no hooks	2 sucking grooves	4 suckers, hooks	4 suckers, hooks
Distinguishing features	Proglottids with 5–13 uterine branches	Proglottids with 15–30 uterine branches	Wide proglottids egg with operculum	Only 3 proglottids	Egg has a 6-hooked embryo
Main route of transmission	Undercooked pork	Under-cooked beef	Under-cooked or pickled fish	Canine fecal–human oral	Fecal-oral

- **d.** If humans ingest *T solium* eggs, larvae invade the bloodstream and embed in many different tissues, including muscle, lung, brain, and the eye.

4. **Laboratory diagnosis:** Adult tapeworm infections are diagnosed by finding proglottids with 5–13 uterine branches in the stool. Cysticerci often calcify and can be seen by x-ray, computed tomography, or magnetic resonance imaging.
5. **Treatment:** Current guidelines should be consulted, but in general, adult *T solium* infections are treated with **praziquantel** and cysticercosis treated with surgical excision, praziquantel, or albendazole.
6. **Prevention:** Infection is best prevented by not eating undercooked pork, proper waste management, and sanitary measures to prevent fecal-oral spread and autoinfection.

B. ***T saginata*** is also known as the **beef tapeworm.**

1. **Clinical manifestations:** Like *T solium,* most adult tapeworm infections are asymptomatic, with only mild gastrointestinal symptoms.
2. **Transmission/epidemiology:** Infection occurs after ingestion of raw or undercooked beef.
   - **a. Cysticercosis does *not* occur** with *T saginata* infection.
   - **b.** *T saginata* is one of the more common tapeworm infections in the United States.
3. **Pathogenesis/virulence factors:** The life cycle is similar to that of *T solium* and is diagrammed in Figure 23–1. Physical properties are summarized in Table 23–1.

4. **Laboratory diagnosis:** *T saginata* tapeworm infections are diagnosed by finding proglottids with 15–30 uterine branches in the stool.
5. **Treatment:** Current guidelines should be consulted, but **praziquantel** generally is used for treatment.
6. **Prevention:** Infection is best prevented by not eating undercooked beef and by proper disposal of human waste.

C. ***D latum*** is also known as the **broad fish tapeworm.**
1. **Clinical manifestations:** As with *T solium* and *T saginata,* most infections are asymptomatic.
   a. Competition for vitamin B_{12} can lead to a $\mathbf{B_{12}}$ **deficiency.**
   b. Manifestations include **megaloblastic anemia** and **neurologic symptoms,** including numbness and paresthesia.
2. **Transmission/epidemiology:** Infections result from ingestion of undercooked, raw, or pickled freshwater fish. *D latum* has 2 intermediate hosts: freshwater crustaceans and freshwater fish.
3. **Pathogenesis/virulence factors:** Physical properties are summarized in Table 23–1, and the life cycle is diagrammed in Figure 23–1.
   a. Eggs are released through a genital pore and passed in the stool in large numbers.
   b. Embryos emerge in freshwater, are eaten by the crustacean intermediate host, which is in turn eaten by a freshwater fish.
   c. Larvae reside in the muscles of fish, which are then eaten by humans.
   d. Larvae attach to the intestine and grow into adults as long as 13 m.
4. **Laboratory diagnosis:** The presence, in stool, of elongated eggs with a lidlike **operculum** is diagnostic. Proglottids are wider than they are long and have a **rosette pattern** of uterine branches.
5. **Treatment:** Current guidelines should be consulted, but **praziquantel** is generally used for treatment.
6. **Prevention:** Infection is prevented by avoiding undercooked fish and by proper sanitation to keep human waste out of freshwater lakes.

D. ***E granulosus*** is very small, with a scolex and only 3 proglottids.
1. **Clinical manifestations:** *E granulosus* causes **hydatid cyst disease,** which can be asymptomatic or can exhibit a variety of liver, lung, and brain manifestations, depending on the site of growth. **Anaphylaxis** is induced by rupture of the cyst, which also results in dissemination of infectious protoscoleces.
2. **Transmission/epidemiology:** Infection in humans is by ingestion of eggs in food or water contaminated with dog feces.
   a. Dogs are the definitive host.
   b. Sheep are intermediate hosts, and humans are dead-end accidental hosts (Figure 23–2).
   c. Dogs become infected by eating sheep viscera.
3. **Pathogenesis/virulence factors** (Figure 23–2): Once eggs are ingested, embryos invade intestinal cells and are spread in the bloodstream.
   a. Larvae develop in tissue and form a fluid-filled, unilocular hydatid cyst in a variety of tissues, including lung, liver, brain, and bone.
   b. The large size of the hydatid cysts, up to 20 cm in diameter, accounts for much of its pathogenesis.
      (1) The hydatid cysts contain **brood capsules** filled with **protoscoleces.**

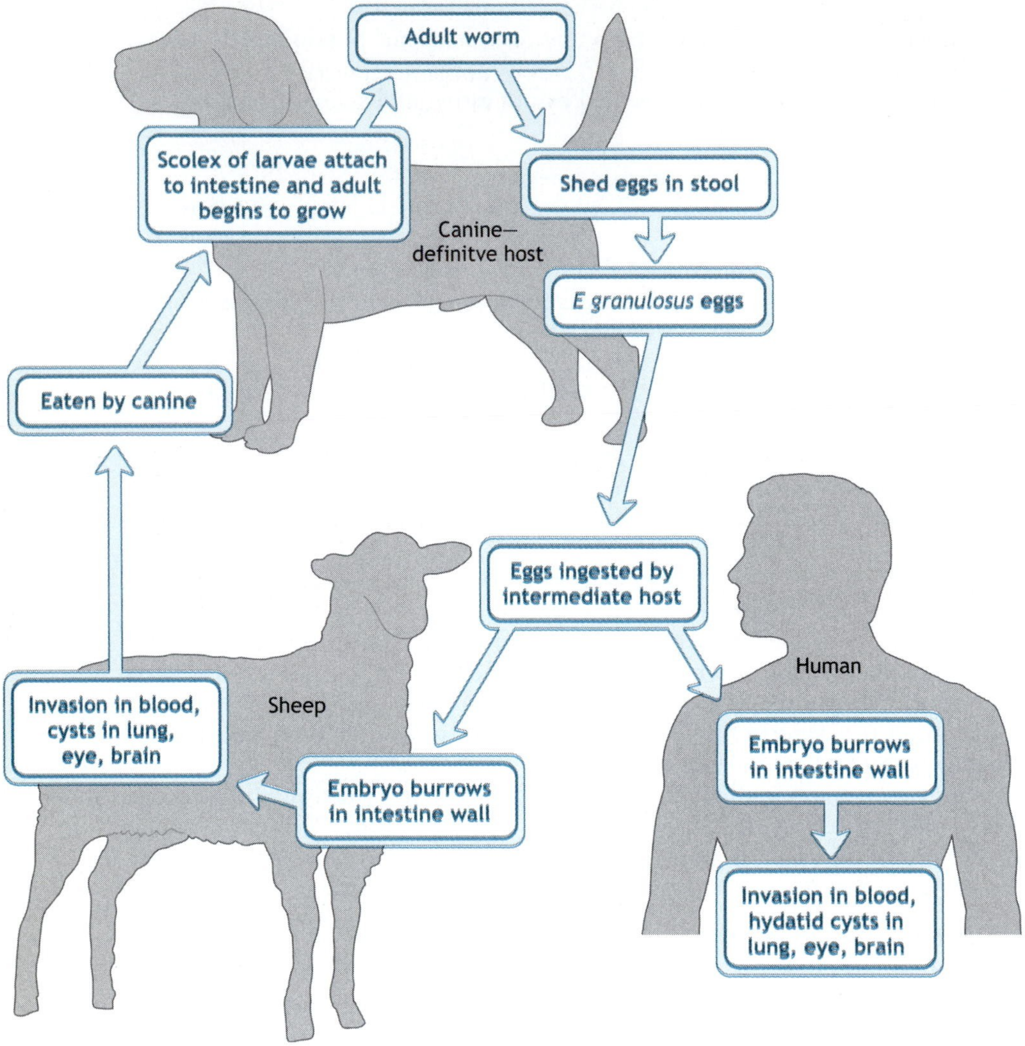

Figure 23–2. Life cycle of *E granulosus.*

(2) If the cyst ruptures, the protoscoleces can disseminate, spreading infection, and the fluid acts like an anaphylatoxin.

c. Adult worms do not develop in humans.

4. **Laboratory diagnosis:** Fluid-filled hydatid cysts can be visualized by x-ray or computed tomography. Serologic tests are available.
5. **Treatment:** Current guidelines should be consulted, but treatment generally consists of albendazole and surgical removal of the cyst. Surgical removal must be done with care because of the risk of anaphylactic reactions and dissemination of protoscoleces.

6. **Prevention:** Dogs should be dewormed and should not be fed sheep viscera. Good personal hygiene can help prevent spread by fecal-oral contamination.

E. ***H nana*** is also called the **dwarf tapeworm.**

1. **Clinical manifestations:** With small worm burdens, infection is usually asymptomatic. However, with large worm burdens, more gastrointestinal symptoms develop.
2. **Transmission/epidemiology:** Infection results from fecal-oral spread.
   - **a.** *H nana* infections are one of the most common tapeworm infections in the United States, especially the southeastern United States.
   - **b.** Humans are the definitive host, and no intermediate hosts are required in the life cycle.
3. **Pathogenesis/virulence factors:** Eggs are directly infectious to humans.
   - **a.** Once ingested, eggs hatch and larvae attach to the intestine.
   - **b.** Adult worms grow to 2–5 cm long and produce eggs that pass in stool or autoinfect the host.
   - **c.** One person can have hundreds of worms.
4. **Laboratory diagnosis:** Stool examination for *H nana* eggs (Table 23–1) is diagnostic.
5. **Treatment:** Current guidelines should be consulted, but praziquantel is typically used for treatment.
6. **Prevention:** Infection is best prevented by measures to limit fecal-oral transmission.

III. Trematodes: *Schistosoma*

A. The **blood flukes,** causing the majority of human disease, include 3 different species of ***Schistosoma:*** *S mansoni, S japonicum,* and *S haematobium.*

1. **Clinical manifestations:** Schistosomes manifest 3 different phases of disease.
   - **a.** Early infection **dermatitis** ("swimmer's itch") is seen after skin penetration.
   - **b.** Acute disease (**Katayama's syndrome**) is a febrile illness associated with the onset of **oviposition** and characterized by fever, chills, and other symptoms associated with circulating immune complexes.
   - **c.** Chronic disease symptoms (**schistosomiasis**) vary depending on the location of egg-induced host inflammation.
     - *(1)* **Intestinal schistosomiasis,** caused by *S mansoni* and *S japonicum,* includes abdominal pain, diarrhea, blood in the stool, and hepatosplenomegaly.
     - *(2)* **Vesicular schistosomiasis,** caused by *S haematobium,* includes hematuria, dysuria, obstruction, frequency, and an association with development of **bladder carcinoma.**
     - *(3)* **Neurologic schistosomiasis** resulting from eggs migrating to the brain is more frequent with *S japonicum.*
2. **Transmission/epidemiology:** The life cycle and important properties of schistosomes are summarized in Table 23–2 and Figure 23–3.
   - **a.** Eggs hatch into **miracidia** in freshwater and infect the snail intermediate host.
   - **b.** Inside the snail, miracidia replicate and develop into free-swimming **cercariae.**
   - **c.** **Cercariae penetrate skin** of humans or other reservoir hosts, where they eventually develop into egg-laying adults.
   - **d.** Eggs are shed in urine (*S haematobium*) or stool (*S mansoni* and *S japonicum*).

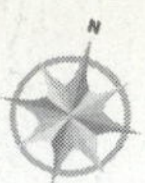

Table 23–2. Properties of schistosomes.

	S mansoni	*S japonicum*	*S haematobium*
World distribution	Africa, South America, Middle East, West Indies, Puerto Rico	Far East: China, Japan, Philippines	Africa, Middle East, India
Egg characteristics	Sharp lateral spine	Inconspicuous spine	Terminal spine
Adult location	Mesenteric veins (colon)	Mesenteric veins (small intestine, colon)	Veins around bladder and pelvic organs
Egg transmission	Feces	Feces	Urine

3. **Pathogenesis/virulence factors:** The life cycle of schistosomes is diagrammed in Figure 23–3.
   a. After cercariae penetrate skin, they enter the circulation and migrate through the heart and lungs to the portal veins, where they develop into male and female adults.
   b. The adults evade the immune system by coating themselves with host substances.
   c. Male and female adults pair together and become attached in permanent copulation.
   d. These adults then migrate to their final location (mesenteric veins for *S mansoni* and *S japonicum* or veins around the bladder for *S haematobium*) and begin oviposition (producing massive quantities of eggs).
   e. Eggs can be carried in the circulation to distant sites (liver, lung, and brain).
   f. Pathogenesis results from the immune response to the eggs manifested by microabscesses, granulomas, fibrosis, and scarring with clinical consequences depending on the location.
   g. Eggs also produce enzymes that destroy tissue, allowing them to enter the lumen of the bowel or bladder and be passed in stool (*S mansoni* and *S japonicum*) or urine (*S haematobium*).
4. **Laboratory diagnosis:** The presence of characteristic eggs in stool or urine (Table 23–2) is diagnostic.
5. **Treatment:** Current guidelines should be consulted, but, in general, **praziquantel** is used for treatment.
6. **Prevention:** Infection is prevented by avoiding swimming in freshwater in endemic areas, eradicating snail populations, and observing proper waste management.

SWIMMER'S ITCH IN THE UNITED STATES

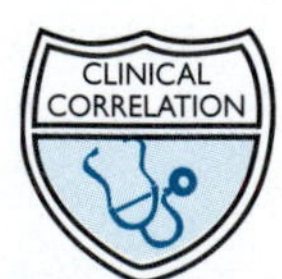

- *Although human schistosomes are not endemic to the United States, schistosomes of many avian species are present in many states, especially around the Great Lakes.*
- *Skin penetration by avian schistosomes results in a localized erythematous rash that can become papular at the site of penetration and can last for 4 or 5 days.*
- *Unlike the human schistosomes, these avian schistosomes do not develop further in humans.*

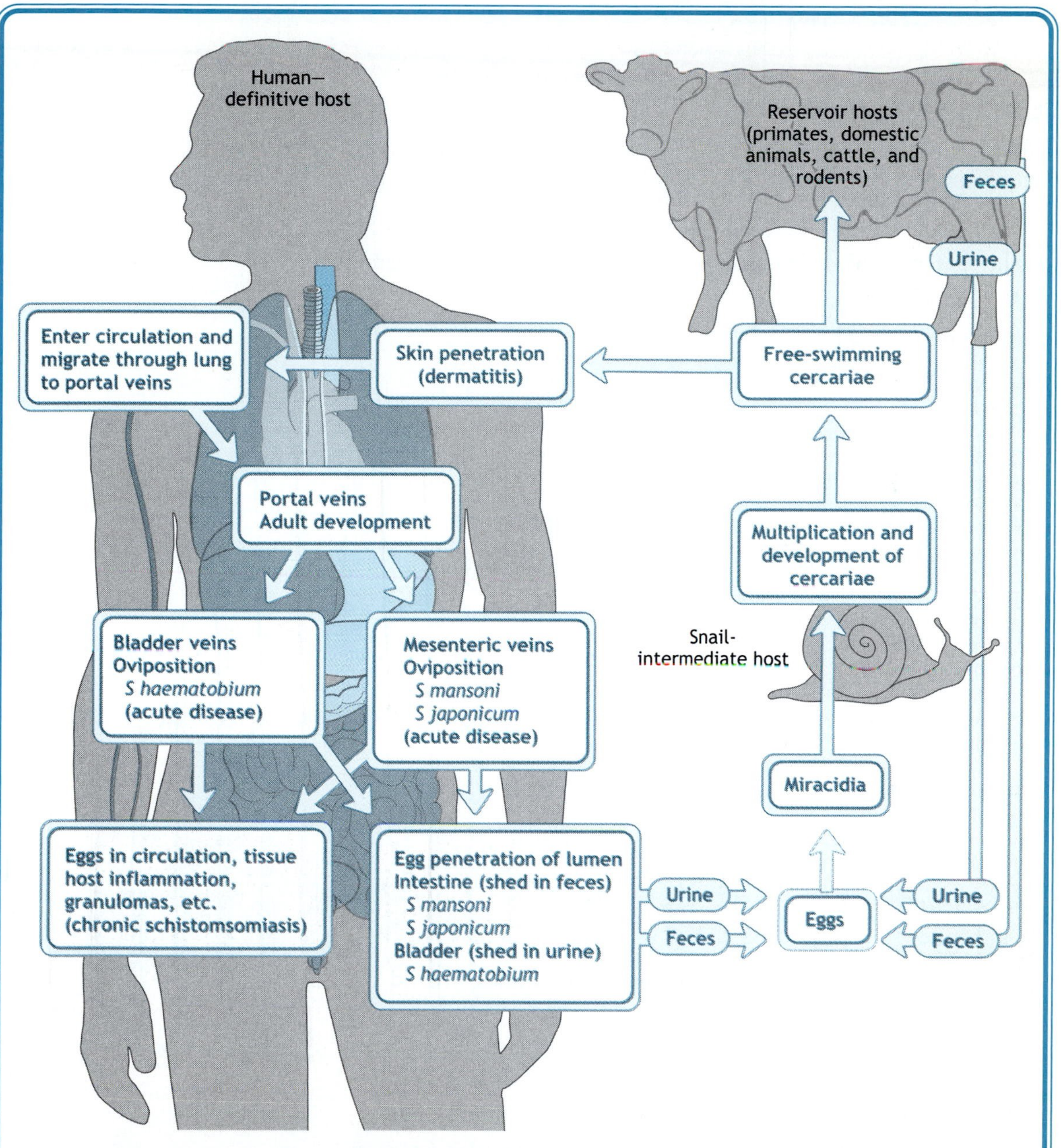

Figure 23–3. Life cycle of schistosomes.

 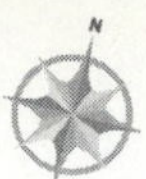

CLINICAL PROBLEMS

A 30-year-old man experiences mild gastrointestinal discomfort and is asked to provide a stool sample. On examination, a proglottid with an intricate pattern of 28 uterine branches is detected.

1. This man most likely acquired this tapeworm infection by eating:
   A. Undercooked pork
   B. Undercooked beef
   C. Undercooked fish
   D. Vegetables contaminated with dog feces

A 48-year-old Swedish immigrant suspected of having a fish tapeworm infection is found to also have a vitamin B_{12} deficiency.

2. A stool sample sent to the laboratory is expected to contain:
   A. Proglottids with between 3 and 15 uterine branches
   B. Round eggs
   C. Elongated eggs with an operculum
   D. Eggs containing 6 hooked embryos

Calcified cysticerci are seen on magnetic resonance imaging of a 29-year-old woman with meningoencephalitis.

3. The most likely organism to have caused these cysticerci is:
   A. *T solium*
   B. *T saginata*
   C. *D latum*
   D. *H nana*

Computed tomography reveals a 5-cm-wide, fluid-filled hydatid cyst in the liver of a 30-year-old man.

4. The adult form of the organism most likely to have caused this cyst contains a scolex with:
   A. 4 suckers, hooks, and a strobila approaching 5 m in length
   B. 4 suckers, no hooks, and a strobila approaching 10 m in length
   C. 2 sucking grooves and a strobila approaching 13 m in length
   D. 4 suckers, hooks, and a strobila of only 3 proglottids

After swimming in a freshwater pond in Puerto Rico, a 14-year-old boy develops intense itching, edema, and a rash. Three months later, he experiences abdominal pain, diarrhea, and blood in the stool. Examination of stool revealed eggs with a prominent lateral spine.

5. What organism is most likely responsible for this child's illness?
   A. *Balantidium coli*
   B. *Entamoeba histolytica*
   C. *S mansoni*
   D. *H nana*

ANSWERS

1. The answer is B. The proglottid described is characteristic of *T saginata,* the beef tapeworm.
2. The answer is C. The fish tapeworm is caused by *D latum,* which has characteristic proglottids that are wider than they are long with uterine branches in a rosette pattern. Eggs in stool are diagnostic and are elongated with an operculum.
3. The answer is A. Cysticercosis is characteristic of *T solium* infection after ingestion of eggs.
4. The answer is D. The hydatid cyst is a clinical manifestation of *E granulosus.* The adult form, which does not develop in humans, is small, with only 3 proglottids. The other choices describe the pork, beef, and fish tapeworms, respectively.
5. The answer is C. The symptoms and history are consistent with those of a schistosome infection. The egg described is characteristic of *S mansoni.*

CHAPTER 24
ROLE OF BACTERIA, VIRUSES, FUNGI, AND PARASITES IN INFECTIOUS DISEASES

I. Overview

A. This chapter diagrammatically summarizes the major infectious disease syndromes in the context of the target organ and the role of medically important bacteria, viruses, fungi, and parasites.

B. The material is presented in the form of **concept maps,** which are a visual and spatial way to organize knowledge and relationships between concepts.

C. Because of space constraints, some concept maps are subdivided into 2 or more separate maps. The reader should view the maps together to see "the big picture."

II. Concept Maps

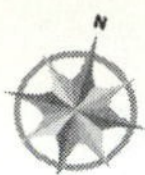

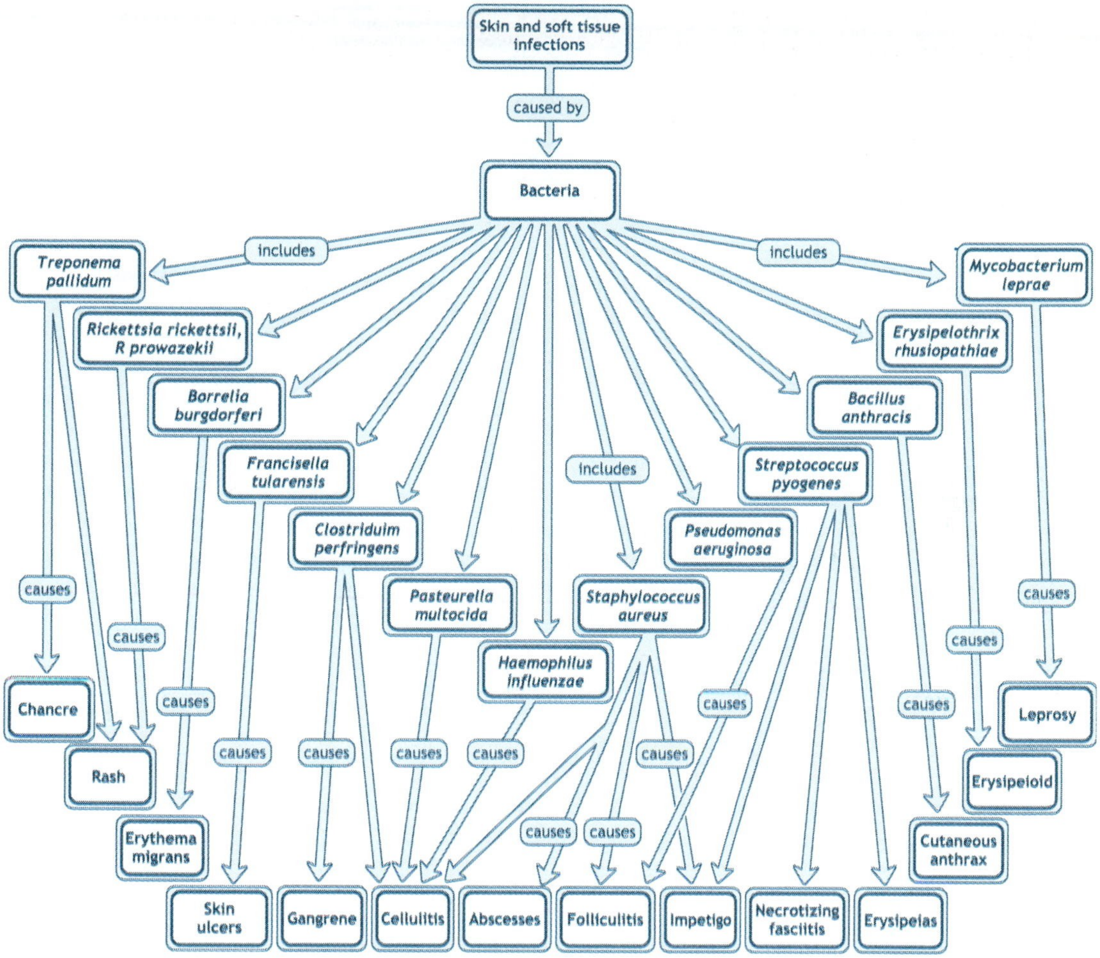

Skin and soft tissue infections
caused by
Bacteria
includes
includes
Treponema pallidum
Mycobacterium leprae
Rickettsia rickettsii, R prowazekii
Erysipelothrix rhusiopathiae
Borrelia burgdorferi
Bacillus anthracis
Francisella tularensis
includes
Streptococcus pyogenes
Clostriduim perfringens
Pseudomonas aeruginosa
Pasteurella multocida
Staphylococcus aureus
Haemophilus influenzae
causes
causes
causes
causes
causes
causes
causes
causes
causes
causes
causes
causes
causes
causes
Chancre
Rash
Erythema migrans
Leprosy
Erysipeloid
Cutaneous anthrax
Skin ulcers
Gangrene
Cellulitis
Abscesses
Folliculitis
Impetigo
Necrotizing fasciitis
Erysipelas

Figure 24–1. Skin and soft tissue infections: bacteria.

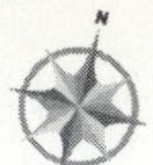

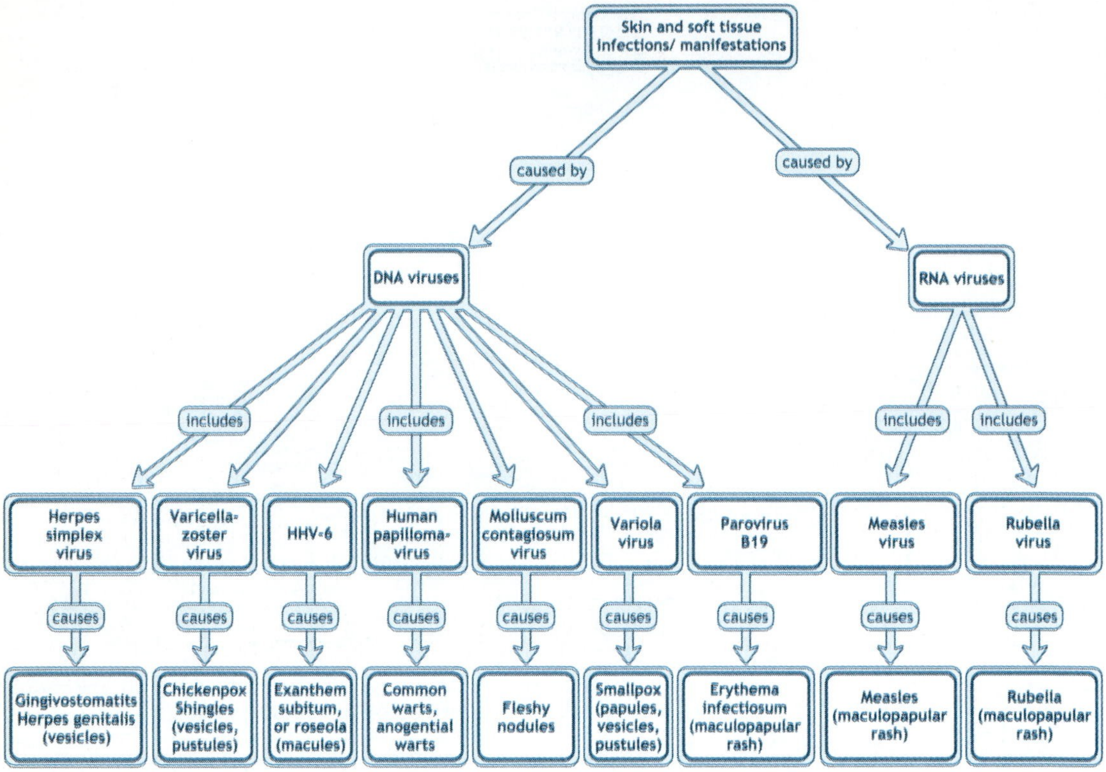

Skin and soft tissue infections/ manifestations

caused by

caused by

DNA viruses

RNA viruses

includes

includes

includes

includes

includes

Herpes simplex virus

Varicella-zoster virus

HHV-6

Human papilloma-virus

Molluscum contagiosum virus

Variola virus

Parovirus B19

Measles virus

Rubella virus

causes

causes

causes

causes

causes

causes

causes

causes

causes

Gingivostomatits Herpes genitalis (vesicles)

Chickenpox Shingles (vesicles, pustules)

Exanthem subitum, or roseola (macules)

Common warts, anogential warts

Fleshy nodules

Smallpox (papules, vesicles, pustules)

Erythema infectiosum (maculopapular rash)

Measles (maculopapular rash)

Rubella (maculopapular rash)

Figure 24–2. Skin and soft tissue infections and manifestations: viruses.

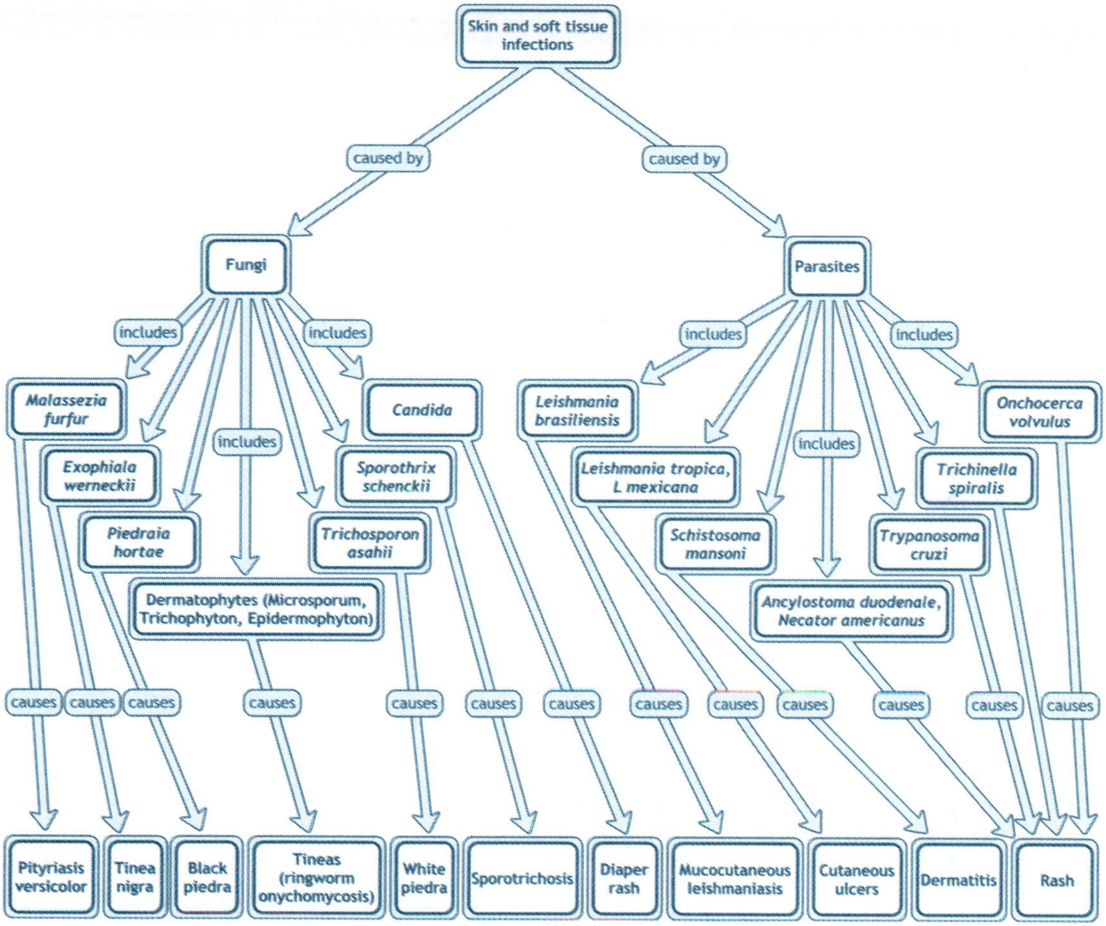

Skin and soft tissue infections
caused by
caused by
Fungi
Parasites
includes
includes
includes
includes
includes
includes
Malassezia furfur
Exophiala werneckii
Piedraia hortae
Dermatophytes (Microsporum, Trichophyton, Epidermophyton)
Trichosporon asahii
Sporothrix schenckii
Candida
Leishmania brasiliensis
Leishmania tropica, L mexicana
Schistosoma mansoni
Ancylostoma duodenale, Necator americanus
Trypanosoma cruzi
Trichinella spiralis
Onchocerca volvulus
causes
causes
causes
causes
causes
causes
causes
causes
causes
causes
causes
causes
causes
Pityriasis versicolor
Tinea nigra
Black piedra
Tineas (ringworm onychomycosis)
White piedra
Sporotrichosis
Diaper rash
Mucocutaneous leishmaniasis
Cutaneous ulcers
Dermatitis
Rash

Figure 24–3. Skin and soft tissue infections: fungi and parasites.

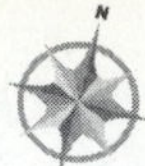

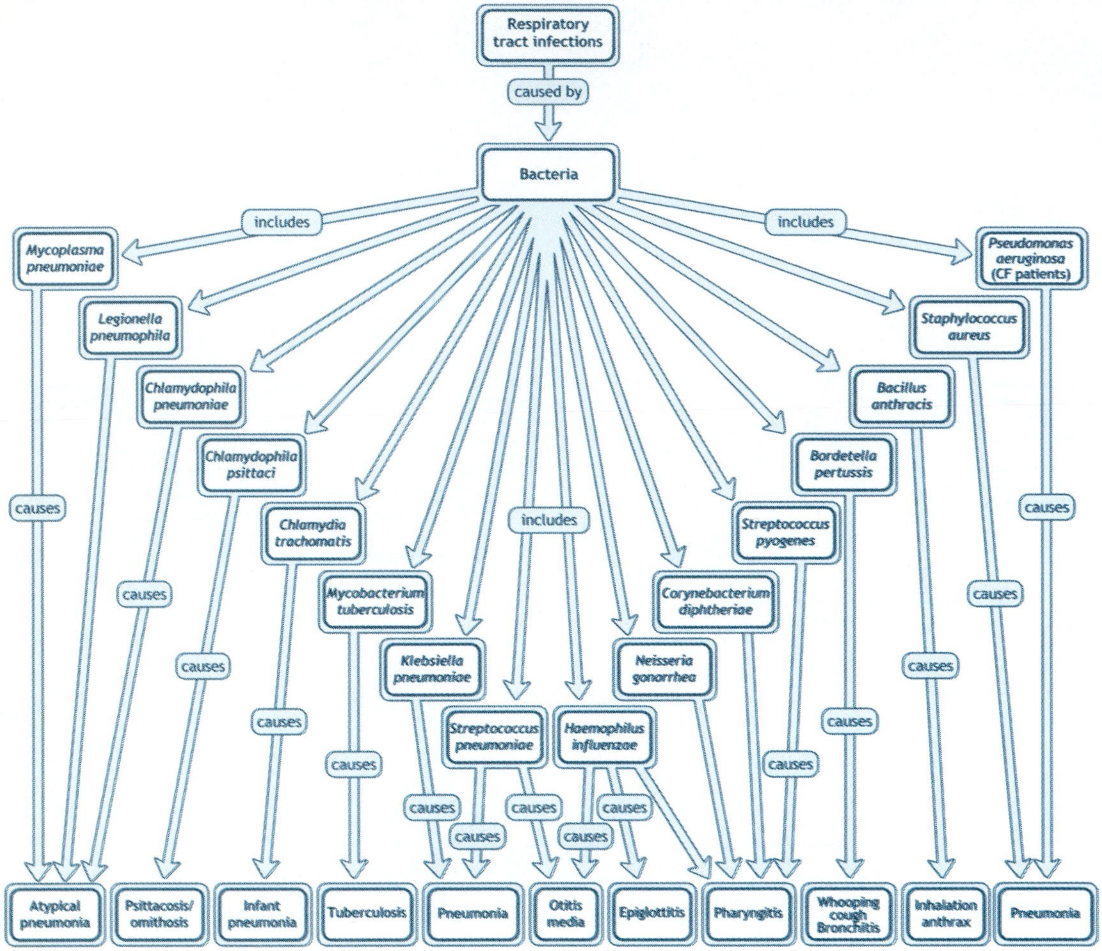

Respiratory tract infections

caused by

Bacteria

includes

includes

Mycoplasma pneumoniae

Pseudomonas aeruginosa (CF patients)

Legionella pneumophila

Staphylococcus aureus

Chlamydophila pneumoniae

Bacillus anthracis

Chlamydophila psittaci

Bordetella pertussis

causes

includes

causes

Chlamydia trachomatis

Streptococcus pyogenes

causes

Mycobacterium tuberculosis

Corynebacterium diphtheriae

causes

causes

Klebsiella pneumoniae

Neisseria gonorrhea

causes

causes

causes

Streptococcus pneumoniae

Haemophilus influenzae

causes

causes

causes

causes

causes

causes

causes

causes

Atypical pneumonia

Psittacosis/ omithosis

Infant pneumonia

Tuberculosis

Pneumonia

Otitis media

Epiglottitis

Pharyngitis

Whooping cough Bronchitis

Inhalation anthrax

Pneumonia

Figure 24–4. Respiratory tract infections: bacteria.

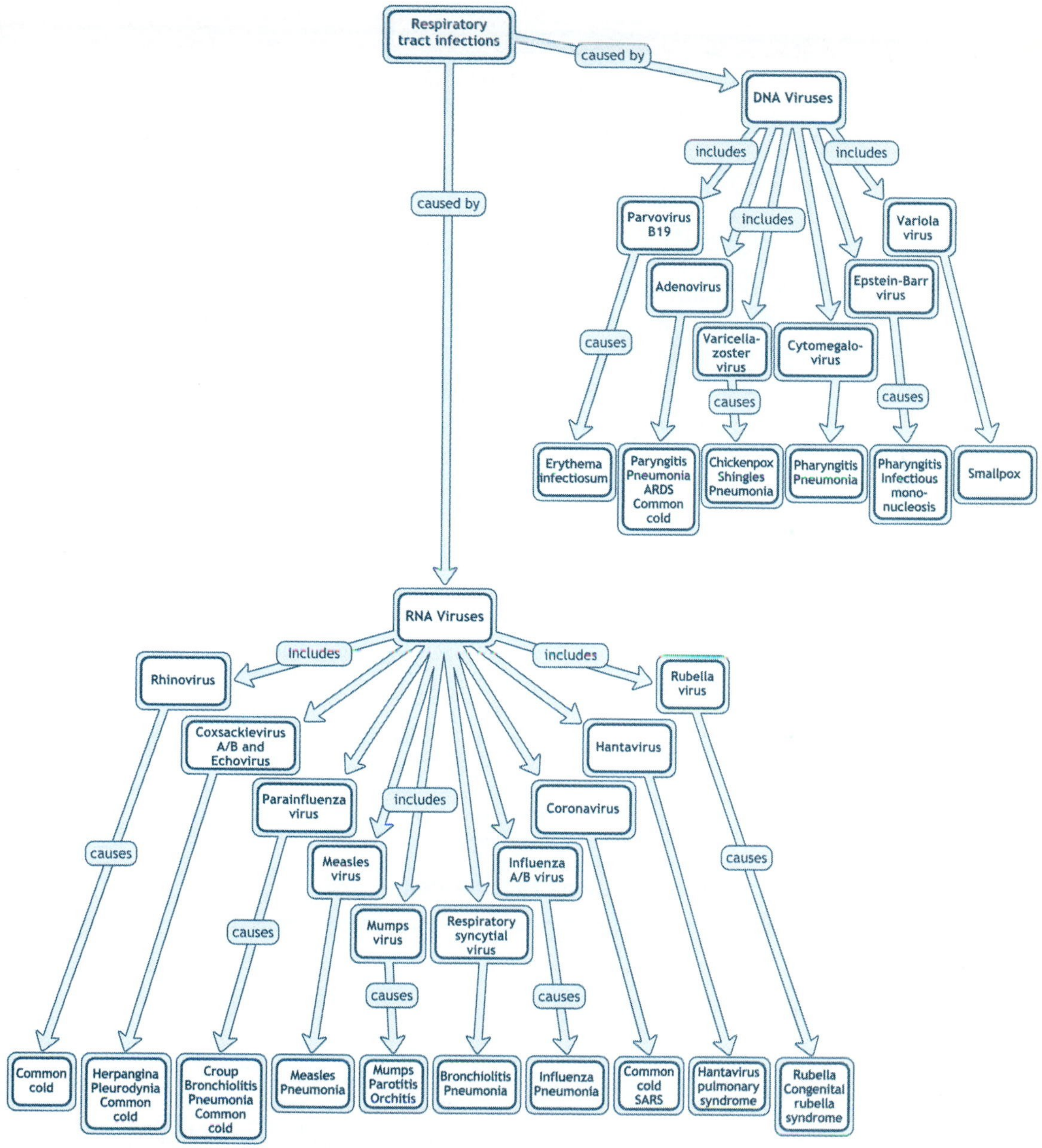

Respiratory tract infections
caused by
DNA Viruses
includes
includes
includes
Parvovirus B19
Variola virus
Adenovirus
Epstein-Barr virus
Varicella-zoster virus
Cytomegalo-virus
causes
causes
causes
Erythema infectiosum
Paryngitis Pneumonia ARDS Common cold
Chickenpox Shingles Pneumonia
Pharyngitis Pneumonia
Pharyngitis Infectious mono-nucleosis
Smallpox
caused by
RNA Viruses
includes
includes
Rhinovirus
Rubella virus
Coxsackievirus A/B and Echovirus
Hantavirus
Parainfluenza virus
includes
Coronavirus
Measles virus
Influenza A/B virus
Mumps virus
Respiratory syncytial virus
causes
causes
causes
causes
causes
Common cold
Herpangina Pleurodynia Common cold
Croup Bronchiolitis Pneumonia Common cold
Measles Pneumonia
Mumps Parotitis Orchitis
Bronchiolitis Pneumonia
Influenza Pneumonia
Common cold SARS
Hantavirus pulmonary syndrome
Rubella Congenital rubella syndrome

Figure 24–5. Respiratory tract infections: viruses.

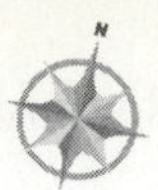

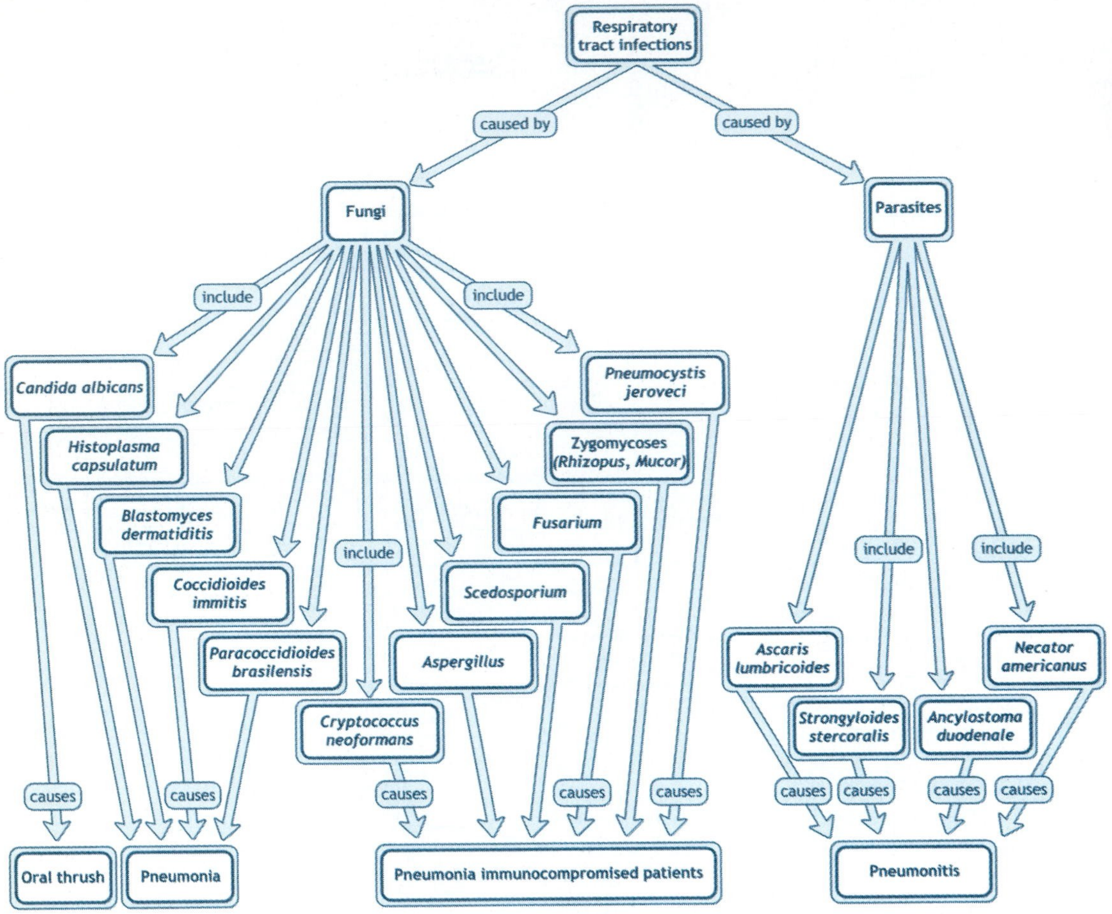

Respiratory tract infections
caused by
Fungi
caused by
Parasites

include
include
Candida albicans
Histoplasma capsulatum
Blastomyces dermatiditis
Coccidioides immitis
Paracoccidioides brasilensis
include
Cryptococcus neoformans
Aspergillus
Scedosporium
Fusarium
Zygomycoses (Rhizopus, Mucor)
Pneumocystis jeroveci

include
include
Ascaris lumbricoides
Strongyloides stercoralis
Ancylostoma duodenale
Necator americanus

causes
causes
causes
causes
causes
causes
causes
causes
causes
Oral thrush
Pneumonia
Pneumonia immunocompromised patients
Pneumonitis

Figure 24–6. Respiratory tract infections: fungi and parasites.

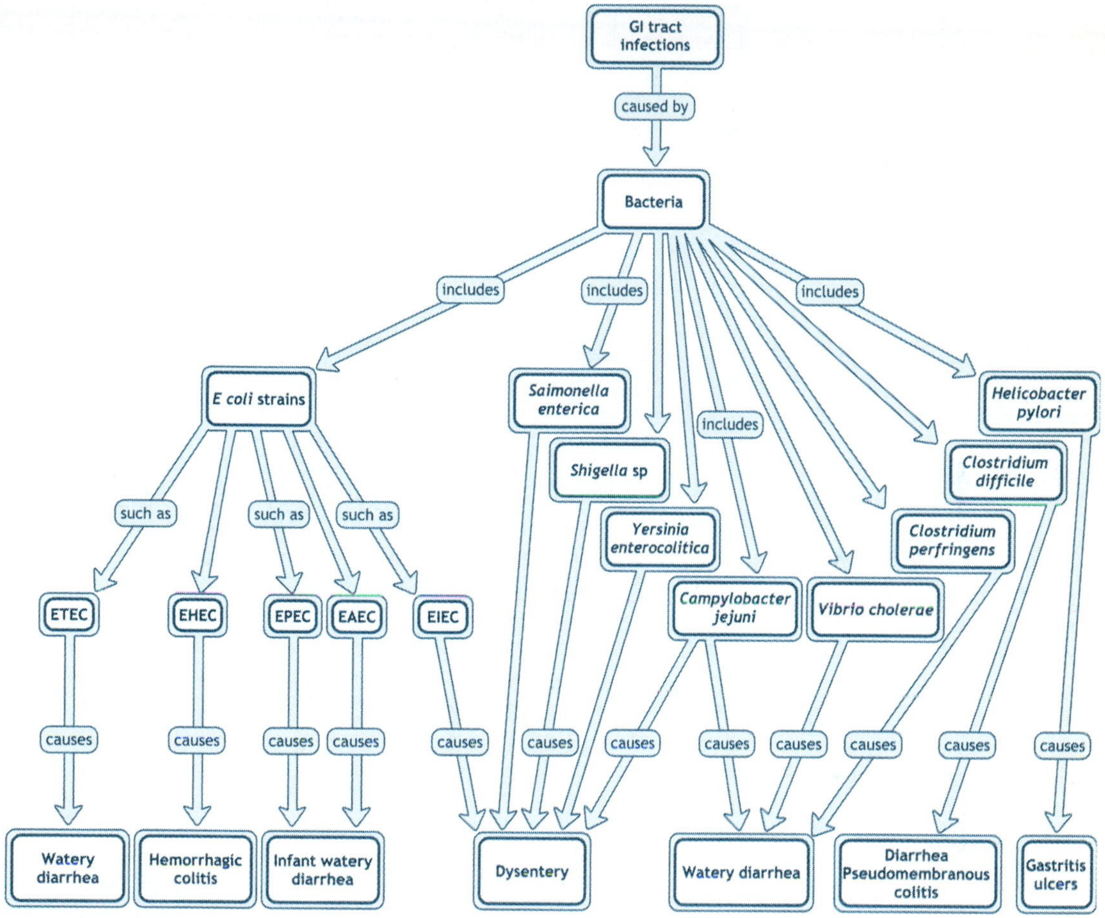

GI tract infections

caused by

Bacteria

includes

E coli strains

such as

ETEC

EHEC

EPEC

EAEC

EIEC

Salmonella enterica

Shigella sp

Yersinia enterocolitica

Campylobacter jejuni

Vibrio cholerae

Clostridium perfringens

Clostridium difficile

Helicobacter pylori

causes

Watery diarrhea

Hemorrhagic colitis

Infant watery diarrhea

Dysentery

Watery diarrhea

Diarrhea Pseudomembranous colitis

Gastritis ulcers

Figure 24–7. Gastrointestinal tract infections: bacteria.

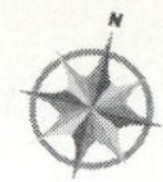

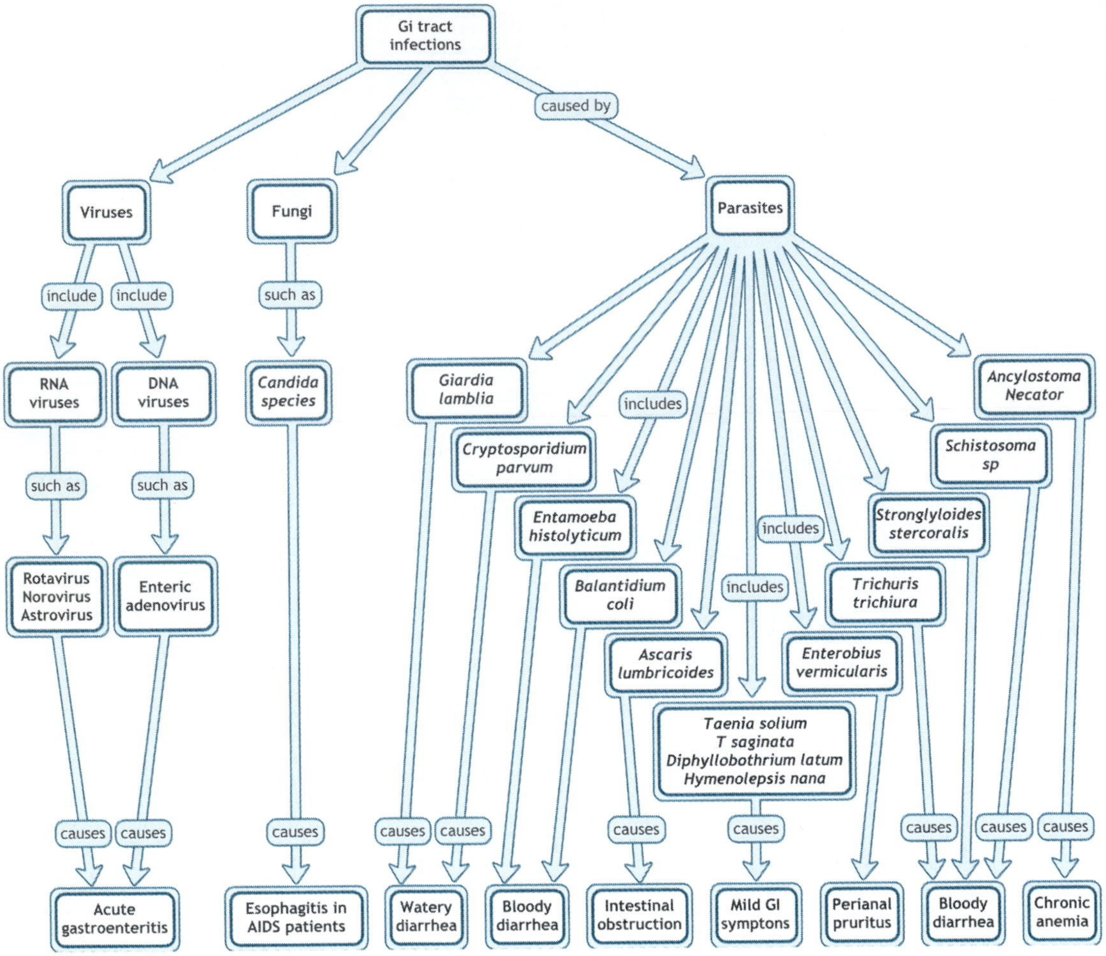

Gi tract infections — caused by:

- Viruses
  - include → RNA viruses — such as → Rotavirus, Norovirus, Astrovirus — causes → Acute gastroenteritis
  - include → DNA viruses — such as → Enteric adenovirus — causes → Acute gastroenteritis
- Fungi
  - such as → *Candida species* — causes → Esophagitis in AIDS patients
- Parasites — includes:
  - *Giardia lamblia* — causes → Watery diarrhea
  - *Cryptosporidium parvum* — causes → Watery diarrhea
  - *Entamoeba histolyticum* → Bloody diarrhea
  - *Balantidium coli* → Bloody diarrhea
  - *Ascaris lumbricoides* — causes → Intestinal obstruction
  - *Taenia solium*, *T saginata*, *Diphyllobothrium latum*, *Hymenolepsis nana* — causes → Mild GI symptons
  - *Enterobius vermicularis* → Perianal pruritus
  - *Trichuris trichiura* — causes → Bloody diarrhea
  - *Stronglyloides stercoralis* → Bloody diarrhea
  - *Schistosoma sp* — causes → Bloody diarrhea
  - *Ancylostoma Necator* — causes → Chronic anemia

Figure 24–8. Gastrointestinal tract infections: viruses, fungi, and parasites.

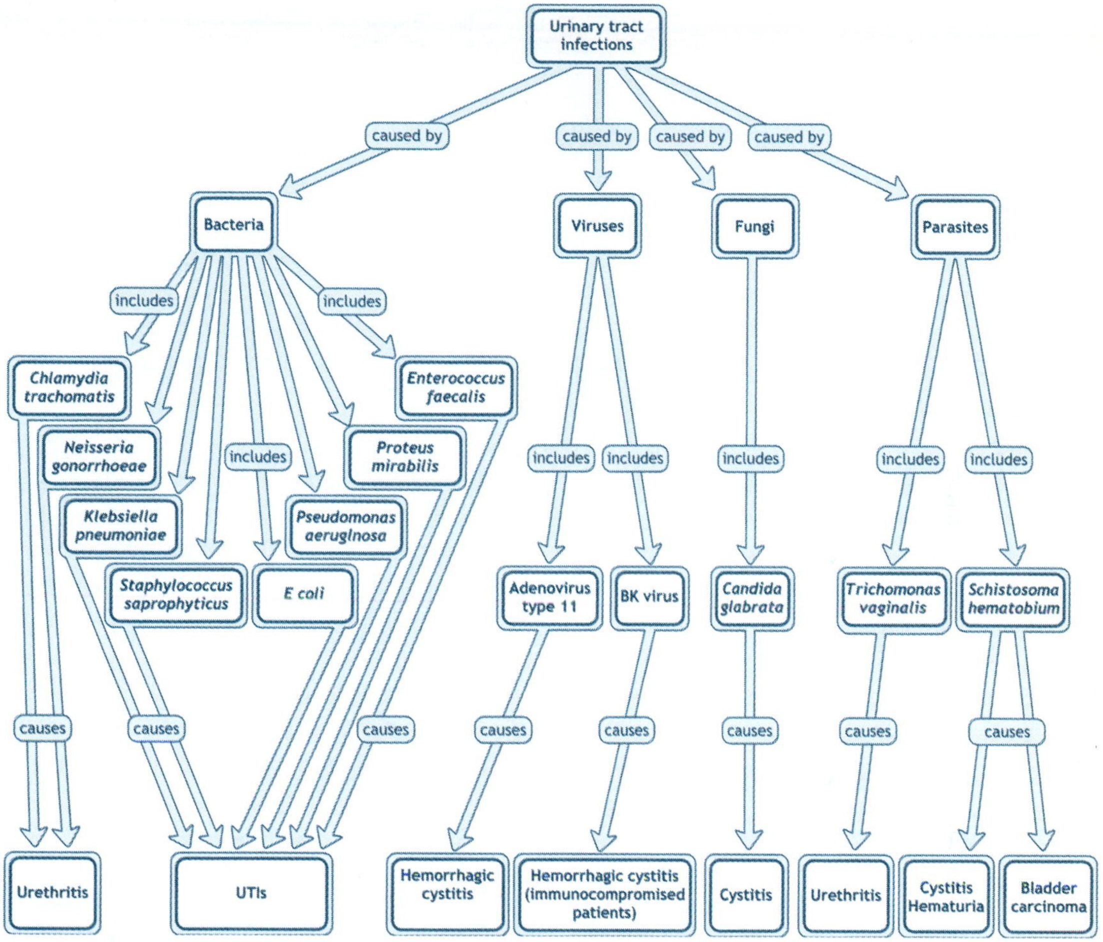

Urinary tract infections
caused by
caused by
caused by
caused by
Bacteria
Viruses
Fungi
Parasites
includes
includes
Chlamydia trachomatis
Enterococcus faecalis
Neisseria gonorrhoeae
includes
Proteus mirabilis
includes
includes
includes
includes
includes
Klebsiella pneumoniae
Pseudomonas aeruginosa
Staphylococcus saprophyticus
E coli
Adenovirus type 11
BK virus
Candida glabrata
Trichomonas vaginalis
Schistosoma hematobium
causes
causes
causes
causes
causes
causes
causes
causes
Urethritis
UTIs
Hemorrhagic cystitis
Hemorrhagic cystitis (immunocompromised patients)
Cystitis
Urethritis
Cystitis Hematuria
Bladder carcinoma

Figure 24–9. Urinary tract infections: bacteria, viruses, fungi, and parasites.

 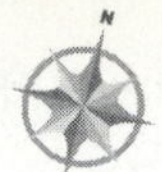

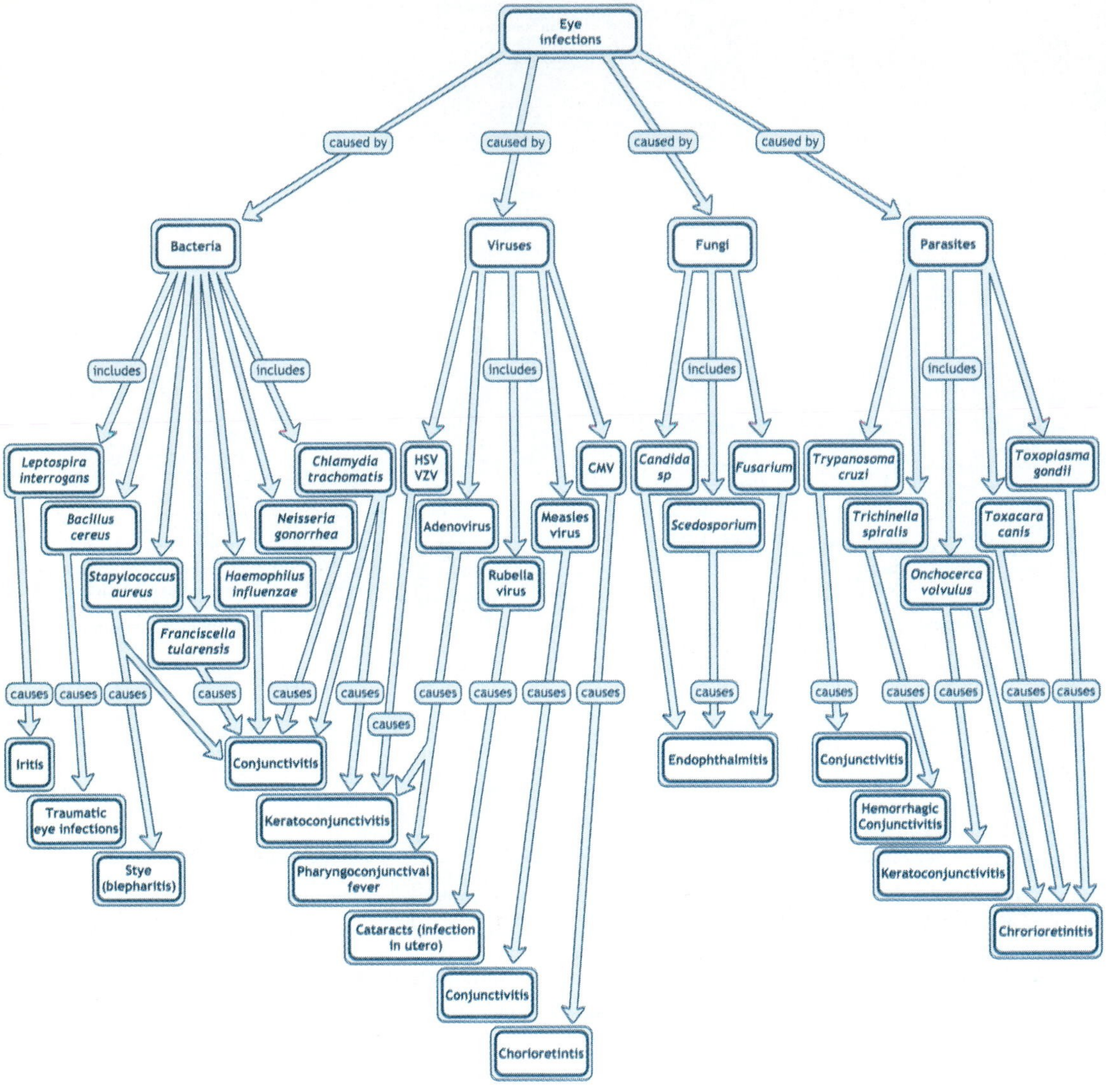

- Eye infections
  - caused by → Bacteria
    - includes → *Leptospira interrogans* — causes → Iritis
    - includes → *Bacillus cereus* — causes → Traumatic eye infections
    - includes → *Stapylococcus aureus* — causes → Stye (blepharitis); Conjunctivitis
    - includes → *Franciscella tularensis* — causes → Conjunctivitis
    - includes → *Haemophilus influenzae* — causes → Conjunctivitis
    - includes → *Neisseria gonorrhea* — causes → Conjunctivitis
    - includes → *Chlamydia trachomatis* — causes → Conjunctivitis; Keratoconjunctivitis
  - caused by → Viruses
    - includes → HSV VZV — causes → Keratoconjunctivitis
    - includes → Adenovirus — causes → Keratoconjunctivitis; Pharyngoconjunctival fever
    - includes → Rubella virus — causes → Cataracts (infection in utero)
    - includes → Measles virus — causes → Conjunctivitis
    - includes → CMV — causes → Chorioretintis
  - caused by → Fungi
    - includes → *Candida sp*; *Scedosporium*; *Fusarium* — causes → Endophthalmitis
  - caused by → Parasites
    - includes → *Trypanosoma cruzi* — causes → Conjunctivitis
    - includes → *Trichinella spiralis* — causes → Hemorrhagic Conjunctivitis
    - includes → *Onchocerca volvulus* — causes → Keratoconjunctivitis; Chroriorentinitis
    - includes → *Toxacara canis* — causes → Chroriorentinitis
    - includes → *Toxoplasma gondii* — causes → Chroriorentinitis

Figure 24–10. Eye infections: bacteria, viruses, fungi, and parasites.

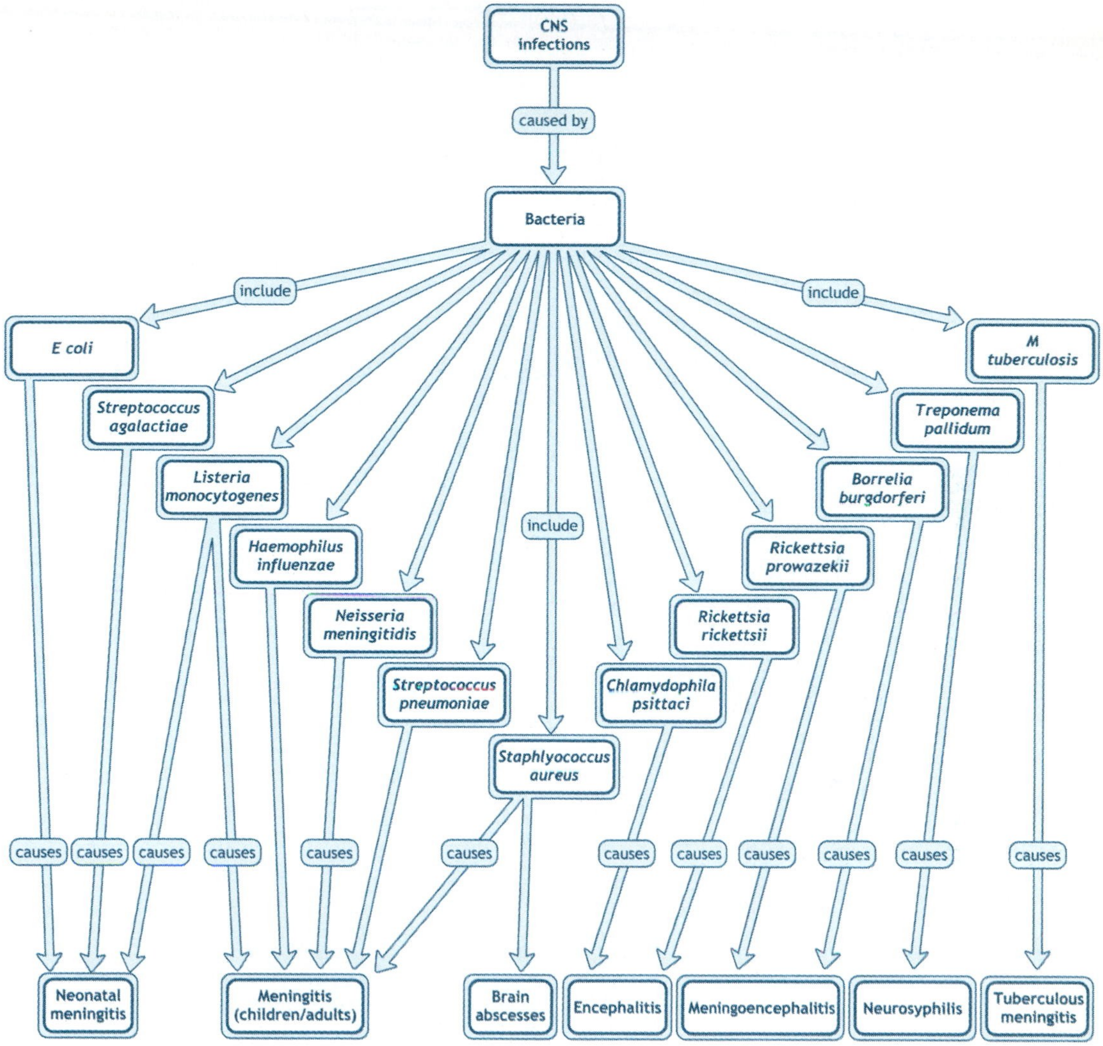

CNS infections
caused by
Bacteria
include
E coli
Streptococcus agalactiae
Listeria monocytogenes
Haemophilus influenzae
Neisseria meningitidis
Streptococcus pneumoniae
Staphlyococcus aureus
Chlamydophila psittaci
Rickettsia rickettsii
Rickettsia prowazekii
Borrelia burgdorferi
Treponema pallidum
M tuberculosis
causes
Neonatal meningitis
Meningitis (children/adults)
Brain abscesses
Encephalitis
Meningoencephalitis
Neurosyphilis
Tuberculous meningitis

Figure 24–11. Central nervous system infections: bacteria.

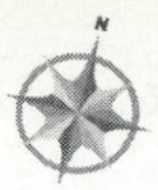

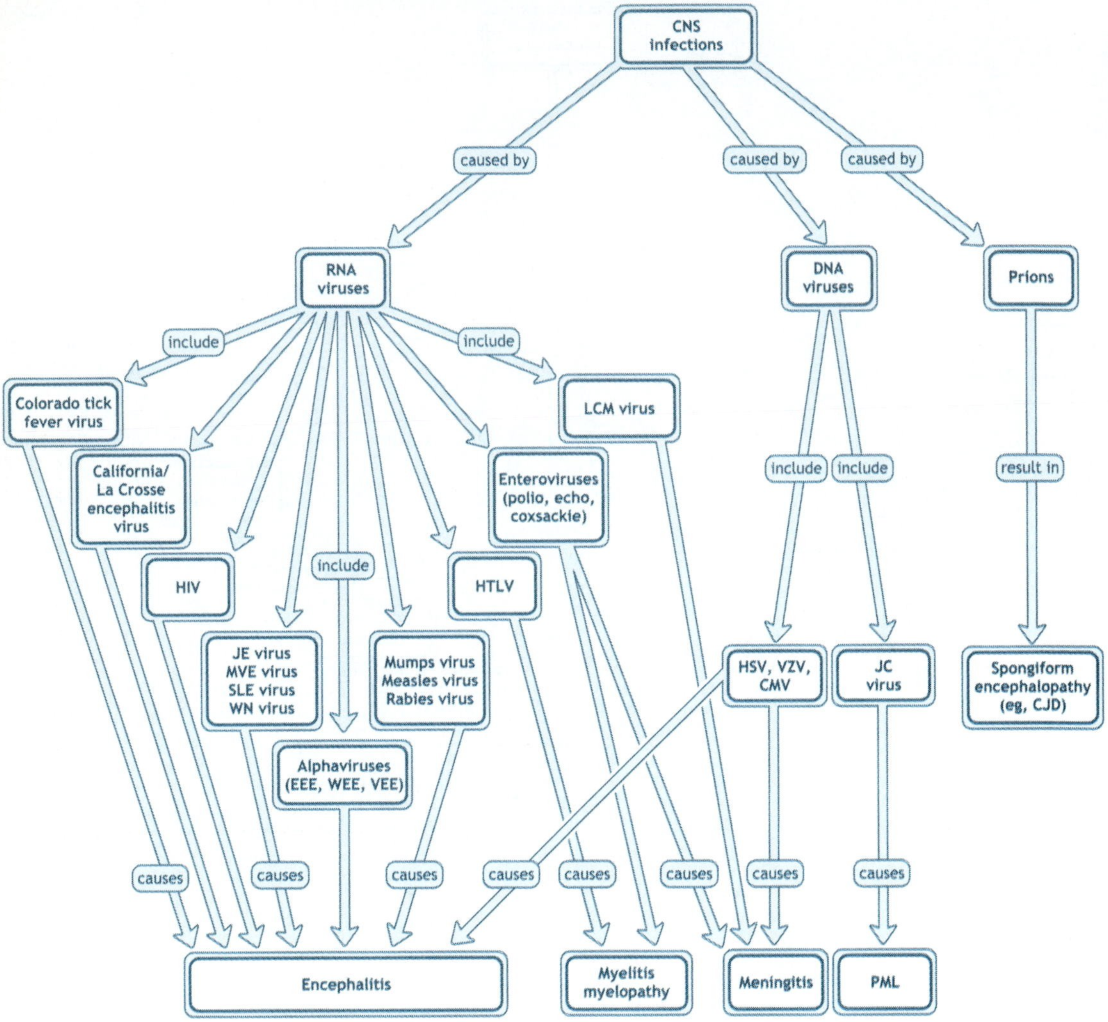

Figure 24–12. Central nervous system infections: viruses.

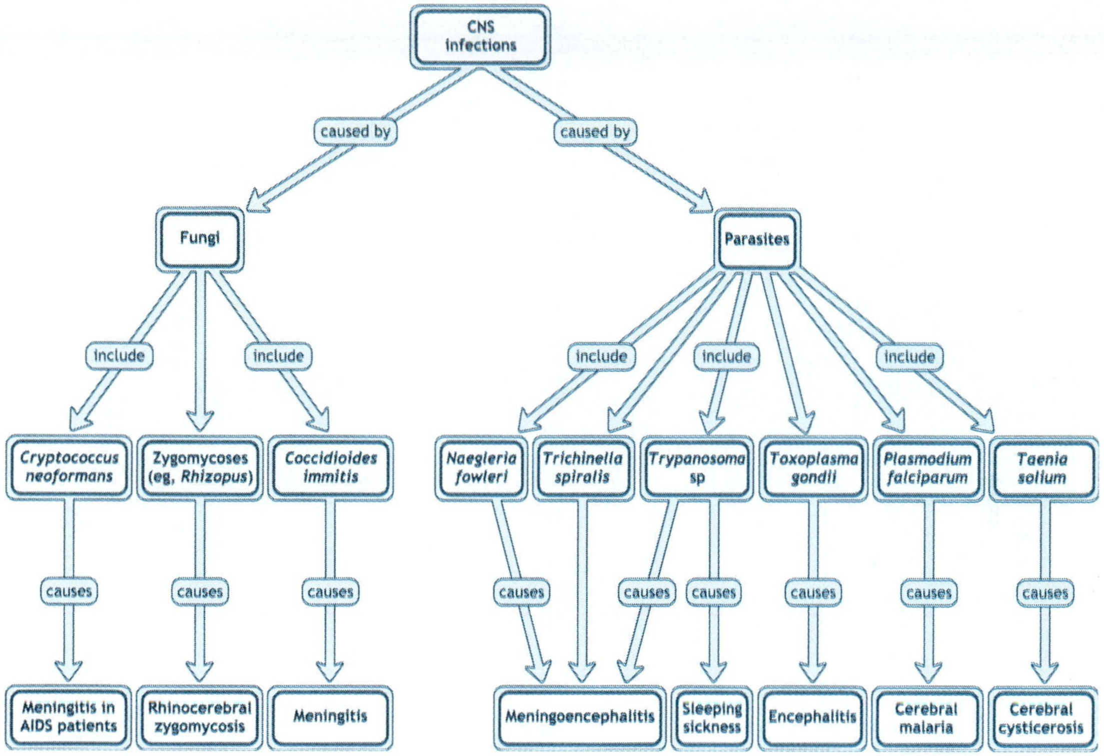

CNS infections
caused by
caused by
Fungi
Parasites
include
include
include
include
include
Cryptococcus neoformans
Zygomycoses (eg, *Rhizopus*)
Coccidioides immitis
Naegleria fowleri
Trichinella spiralis
Trypanosoma sp
Toxoplasma gondii
Plasmodium falciparum
Taenia solium
causes
causes
causes
causes
causes
causes
causes
causes
causes
Meningitis in AIDS patients
Rhinocerebral zygomycosis
Meningitis
Meningoencephalitis
Sleeping sickness
Encephalitis
Cerebral malaria
Cerebral cysticerosis

Figure 24–13. Central nervous system infections: fungi and parasites.

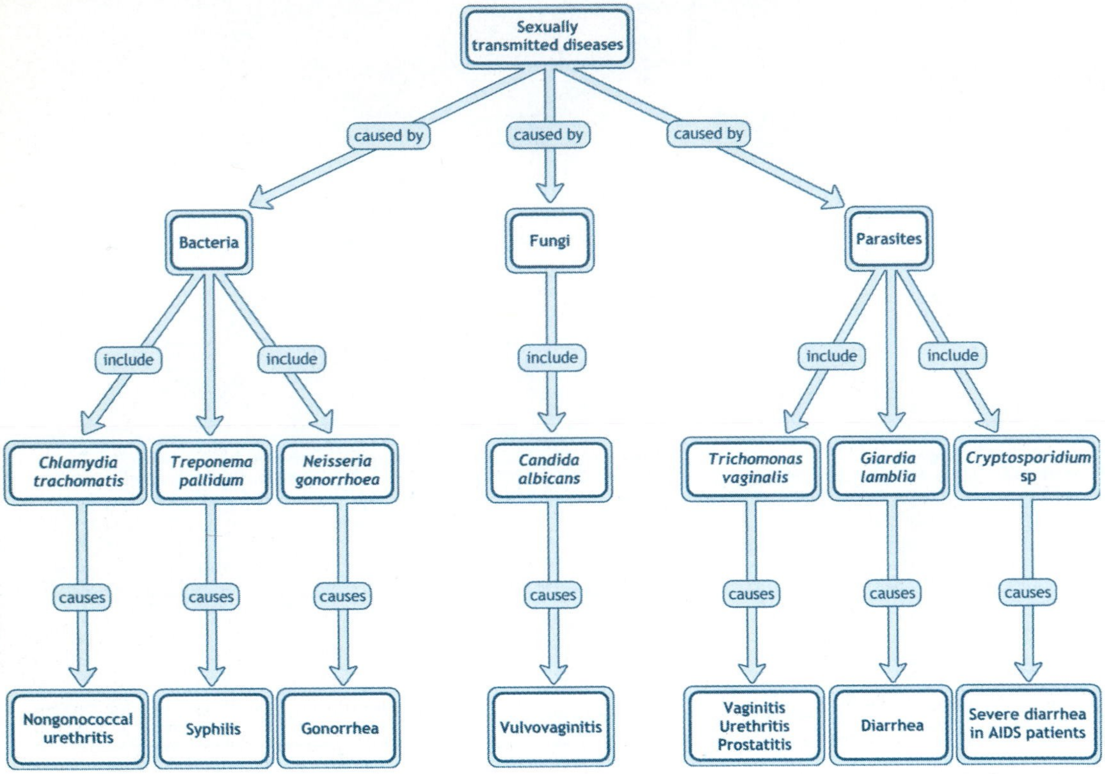

Figure 24–14. Sexually transmitted diseases: bacteria, fungi, and parasites.

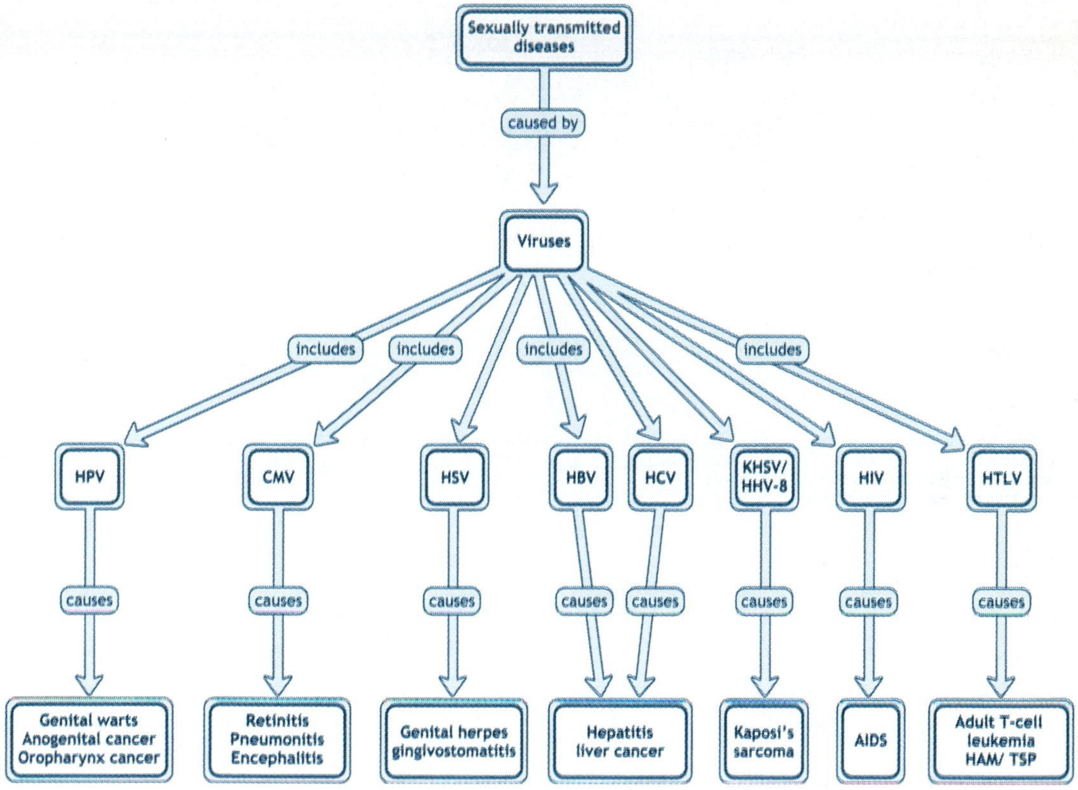

Sexually transmitted diseases
caused by
Viruses
includes
includes
includes
includes
HPV
CMV
HSV
HBV
HCV
KHSV/ HHV-8
HIV
HTLV
causes
causes
causes
causes
causes
causes
causes
causes
Genital warts Anogenital cancer Oropharynx cancer
Retinitis Pneumonitis Encephalitis
Genital herpes gingivostomatitis
Hepatitis liver cancer
Kaposi's sarcoma
AIDS
Adult T-cell leukemia HAM/ TSP

Figure 24–15. Sexually transmitted diseases: viruses.

 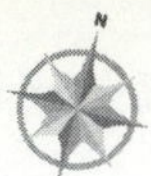

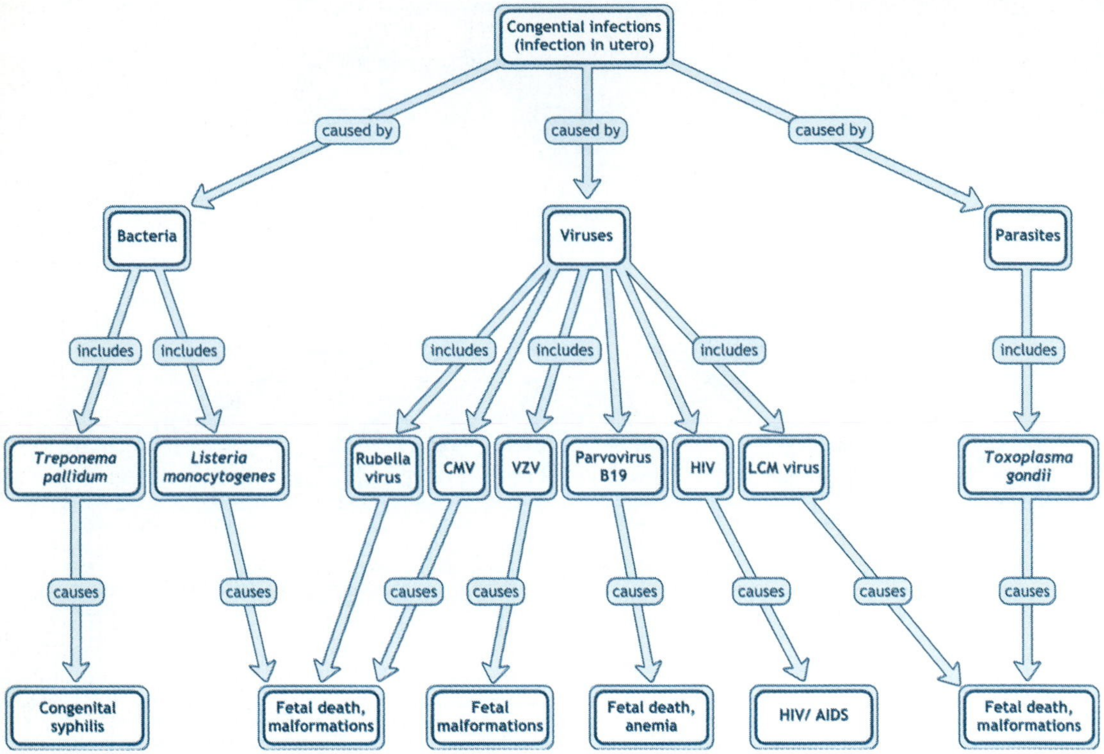

Congential infections (infection in utero)

caused by → Bacteria
- includes → *Treponema pallidum* → causes → Congenital syphilis
- includes → *Listeria monocytogenes* → causes → Fetal death, malformations

caused by → Viruses
- includes → Rubella virus → Fetal death, malformations
- CMV → causes → Fetal death, malformations
- includes → VZV → causes → Fetal malformations
- Parvovirus B19 → causes → Fetal death, anemia
- HIV → causes → HIV/ AIDS
- includes → LCM virus → causes → Fetal death, malformations

caused by → Parasites
- includes → *Toxoplasma gondii* → causes → Fetal death, malformations

Figure 24–16. Congenital infections: bacteria, viruses, and parasites.

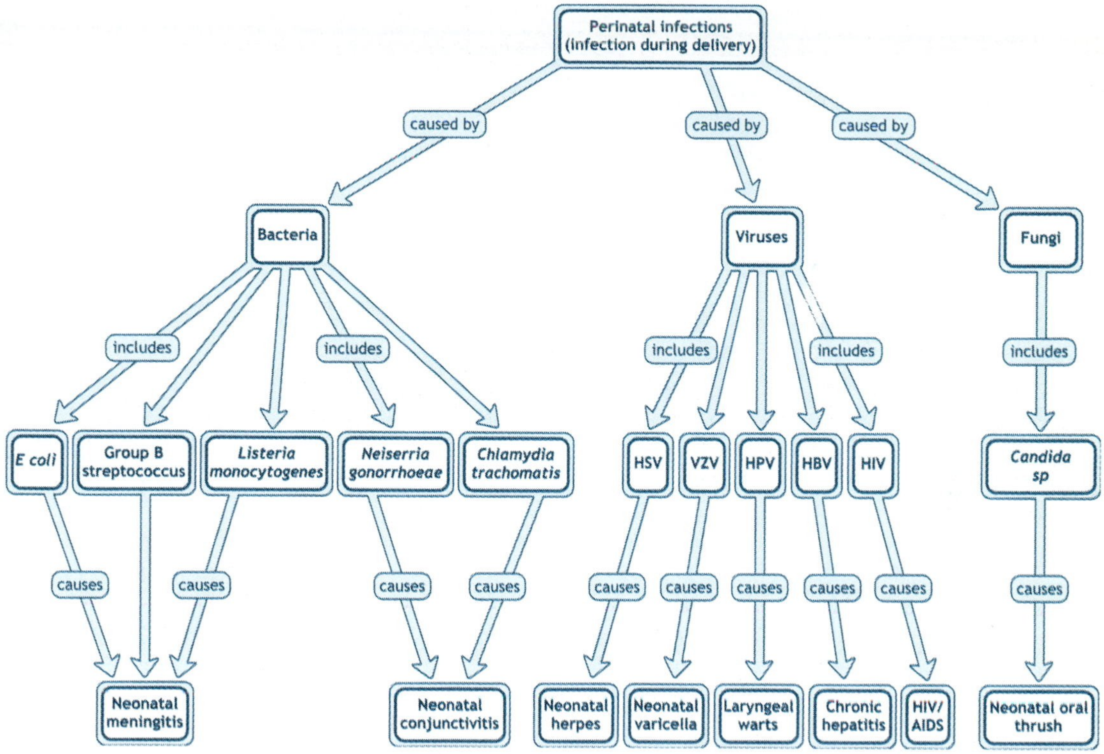

Perinatal infections
(infection during delivery)
caused by
caused by
caused by
Bacteria
Viruses
Fungi
includes
includes
includes
includes
includes
E coli
Group B streptococcus
Listeria monocytogenes
Neiserria gonorrhoeae
Chlamydia trachomatis
HSV
VZV
HPV
HBV
HIV
Candida sp
causes
causes
causes
causes
causes
causes
causes
causes
causes
causes
Neonatal meningitis
Neonatal conjunctivitis
Neonatal herpes
Neonatal varicella
Laryngeal warts
Chronic hepatitis
HIV/AIDS
Neonatal oral thrush

Figure 24–17. Perinatal infections: bacteria, viruses, and fungi.

INDEX

Page numbers followed by italic *f* or *t* indicate figures or tables, respectively.

 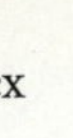

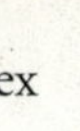

 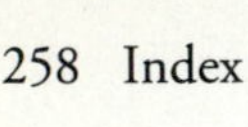